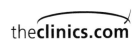

A. Simon Turner, BVSc, MS
CONSULTING EDITOR

VETERINARY CLINICS

OF NORTH AMERICA

Equine Practice

Medical Case Management

GUEST EDITOR
Jennifer M. MacLeay, DVM, PhD

April 2006 • Volume 22 • Number 1

SAUNDERS

An Imprint of Elsevier, Inc.
PHILADELPHIA   LONDON   TORONTO   MONTREAL   SYDNEY   TOKYO

W.B. SAUNDERS COMPANY
A Division of Elsevier Inc.

Elsevier, Inc., 1600 John F. Kennedy Blvd., Suite 1800, Philadelphia, PA 19103-2899

http://www.vetequine.theclinics.com

VETERINARY CLINICS OF NORTH AMERICA:	Volume 22, Number 1
EQUINE PRACTICE	**ISSN 0749-0739**
April 2006	**ISBN 1-4160-3579-6**
Editor: John Vassallo	

The ideas and opinions expressed in *Veterinary Clinics of North America: Equine Practice* do not necessarily reflect those of the Publisher. The Publisher does not assume any responsibility for any injury and/or damage to persons or property arising out of or related to any use of the material contained in this periodical. The reader is advised to check the appropriate medical literature and the product information currently provided by the manufacturer of each drug to be administered to verify the dosage, the method and duration of administration, or contraindications. It is the responsibility of the treating physician or other health care professional, relying on independent experience and knowledge of the patient, to determine drug dosages and the best treatment for the patient. Mention of any product in this issue should not be construed as endorsement by the contributors, editors, or the Publisher of the product or manufacturers' claims.

Veterinary Clinics of North America: Equine Practice (ISSN 0749-0739) is published in April, August, and December by W.B. Saunders, 360 Park Avenue South, New York, NY 10010-1710. Business and Editorial Offices: 1600 John F. Kennedy Blvd., Suite 1800, Philadelphia, PA 19103-2899. Accounting and circulation offices: 6277 Sea Harbor Drive, Orlando, FL 32887-4800. Subscription prices are $150.00 per year for US individuals, $245.00 per year for US institutions, $75.00 per year for US students and residents, $175.00 per year for Canadian individuals, $300.00 per year for Canadian institutions, $190.00 per year for international individuals, $300.00 per year for international institutions and $95.00 per year for Canadian and foreign students/residents. To receive student/resident rate, orders must be accompanied by name of affiliated institution, date of term, and the *signature* of program/residency coordinator on institution letterhead. Orders will be billed at individual rate until proof of status is received. Foreign air speed delivery is included in all *Clinics* subscription prices. All prices are subject to change without notice. **POSTMASTER:** Send address changes to *Veterinary Clinics of North America: Equine Practice*, Elsevier Periodicals Customer Service, 6277 Sea Harbor Drive, Orlando, FL 32887-4800, USA; phone: 1-800-654-2452 [toll free number for US customers], or 1-407-345-4000 [customers outside US]; fax: 1-407-363-1354; e-mail: usjcs@elsevier.com

Reprints. For copies of 100 or more, of articles in this publication, please contact the Commercial Reprints Department, Elsevier Inc., 360 Park Avenue South, New York, New York 10010-1710. Tel. (212) 633-3813, Fax: (212) 462-1935 email: reprints@elsevier.com.

Veterinary Clinics of North America: Equine Practice is covered in *Index Medicus, Excerpta Medica, Current Contents/Agriculture, Biology and Environmental Sciences, and ISI.*

Printed in the United States of America.

CONSULTING EDITOR

A. SIMON TURNER, BVSc, MS, Diplomate, American College of Veterinary Surgeons; Professor, Department of Clinical Sciences, College of Veterinary Medicine and Biomedical Sciences, Colorado State University, Fort Collins, Colorado

GUEST EDITOR

JENNIFER M. MACLEAY, DVM, PhD, Diplomate, American College of Veterinary Internal Medicine; Department of Clinical Sciences, College of Veterinary Medicine and Biomedical Sciences, Colorado State University, Fort Collins, Colorado

CONTRIBUTORS

BONNIE S. BARR, VMD, Internal Medicine Clinician, Rood and Riddle Equine Hospital, Lexington, Kentucky

JOSEPH J. BERTONE, DVM, MS, Diplomate, American College of Veterinary Internal Medicine; Professor, Equine Medicine, College of Veterinary Medicine, Western University of Health Sciences, Pomona, California

MICHAEL BRASHIER, DVM, MS, Diplomate, American College of Veterinary Internal Medicine; Associate Professor, College of Veterinary Medicine, Mississippi State University, Mississippi

SUSANNE DYKGRAAF, BVSc, MVSc, Large Animal Clinic, Veterinary Medical Teaching Hospital, University of California at Davis, Davis, California

EMILY A. GRAVES, VMD, MS, Equine Consulting of the Rockies, Fort Collins, Colorado

TAMARA GULL, DVM, Diplomate, American College of Veterinary Internal Medicine; Department of Veterinary Pathobiology, Texas A&M University, College Station, Texas

JAMES HART, BVSc, University Veterinary Centre Camden, Faculty of Veterinary Science, University of Sydney, Camden, Australia

LISA KATZ, DVM, MS, PhD, MRCVS, Diplomate, American College of Veterinary Internal Medicine; Diplomate, European College of Equine Internal Medicine, University Veterinary Hospital, School of Agriculture, Food Science and Veterinary Medicine, University College Dublin, Belfield, Dublin, Ireland

JENNIFER M. MACLEAY, DVM, PhD, Diplomate, American College of Veterinary Internal Medicine; Department of Clinical Sciences, College of Veterinary Medicine and Biomedical Sciences, Colorado State University, Fort Collins, Colorado

JONATHAN H. MAGID, DVM, MS, Diplomate, American College of Veterinary Internal Medicine; Dr. T's Equine Clinic, Salado, Texas

TONY D. MOGG, BVSc(HONS), PhD, FACVSc, Diplomate, American College of Veterinary Internal Medicine; Diplomate, American College of Veterinary Clinical Pharmacology; University Veterinary Centre Camden, Faculty of Veterinary Science, University of Sydney, Camden, Australia

JONATHAN M. NAYLOR, BVSc, PhD, Diplomate, American College of Veterinary Internal Medicine; Diplomate, American College of Veterinary Nutrition; Professor, Ross University School of Veterinary Medicine, Basseterre, St. Kitts, West Indies; formerly, Department of Large Animal Clinical Sciences, Western College of Veterinary Medicine, University of Saskatchewan, Saskatoon, Saskatchewan, Canada

OLIMPO E. OLIVER, DVM, MSc, DVSc, Profesor Asociado, Clinica de Grandes Animales, Departamento de Salud Animal, Facultad de Medicina Veterinaria y de Zootecnia, Universidad Nacional de Colombia, Bogota, Colombia

PAUL J. PLUMMER, DVM, Diplomate, American College of Veterinary Internal Medicine; Veterinary Microbiology and Preventative Medicine, Iowa State University Ames, Iowa

DAVID J. RUTHERFORD, BVM&S, Resident in Equine Studies, Institute of Veterinary, Animal and Biomedical Sciences, Massey University, Palmerston North, New Zealand

W. KENT SCARRATT, DVM, Diplomate, American College of Veterinary Internal Medicine; Department of Large Animal Clinical Sciences, Virginia-Maryland Regional College of Veterinary Medicine, Virginia Tech, Blacksburg, Virginia

HAROLD C. SCHOTT II, DVM, PhD, Diplomate, American College of Veterinary Internal Medicine; Associate Professor, Equine Internal Medicine; Department of Large Animal Clinical Sciences, Michigan State University, East Lansing, Michigan

JANYCE SEAHORN, DVM, MS, Diplomate, American College of Veterinary Anesthesiologists; Diplomate, American College of Veterinary Internal Medicine; Diplomate, American College of Veterinary Emergency and Critical Care; Equine Veterinary Specialists, Georgetown, Kentucky

HENRY STÄMPFLI, DVM, Dr Med Vet, Diplomate, American College of Veterinary Internal Medicine; Professor, Large Animal Medicine, Department of Clinical Studies, Ontario Veterinary College, University of Guelph, Guelph, Ontario, Canada

ALLISON J. STEWART, BVSc(HONS), MS, Diplomate, American College of Veterinary Internal Medicine; Assistant Professor, Department of Clinical Sciences, College of Veterinary Medicine, Auburn University, Alabama

JAMIE WEARN, BVSc(HONS), University Veterinary Centre Camden, Faculty of Veterinary Science, University of Sydney, Camden, Australia

PAMELA A. WILKINS, DVM, MS, PhD, Diplomate, American College of Veterinary Internal Medicine; Diplomate, American College of Veterinary Emergency and Critical Care; Chief, Section of Emergency Critical Care and Anesthesia, University of Pennsylvania School of Veterinary Medicine, Kennett Square, Pennsylvania

DAVID WONG, DVM, MS, Diplomate, American College of Veterinary Medicine; Veterinary Clinical Sciences, College of Veterinary Medicine, Iowa State University, Ames, Iowa

CONTENTS

and distal reflux esophagitis. Contrast gastrointestinal radiography revealed delayed gastric emptying. Initially, medical management was instituted including antiulcer medication, gastric decompression, and intravenous fluids. Because of poor response to medical therapy, an exploratory celiotomy was performed, and a duodenal stricture was identified.

Neonatal Diarrhea and Septicemia in an American Miniature Horse
Jonathan H. Magid

A 1-day-old American Miniature Horse colt was presented for mild diarrhea and a scrotal hernia. A working diagnosis of neonatal septicemia was made through a physical examination, complete blood cell count, serum chemistry, and sepsis scoring. Supportive care and broad-spectrum antibiotic therapy were initiated. A diagnosis of septicemia was confirmed by blood cultures. Antibiotic therapy was validated based on blood cultures. The colt made a complete recovery.

Chronic Hyperproteinemia Associated with a Probable Abdominal Abscess in an Appaloosa Stallion
Jonathan H. Magid

A 12-year-old Appaloosa stallion was presented with a 3-month history of weight loss and reluctance to move. Repeated laboratory work during this time by the referring veterinarian consistently showed elevated serum total protein and mild anemia. A presumptive diagnosis of an abdominal abscess was made based on physical examination, neurologic examination, a complete blood cell count, serum chemistry, serum protein electrophoresis, abdominocentesis, and bone marrow aspiration. After a 55-day course of ceftiofur, clinical signs were absent and laboratory values had returned to normal. The horse was reported to be doing well 8 months after initiating treatment.

Postpartum Hemoperitoneum and Septic Peritonitis in a Thoroughbred Mare
Tony D. Mogg, James Hart, and Jamie Wearn

Periparturient hemorrhage and hemoperitoneum in mares has been described secondary to arterial rupture or rupture of the uterus. Septic peritonitis may occur concurrently with hemoperitoneum in cases of uterine rupture. The history, physical examination findings, case assessment, treatment, and outcome of a Thoroughbred mare with postparturient hemoperitoneum and septic peritonitis (suspected to be the result of a uterine tear) are described in this case report.

report describes the diagnosis and supportive management of liver disease in a mature Arabian stallion.

Diseases of Muscle

Clostridial Myositis and Collapse in a Standardbred Filly
Allison J. Stewart

A 2-year-old Standardbred filly presented with a 5-day history of progressive neck and head swelling following an intramuscular vaccination. The filly was weak and disoriented and collapsed during initial evaluation. A presumptive diagnosis of clostridial myositis was made by clinical examination, radiology, ultrasonography, and Gram's stain. The filly responded well to antimicrobial, anti-inflammatory, and supportive therapy.

Polysaccharide Storage Myopathy in a 4-Year-Old Holsteiner Gelding
Jennifer M. MacLeay

This case report describes the diagnosis and management of a Holsteiner gelding with polysaccharide storage myopathy. Attention is also paid to the common differential diagnosis for muscle cramping in horses.

Neurologic Diseases

Excessive Drowsiness Secondary to Recumbent Sleep Deprivation in Two Horses
Joseph J. Bertone

These two cases represent an array of etiologies for excessive drowsiness secondary to recumbent sleep deprivation in horses. The first case represents excessive drowsiness secondary to abdominal cavity pain on becoming recumbent. The second case represents herd-deprived behavioral excessive drowsiness. Monotony-induced and musculoskeletal pain-induced excessive drowsiness and narcolepsy cataplexy are discussed in brief.

Left Otitis Media/Interna and Right Maxillary Sinusitis in a Percheron Mare
Lisa Katz

This case report describes the diagnosis and management of a 6-year-old Percheron mare with otitis media/interna and maxillary sinusitis on the contralateral side. The etiology and prognosis for horses with this condition are also discussed.

thin, 102-kg, 5-month-old weanling Quarter Horse colt. This diagnosis was based on laboratory values derived during baseline observation, water deprivation, antidiuretic hormone supplementation, and a Hickey-Hare test. With moderate water and sodium restriction, proper nutrition, and appropriate anthelmintic therapy, the colt began to grow at a more normal rate, gaining 68 kg in 90 days or 0.76 kg/d (1.66 lb/d).

An 11-year-old Quarter Horse mare was diagnosed with type 1 (distal) renal tubular acidosis based on physical and laboratory examination. Treatment focused on correction of electrolyte and acid-base abnormalities, including long-term bicarbonate therapy. The recognition, diagnosis, and treatment of renal tubular acidosis are reviewed.

Respiratory Diseases

A 3-month-old Thoroughbred colt was evaluated for fevers and tachypnea. Thoracic radiographs identified diffuse, patchy opacities. *Rhodococcus equi* was cultured from the percutaneous transtracheal aspirate. The foal responded well to a 4-week treatment course with azithromycin and rifampin.

A 3-year-old Appaloosa mare was presented with a 6-day history of coughing and fever. A diagnosis of pleuropneumonia was made based on clinical signs, laboratory tests, ultrasonography, radiography, transtracheal wash, and thoracocentesis. Antimicrobial treatment, supportive care, and pleural drainage were instituted. Antimicrobial treatment was altered based on culture and sensitivity testing results. The case was followed for 4 months with repeated radiographs and ongoing antimicrobial therapy. The mare made a full recovery and was returned to training.

This case report describes the clinical presentation, diagnostic findings, and management of a 19-year-old late-term pregnant Thoroughbred broodmare with a diaphragmatic hernia. Differential diagnoses for respiratory disease in older horses are discussed, as is management of a high-risk pregnancy. The mare was followed for 7 years after discharge from the hospital.

The following articles appear only online. Subscribers may access these articles by visiting www.vetequine.theclinics.com and clicking on the April 2006 issue, "Medical Case Management."

@ Additional material available online.

Respiratory Diseases

Fever of Unknown Origin Secondary to Occult Pleuropneumonia @

Joseph J. Bertone

This case represents what clinical impression indicates is the most common form of pleuropneumonia seen in equine practice, which presents with fever of unknown origin with few, if any, signs referable to the respiratory system. This form of pleuropneumonia rarely is discussed in the literature. The more severe form of pleuropneumonia (with extensive purulence and exudation, lung infarction, and so forth) is the focus of most literature discussion, likely because of referral filter bias and the unlikelihood that cases of occult or mild pleuropneumonia are referred for evaluation. Theoretically, many are likely to respond spontaneously or with empiric antimicrobial treatment without a specific diagnosis of pleuritis.

Actinobacillus Pleuritis and Peritonitis in a Quarter Horse Mare @

Allison J. Stewart

A 26-year-old Quarter Horse mare presented with a 7-day history of worsening ataxia, inappetance, and depression. Peritonitis and pleuritis were diagnosed by clinical examination and laboratory diagnostics. The mare responded well to antimicrobial therapy after pleural drainage. No underlying etiology was determined, and the mare made an uneventful recovery.

GOAL STATEMENT

The goal of the *Veterinary Clinics of North America: Equine Practice* is to keep practicing veterinarians up to date with current clinical practice in equine medicine by providing timely articles reviewing the state of the art in equine care.

ACCREDITATION

The *Veterinary Clinics of North America: Equine Practice* offers continuing education credits, awarded by Cummings School of Veterinary Medicine at Tufts University, Office of Continuing Education.

Cummings School of Veterinary Medicine at Tufts University is a designated provider of continuing veterinary medical education. Veterinarians participating in this learning activity may earn up to 6 credits per issue up to a maximum of 18 credits per year. Credits awarded may not apply toward license renewal in all states. It is the responsibility of each participant to verify the requirements of their state licensing board.

Credit can be earned by reading the text material, taking the examination online at *http://www.theclinics.com/home/cme*, and completing the program evaluation. Following your completion of the test and program evaluation, and review of any and all incorrect answers, you may print your certificate.

TO ENROLL

To enroll in the *Veterinary Clinics of North America: Equine Practice* Continuing Veterinary Medical Education Program, call customer service at 1-800-654-2452 or sign up online at *http://www.theclinics.com/home/cme*. The CVME program is now available at a special introductory rate of $49.95 for a year's subscription.

FORTHCOMING ISSUES

RECENT ISSUES

The Clinics are now available online!

Access your subscription at:
www.theclinics.com

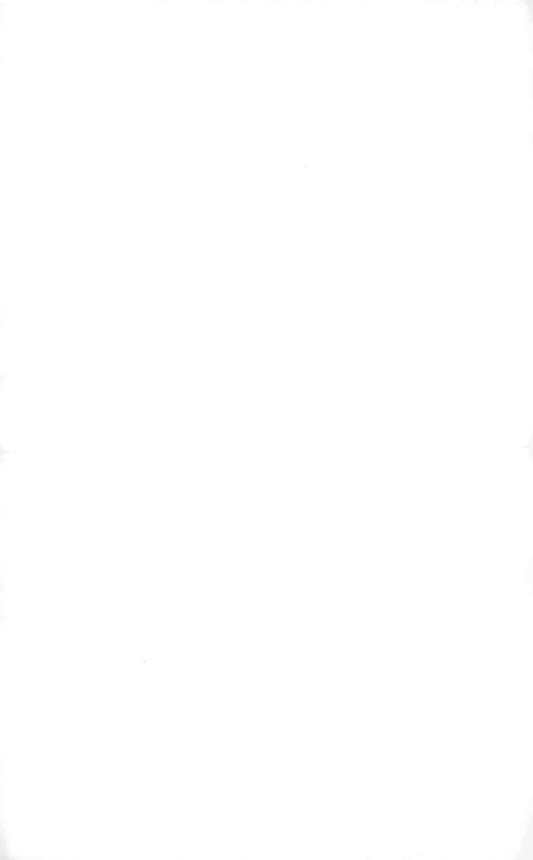

ELSEVIER
SAUNDERS

VETERINARY
CLINICS
Equine Practice

Vet Clin Equine 22 (2006) xix–xx

Preface

Medical Case Management

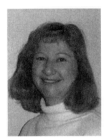

Jennifer M. MacLeay, DVM, PhD
Guest Editor

This issue represents a break from the traditional format. Instead of reviews, we are presenting case reports. Although many journals include unique case reports that have not been previously published, the goal of this issue was to present some of the more common yet challenging medical cases that the practitioner might encounter. The American College of Veterinary Internal Medicine has required case reports as part of the certification process for its diplomates. The reports presented here, with the exception of those concerning fluid therapy, are similar to those reports but have been expanded on by their authors to discuss the differential diagnosis and pathophysiology more fully. A goal of this format is to provide the reader with some insight into the thought process of the internist as he or she works through a medical case.

As you read through the cases, the authors also provide background information concerning the differential diagnosis, pathophysiology, and pharmaceutic choices. The issue begins with a review of fluid therapy, because effective use of fluid therapy is a common component of medical management and because its implementation can be an art form in and of itself.

One of the great aspects of our profession is the camaraderie we enjoy from sharing how we manage cases. Requests for input on case management are common on the equine and large animal LISTSERVs that many practitioners and specialists participate in. We are a generous profession, happy to share information and egoless in requesting help when we need to. This camaraderie was exemplified by the author response to my requests for cases to include in this issue. The response was so overwhelming that we simply

doi:10.1016/j.cveq.2005.12.033   *vetequine.theclinics.com*

could not fit them all in this volume. As a result, the reader is directed to additional cases accessible on-line (www.vetequine.theclinics.com) under the April 2006 issue banner (you must be a subscriber to access them).

Because of their enthusiastic support, I must thank all the internists who participated in this issue. I would also like to thank Simon Turner and John Vassallo for supporting this format for this issue. I hope that you will be as pleased with it as I am.

Jennifer M. MacLeay, DVM, PhD
Department of Clinical Sciences
College of Veterinary Medicine and Biomedical Sciences
Colorado State University
300 West Drake Road
Fort Collins, CO 80523, USA

E-mail address: jmacleay@colostate.edu

VETERINARY
CLINICS
Equine Practice

Vet Clin Equine 22 (2006) 1–14

Fluid Therapy: A Primer for Students, Technicians, and Veterinarians in Equine Practice

Harold C. Schott II, DVM, PhD

*Department of Large Animal Clinical Sciences, D-202 Veterinary Medical Center,
Michigan State University, East Lansing, MI 48824, USA*

Attention to hydration and, when necessary, use of fluid therapy is the mainstay of supportive care for equine patients with a variety of medical and surgical problems. Correction of dehydration and maintenance of adequate hydration are paramount for recovery from disease as well as for minimizing adverse effects of many commonly used medications. Nevertheless, it is sometimes unclear whether a patient needs fluid therapy and, if so, what the best route of administration may be.

Body fluid and electrolyte balance

Before specific aspects of fluid therapy are discussed, it is important to review normal water and electrolyte balance in the healthy horse. Under mild ambient conditions as would be found in most hospital settings, adult horses have a water requirement of about 50 mL/kg/day or about 25 L (or 6 gallons)/day for a typical 500-kg horse that is eating normally. In horses fed a typical hay and grain diet, most of this water (> 90%) is taken in by periprandial drinking with the remainder coming from feed. This water is subsequently eliminated through feces, urine, and insensible routes (across the skin and humidification of inspired air). When a horse is off feed, water requirements and intake may drop by more than 50% without development of significant dehydration because of a similar decrease in water output in feces and urine. Further, the type of feed ingested may have a profound effect on water intake by drinking. For example, many horse owners recognize that they fill the water tank much less often when horses

E-mail address: schott@cvm.msu.edu

doi:10.1016/j.cveq.2005.12.021   *vetequine.theclinics.com*

are turned out to pasture. Because most pasture grasses are more than 90% water, little further water intake by drinking is needed on a pasture-based diet. More subtle dietary factors that can affect water intake include protein, calcium, and fiber content of the feed; water intake may increase mildly with increased amounts of all of these factors. These dietary factors also affect water output: a diet high in protein and calcium will increase urine production and water loss by this route, whereas a diet high in fiber will increase fecal water output and decrease urine volume. Next, daily water requirements are increased in exercising horses (to replace sweat losses), horses with chronic diarrhea, and in horses stabled under conditions of high heat and humidity.

A comment about water intake by foals is also warranted: foals less than 30 days of age are rarely observed to drink water because they often ingest a volume of milk in excess of 20% of their body mass daily. This intake equates to a fluid intake approaching 250 mL/kg/day, five times that of the adult horse. To eliminate this considerable water intake, healthy foals urinate almost every time they get up to nurse, and their urine is so dilute (specific gravity around 1.005) that it looks like water. Horses are also different from small animals in body fluid stores: healthy horses have a substantial reserve of water and electrolytes in the lumen of the intestinal tract (10%–12% of total body mass is gut contents) that can initially be used to replace some types of fluid loss (eg, sweating during prolonged exercise or transport). This reserve becomes useless with other problems (eg, profuse diarrhea), however, and has probably already been depleted in horses that have been off feed for 2 to 4 days.

Body fluid is distributed in two compartments as illustrated in Fig. 1. Water is the most abundant molecule in the body (total body water accounts for 60%–65% of body mass). Because the body is made up of cells, most water (two thirds of total body water) is found inside cells, collectively called the intracellular fluid space (ICF). The remaining one third of total body water is outside cells, in the extracellular fluid space (ECF), which can be further subdivided into the plasma space (25–30 L), the interstitial spaces between cells (40–45 L), and the transcellular space (about 30 L, primarily in the lumen of the gastrointestinal tract but to a lesser extent in cerebrospinal fluid, pleural fluid, peritoneal fluid, and within joints). In addition to water, body fluids are rich in electrolytes, but the electrolyte composition varies greatly between ICF and ECF (see Fig. 1).

As with water balance, diet can affect electrolyte balance. Most hays are rich in potassium (K^+) but contain little sodium (Na^+). Thus, horses typically consume diets that are excessive in K^+ and marginal in Na^+. This diet is reflected in the urine of normal, hydrated horses, which usually contains high concentrations of K^+ (200–400 mEq/L) and low concentrations of Na^+ (0–50 mEq/L). Further, with disorders causing inappetence and dehydration, the ability of the kidneys to conserve (reabsorb) Na^+ is much greater than that for K^+. This point is particularly important to remember

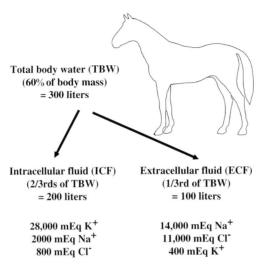

Total body water (TBW)
(60% of body mass)
= 300 liters

Intracellular fluid (ICF)
(2/3rds of TBW)
= 200 liters

28,000 mEq K^+
2000 mEq Na^+
800 mEq Cl^-

Extracellular fluid (ECF)
(1/3rd of TBW)
= 100 liters

14,000 mEq Na^+
11,000 mEq Cl^-
400 mEq K^+

Fig. 1. Body fluid distribution.

for two reasons: (1) most crystalloid fluids that are administered intravenously are similar in electrolyte composition to plasma; that is, they are high in Na^+ but contain little K^+; (2) horses that are off feed will have continued obligate losses of K^+ in urine. Without adequate supplementation of K^+ orally or in fluids, horses that are receiving intravenous fluids for more than a couple of days are at risk of depletion of K^+ from body stores, and this depletion could contribute to muscle weakness (eg, another complicating factor for postoperative ileus). Another electrolyte that can be significantly affected by diet is calcium (Ca^{++}). Horses are somewhat unique among the large domestic species in that Ca^{++} metabolism is not well regulated at the gut. As a consequence, horses absorb excessive amounts of Ca^{++} from feed, and this excess is eliminated in the form of calcium carbonate crystals in the urine (a major cause for the turbid appearance of normal equine urine). Thus, inappetence in horses is almost always accompanied by a modest decrease in total serum Ca^{++} concentration (eg, from a normal value of 12 mg/dL to 10 mg/dL) and decreased turbidity of urine.

Fortunately, this trend toward mild hypocalcemia rarely complicates the primary disease process, although it can exacerbate muscle weakness and decrease cardiac contractility. It does provide the rationale for supplementing intravenous fluids with Ca^{++}, especially when fluids are administered for more than a day. Although not as important for initial rehydration of a dehydrated horse, a working knowledge of normal electrolyte balance becomes more useful when customizing a fluid therapy plan for individual patients that may need fluid supplementation for several days.

Determining when and what type of fluid therapy is needed

Assessment of hydration status

To determine whether a sick horse needs fluid therapy, hydration status must first be assessed and an estimate of dehydration made. Unfortunately, clinical examination findings do not become abnormal until a horse becomes 3% to 5% dehydrated, with the percent value referring to percentage decrement in body mass caused by fluid loss. For example, an estimate of 3% to 5% dehydration would lead to an estimated 15- to 25-L fluid deficit in a 500-kg horse. Abnormal clinical findings supporting dehydration may include tacky oral membranes; a cool nose, ears, and extremities; poor distensibility of jugular veins (noticed when collecting blood samples or inserting a catheter); and delayed recovery of tented skin. In the author's experience, noting the temperature of the nose, ears, and extremities (eg, whether the limbs are cool from the fetlocks down or from the carpi and tarsi down) is one of the more useful indicators of hydration status, especially in neonates. The most severely dehydrated horses rarely have a fluid deficit greater than 15% (a 75-L fluid deficit in a 500-kg horse), and dehydration is estimated between 5% and 15% on the basis of severity of changes in clinical parameters of hydration status. In addition to examination findings, these parameters also include packed cell volume (PCV) and plasma total solids (TS, measured with a refractometer). They must always be interpreted in combination with examination findings, however, because markedly dehydrated horses may have laboratory data altered by disease (eg, despite severe dehydration, TS may actually be decreased in horses with profuse diarrhea as a result of protein loss in feces). In a hospital setting, the ideal measurement for assessing hydration is body mass. Although weighing the horse at admission does not provide immediate information about the magnitude of dehydration, because the body mass in the euhydrated state is not available, monitoring weight gain by serial measurement of body mass is the single best method of assessing dehydration, albeit in a retrospective fashion. Further, recent studies of human and small animal patients admitted to critical care units have revealed that the commonly assessed clinical parameters of hydration described previously are not highly accurate; thus, body mass should be determined when scales are easily accessible. In addition, serial measurement of body mass is useful to detect inappropriate increases in body mass, as may accompany development of uroperitoneum or oliguric acute renal failure.

As a rule of thumb, all horses that show clinical evidence of dehydration are candidates to receive fluid therapy. In addition, horses that show marginal evidence of dehydration would probably also benefit from an initial period of fluid therapy if they are azotemic (increased serum concentrations of urea nitrogen and creatinine) at admission or have a history of use of nephrotoxic medications (eg, nonsteroidal anti-inflammatory drugs or gentamicin) for several days.

Route of administration

With the development of 5-L intravenous fluid bags and systems designed to hang multiple bags (eg, 20–25 L at a time), use of intravenous fluids in equine practice has expanded considerably over the past 10 to 20 years. A consequence of this advance in treatment capability seems to have been a decrease in the use of enteral fluid therapy (ie, fluids administered by a nasogastric tube). This development is somewhat unfortunate, because enteral fluids are rapidly absorbed across the stomach wall and in the upper small intestine, as long as that portion of bowel remains functional. In fact, a larger volume of fluids can often be given by this route (eg, 10–12 L every 30–60 minutes through an indwelling nasogastric tube) than can be administered through a single intravenous catheter. Recent work indicates that the enteral route may have an additional benefit—specifically, stimulation of intestinal motility. This stimulation would be an advantage in a horse with impaction colic, but it may occasionally be accompanied by exacerbation of colic signs during the 10- to 15-minute period after fluid administration. The only real contraindications for use of enteral fluids are presence of gastric reflux when a stomach tube is passed or severe resistance by the horse when the tube is being passed. Further, enteral fluid solutions can easily be made when needed and are inexpensive. For example, 30 g of salt, either iodized or noniodized, or "lite" salt (a 1:1 mix of sodium chloride [NaCl] and potassium chloride [KCl]) can be added to each gallon of water. For further convenience, premeasured amounts of salt or lite salt can be prepared by pharmacy staff, or a permanent marker can be used to draw a line on a plastic container (eg, a 60-mL syringe case or a urine specimen cup) that can be used for stall-side measurement of the appropriate amount of electrolytes to administer. All in all, enteral fluids are ideal for horses with mild-to-moderate dehydration (5%–7%) as long as the intestinal tract is healthy enough to absorb the fluids administered (usually determined by checking for gastric reflux before administration of enteral fluids).

With more severe dehydration (7%–15%), enteral fluids must be administered with caution because absorption may be compromised by decreased blood flow to the intestinal tract. Thus, more severely dehydrated horses are usually initially treated with intravenous fluids although administration of enteral fluids and electrolytes in the form of oral pastes are often useful components of the fluid therapy plan that can decrease the volume of intravenous fluids used. With a standard intravenous catheter (14 gauge, 5.25 inches in length) placed in the jugular vein, intravenous fluids can be administered at a rate of 5 to 7 L/hour, depending on the height at which fluid bags are hung. Rarely is more than one intravenous catheter required for initial rehydration unless multiple types of products (eg, crystalloid solutions and whole blood or plasma) are being administered. Further, placement of catheters in both jugular veins should be approached with caution at initial presentation, because venous thrombosis can be a significant complication in critically ill patients.

Type of fluid

Although water is the most abundant component of most fluid therapy solutions administered intravenously or by a nasogastric tube, these solutions also contain electrolytes or nutrients (glucose). The most important electrolytes to consider are Na^+, K^+, chloride (Cl^-), and Ca^{++}. As illustrated in Fig. 1, Na^+, K^+, and Cl^- are quantitatively of greatest importance. Cl^- is the major exchangeable anion and typically follows losses of the major cations, Na^+ and K^+.

Essentially all commercially available crystalloid fluids have an electrolyte composition similar to plasma. Thus, they are rehydration fluids designed to replace acute losses of fluid from the ECF. As a result, most of these solutions are appropriate choices for initial treatment of dehydrated horses, and variation in products used between hospitals often reflects different costs and availabilities rather that a physiologically preferable solution. Two further comments about initial rehydration of neonatal foals are warranted. First, most sick foals are not nursing well and have limited energy reserves. Thus, addition of glucose (5% dextrose solution) is recommended for initial rehydration of foals less than 30 days of age. An approximately 5% dextrose solution can be made by adding 100 mL of 50% dextrose per liter of crystalloid fluid. Second, foals with uroperitoneum from a ruptured bladder or ureter may have significant hyperkalemia, and K^+-free solutions (eg, 0.9% NaCl, also with 5% dextrose added) are most appropriate for treatment of affected foals.

Developing a fluid therapy plan

Initial rehydration plan

Once the hydration status has been assessed, a fluid therapy plan can be developed. Initially, plans are made for 12 to 24 hours and subsequently modified after assessing the patient's response to treatment. The volume of fluid administered should include (1) the amount estimated to correct dehydration; (2) the amount needed for maintenance; and (3) the amount to replace estimated ongoing fluid losses. As well as being rather variable, the last is also the most difficult to predict and is of greatest importance in horses with significant ongoing losses caused by gastric reflux or diarrhea. As an example, assume a 500-kg horse is afflicted with Potomac horse fever. The horse has had diarrhea for 2 days, is off feed, and clinical examination findings result in an estimate of moderate (7%) dehydration.

A plan for the initial 12 hours would be formulated as follows:

1. Rehydration needs: 0.07 (estimated 7% dehydration) × 500 kg = 35 kg ≈ 35 L
2. Maintenance needs: 50 mL/kg/24 hours × 500 kg = (25,000 mL/24 hours)/2 = 12,500 mL = 12.5 L over 12 hours

3. Ongoing losses: estimated at 2 L/hour × 12 h = 24 L
4. TOTAL: 35 + 12.5 + 24 = 71.5 L

Thus, approximately 70 L of fluid needs to be administered over the initial 12 hours of treatment. This administration could be accomplished by hanging 14 5-L bags with an infusion rate of approximately 6 L/hour. As an alternative, a nasogastric tube could be placed, and 10 L of fluid could be administered seven times over the initial 12 hours. A combination of intravenous fluids and enteral fluids is probably the most logical approach in this case. Most commonly, however, such horses are treated almost exclusively with intravenous fluids because most clinicians do not want to pass a nasogastric tube repeatedly in a sick, depressed horse and prefer not to place an indwelling nasogastric tube in horses that they are encouraging to eat. From a physiologic basis, however, enteral fluid therapy alone would be a completely acceptable alternative, and this point should be remembered when treating horses for which owners may not be able to afford intravenous fluid therapy (especially when the alternative may be euthanasia).

In general, selection of almost any of the commercially available crystalloid polyionic solutions would be appropriate for initial intravenous rehydration, because the most important factor is to administer an appropriate volume of fluids. Fine-tuning of the fluid therapy plan is usually performed after initial laboratory data become available and after the response to the initial 3 to 6 hours of treatment is observed. Modifications to the initial plan may include changing the rate of fluid administration, correction of acid–base disorders, and replacement of specific or anticipated electrolyte deficits by adding electrolytes to the base fluid or supplementing needed electrolytes in enteral solutions or as oral pastes.

Additives to the base fluid

At present, limitations of fluid therapy in equine patients are that commercially available intravenous rehydration solutions fail to address K^+ and Ca^{++} deficits, and maintenance fluid solutions (for use once rehydration has been accomplished) are not available. Ideal maintenance solutions would contain less Na^+ and more K^+ and Ca^{++} than rehydration solutions and would also partially supply energy needs (5% dextrose). Another factor to consider is the nature of the dehydration being treated. For example, a horse that has become dehydrated over a period of 2 to 4 days (eg, frozen water source) has a different type of fluid loss from that in a horse that has developed acute diarrhea over the past 12 hours or has been raced under hot, humid conditions after receiving furosemide for prophylaxis against exercise-induced pulmonary hemorrhage. In the horse deprived of water, fluid deficits have developed more slowly, and dehydration involves a loss of both ECF (Na^+-rich fluid) and ICF (K^+-rich fluid). In contrast, sweating and furosemide administration produce more acute losses of fluid that are predominantly from ECF. Thus, the water-deprived horse would have a greater depletion of body K^+ stores, whereas the racehorse would have greater depletion of body Na^+ stores.

Most horses have adequate body reserves of these electrolytes and energy to get them through a couple of days of disease. Therefore additives to crystalloid fluids are not routinely necessary for horses receiving fluid therapy for 12 to 48 hours for supportive treatment for impaction colic or a mild case of diarrhea. This is especially true for patients that, although depressed, continue to eat 25% to 50% of their daily feed ration. Additives to the intravenous fluids are most critical for completely anorectic patients receiving intravenous fluids for more than 48 hours and in patients that are losing large amounts of fluid in the form of ongoing gastric reflux or profuse diarrhea. In these patients, acid–base status and serum electrolyte concentrations often need to be reassessed several times a day, and these results are used to modify the fluid therapy plan.

A common practice to address the anticipated Ca^{++} deficit in anorectic horses is to add 125 mL of a 23% calcium borogluconate solution to each 5-L intravenous fluid bag. This addition of calcium borogluconate provides about 2.7 g of Ca^{++} in each 5-L bag that would replace about one eighth of the exchangeable Ca^{++} pool in a 500-kg horse. Although hypercalcemia may occasionally develop with this type of supplementation, adverse effects of transient hypercalcemia have not been reported, and the problem is rapidly reversed once Ca^{++} supplementation is discontinued. Monitoring for excessive Ca^{++} supplementation is a further reason that follow-up measurement of serum electrolytes should be considered for horses that are receiving fluid therapy for more than 48 hours, especially when initial laboratory results were outside the reference ranges for one or more values.

Most crystalloid rehydration fluids contain relatively modest amount of K^+ (5 mEq/L or less for most polyionic solutions); thus, addition of supplemental K^+ to the base fluid may be needed in some instances. Because K^+ is the most abundant cation in body fluids (see Fig. 1), supplementation is usually not necessary unless horses have been off feed for several days or have been receiving fluid therapy for more than 48 hours. In these instances, depletion of total body K^+ stores can be substantial, but serum K^+ may still be within the normal range because less than 0.5% of exchangeable K^+ is in plasma. Again, with prolonged support ($>$ 48 hours) with fluids designed for rehydration, excessive replacement of body Na^+ stores may increase urine output and further exacerbate K^+ depletion by increasing obligate K^+ loss in urine. Assuming that the fluid therapy plan at the time a decision to add K^+ is made is to administer about 35 L of intravenous fluid over the subsequent 12 hours (1 L/hour for maintenance and 2 L/hour for anticipated losses in diarrhea, after rehydration has been accomplished), only about 175 mEq of K^+ would be replaced using a typical polyionic crystalloid fluid. This amount would represent replacement of less than 1% of body K^+ stores at the same time that urine K^+ losses could result in further depletion of as much as 3% to 4% of body K^+ stores through production of 10 L of urine (an approximate threefold increase in urine flow caused by a Na^+ diuresis) with a K^+ concentration as low as 100 mEq/L. Simply to match this estimated urine K^+ loss, 25 mEq of additional K^+ would need to be added to each 35 L of fluid administered. As can be seen, addition of 20 mEq/L of K^+ per liter of fluid, usually in the form of KCl, is generally safe (with the exception of horses with hyperkalemia accompanying uroperitoneum and acute renal failure) and is often of benefit to horses receiving fluid support for more than a couple of days. An alternative to adding KCl to the intravenous fluids is to administer KCl in enteral fluids or as an oral paste. For example, to provide 1500 mEq of KCl daily ($\approx 5\%$ of body K^+ stores), 110 g of KCl (1 g of KCl provides 13.4 mEq of both K^+ and Cl^-) could be administered as four doses of 25 to 30 g KCl through a nasogastric tube or as an oral paste.

In critically ill patients, most commonly those with profuse diarrhea and poor perfusion, metabolic acidosis (decreased pH with a decrease in serum bicarbonate concentration, $[HCO_3^-]$) may also have to be addressed. Initially, rehydration with crystalloid fluids (administered intravenously and enterally) is the treatment for both dehydration and acidosis. Volume expansion with this treatment alone may improve perfusion and correct the acidosis. When acidosis is severe (pH < 7.2) and unresponsive to initial rehydration, addition of HCO_3^- to the base fluid may be necessary. In general, supplemental HCO_3^- is not needed unless serum HCO_3^- concentration falls below 15 mEq/L (compared with a normal value of 25–30 mEq/L). To estimate the amount of HCO_3^- to add to the base fluid, the base deficit (a calculation made during blood gas analysis that provides a measure of the decrease in HCO_3^- concentration) is multiplied by body mass and a fraction representing the portion of body mass that is composed of fluid containing HCO_3^-. Recommendations for the latter fraction range from 0.3 to 0.6; the author uses a value of 0.5 to represent the entire ECF as well as a portion of the ICF. As an example, the HCO_3^- deficit in a 500-kg horse with profuse diarrhea and a base deficit of 14 mEq/L (serum HCO_3^- concentration of 13 mEq/L in comparison to a normal value of 27 mEq/L) would be estimated as (assuming that 1 kg $\approx$ 1 L):

$$HCO_3^-\ deficit = 14\ mEq/L\ (base\ deficit) \times 500\,kg \times 0.5$$
$$= 3500\ mEq\ HCO_3^-\ deficit$$

This deficit can be corrected, over 6 to 12 hours, by addition of HCO_3^- to the base intravenous fluid or by enteral administration of HCO_3^- by a nasogastric tube. It is important to remember that HCO_3^- must be coupled with a cation, typically Na^+; consequently, it is not possible to add HCO_3^- without also adding Na^+. Further, HCO_3^- should not be added to fluids containing Ca^{++} because there is a slight risk of forming $CaCO_3$ crystals that could precipitate in the fluids. Thus, $NaHCO_3$, available as either a 5% solution (1 mL = 0.6 mEq of HCO_3^-) or an 8.4% solution (1 mL = 1.0 mEq of HCO_3^-), is generally added to a base fluid of 0.9% NaCl. Assuming the same fluid therapy plan used above for K^+ supplementation (35 L of intravenous fluid over the subsequent 12 hours), 100 mEq of $NaHCO_3$ would have to be added to each liter to correct the 3500 mEq deficit estimated previously. As mentioned earlier, 100 mEq of Na^+ would also have to be added to each liter of fluids and would increase the Na^+ concentration of the fluid to 254 mEq/liter because the Na^+ concentration of 0.9% NaCl is already 154 mEq/liter. Because Na^+ continues to be lost in diarrhea, administration of fluids with this high a Na^+ concentration is generally safe in horses with diarrhea. Addition of $NaHCO_3$ to a base fluid of 0.9% NaCl would have to be approached cautiously in horses with an increased plasma Na^+ concentration or with acidosis from other causes. In these instances, addition of $NaHCO_3$ to a base fluid of 0.45% NaCl (half-strength saline) would be a safer choice. Another option to replace the HCO_3^- deficit would be to administer $NaHCO_3$ as a separate enteral solution that ranges from 300 to 600 mOsm/kg in tonicity (concentration). Because 1 g of $NaHCO_3$ has 12 mEq of both Na^+ and HCO_3^- (for a total of 24 mOsm), the 3500 mEq HCO_3^- deficit could be addressed by administering three ≈ 100 g doses of $NaHCO_3$ (baking soda) in 4 to 8 L of water at 4-hour intervals. A third alternative would be to administer $NaHCO_3$ as an oral paste (by mixing 30 g of $NaHCO_3$ with water or corn oil in a 60-mL dosing syringe and administering two syringes every 2 hours). Although generally safe, enteral administration of $NaHCO_3$, either by a nasogastric tube or as an oral paste, could increase gas (CO_2) accumulation in the bowel lumen and contribute to colic signs in an occasional horse. Finally, the Na^+ load accompanying $NaHCO_3$ administration by any route will usually lead to increased urine output and will exacerbate the obligate loss of K^+ in urine. Thus, attention to K^+ balance, by adding KCl to the base intravenous fluid or enteral solutions being administered or by giving KCl as an oral paste, merits consideration in horses receiving supplemental HCO_3^-.

When adding multiple supplements (eg, KCl, $NaHCO_3$, and dextrose) to a base fluid, the tonicity of the final product should be considered. A general rule is that the total osmolality provided by electrolytes should not exceed more than twice the value of plasma osmolality. Because plasma osmolality is normally about 280 mOsm/kg, a final osmolality of about 600 mOsm/kg would be a reasonable limit. The osmotic contribution from dextrose can largely be ignored, because this additive is metabolized and contributes little to the net number of osmoles added to body fluids. For example, in a base fluid of 0.9% NaCl to which 40 mEq of KCl and 100 mEq of $NaHCO_3$ have been added to each liter, the final osmolality would be 588 mOsm/kg (154 mEq of both Na^+ and Cl^- from the base fluid; 40 mEq of both K^+ and Cl^- from added KCl, and 100 mEq of both Na^+ and HCO_3^- from added $NaHCO_3$).

Administering fluids that are hypertonic (have greater osmolality than plasma) may be advantageous in some dehydrated horses. Specifically, initial fluid replacement in most dehydrated horses is in the form of voluntary water drinking. Ingestion of plain water, however, dilutes the electrolytes remaining in body fluids. Because an increase in plasma osmolality is the most potent stimulus for thirst, dilution of remaining plasma electrolytes by water drinking can abolish thirst. As a result, horses that lose considerable amounts of electrolytes with water through prolonged sweating or in diarrhea can remain moderately to severely dehydrated and yet may have little thirst. Thus, providing fluids that are hypertonic, especially with a higher Na^+ content, may stimulate thirst in dehydrated horses. Increasing voluntary water intake is of benefit to the fluid therapy plan because it may reduce the total volume (and cost) of fluids that need to be administered. Clearly, this benefit is limited to horses that have lost both water and electrolytes in the dehydration process, and the use of hypertonic fluids must be approached cautiously in horses that have become dehydrated by water restriction and in all dehydrated foals.

Although not a specific additive to a base fluid, 1 to 2 L of hypertonic saline (7.5% NaCl solution) is sometimes administered intravenously concurrent with isotonic crystalloid fluids during initial rehydration. Hypertonic saline has Na^+ and Cl^- concentrations of 1285.2 mEq/L or an osmolality of 2565 mOsm/kg, a value approximately ninefold greater than plasma. The goal of administering hypertonic saline is to draw water by osmotic forces into the plasma space from the interstitial space and ICF. This treatment is ideally suited for horses experiencing rapid fluid loss from the vascular space resulting in shock (ie, hemorrhagic shock) but can also be useful in patients that have hypovolemic shock as a result of other types of fluid loss. In both types of shock, administration of hypertonic saline may stimulate drinking, but close patient monitoring is warranted because critically ill patients may not respond as expected. A further use for hypertonic saline is in patients that have moderate-to-severe electrolyte depletion in the face of only mild-to-moderate dehydration. Examples include horses that have performed long-distance exercise (with substantial sweat fluid loss) or that have had diarrhea for several days. In both instances, voluntary drinking may have replaced 50% or more of water loss, but this form of fluid replacement was not accompanied by replacement of electrolytes. Judicious use of hypertonic saline in these patients, along with replacement of K^+ deficits through enteral fluids or administration of oral pastes can be a reasonable alternative to administration of large volumes of isotonic fluids.

Electrolyte administration as oral pastes or in drinking water

Use of oral electrolyte pastes has been mentioned several times as an adjunct to intravenous and enteral fluids. Oral pastes have the distinct advantage of replacing needed electrolytes without placing additives in the base intravenous fluid (increasing osmolality and cost) and limiting the number of times that a nasogastric tube has to be passed. When pastes are used to complement the fluid therapy plan, it is important to ensure that horses also drink water in the hours after electrolyte administration. In fact, it is reasonable initially to treat some horses with mild-to-moderate dehydration (3%–7%) with a dose of enteral fluids (12 L through a nasogastric tube would correct approximately 2.5% dehydration) and oral electrolyte pastes. Because the goal of electrolytes administered orally would be to stimulate further drinking, NaCl should be the predominant electrolyte administered. It can be given alone or mixed with KCl in a ratio of 2:1 to 3:1. As for enteral fluids, oral pastes can be made from table salt and lite salt (a 1:1 mixture of NaCl and KCl). KCl can also be obtained in larger quantities from chemical supply companies or in bulk from feed mills.

Administration of 30 g of NaCl (as an oral paste would provide approximately 500 mEq of Na^+ (1 g of NaCl $\approx$ 17.1 mEq of both Na^+ and Cl^-), equal to that in 3 to 4 L of an isotonic polyionic crystalloid fluid. Thus, dosing oral pastes at 6-hour intervals should provide a similar amount of electrolytes as a maintenance rate of intravenous fluids, and more frequent administration could be used to replace electrolytes lost by disorders producing dehydration. Again, use of oral electrolyte pastes will be beneficial only if horses voluntarily drink water to replace the concurrent water need. Although use of oral pastes has both practical (eg, can be administered by a client on the farm) and economical advantages, their administration may be accompanied by transient interruption of feeding, apparently caused by poor palatability of the pastes. In an attempt to lessen this problem, salts can be mixed with corn oil, molasses, applesauce, or yogurt rather than with water.

A final option to increase electrolyte intake is to dissolve NaCl and KCl in drinking water. Adding 30 g of NaCl, or a mix of NaCl and KCl, to each gallon of drinking water would make a nearly isotonic solution that may be consumed by some horses. Voluntary drinking of water containing electrolytes is rather variable between horses, however; thus, plain water should also be made available in addition to water containing electrolytes.

Monitoring response to treatment

As mentioned previously, correction of dehydration can be assessed most accurately by weighing horses at 12- to 24-hour intervals and observing a lack of further increase in body mass. Unfortunately, repeated weighing is rarely performed in hospitalized patients and is impractical for horses housed in isolation stalls for treatment of suspected contagious diseases. Thus, in most hospital settings, response to fluid therapy is monitored by reassessing the patient's attitude and clinical parameters of hydration, including heart rate; moistness of oral membranes; temperature of the nose, ears, and extremities; skin tent response; PCV; and TS. In addition, an obvious but easily overlooked assessment is the frequency of urination. Most horses should be observed to pass substantial amounts of dilute urine within 6 to 12 hours after onset of fluid administration, and horses with mild dehydration (5%–7%) may start to pass urine within 2 hours.

Once an increase in urine output is observed, the rate of fluid administration should be reassessed and usually reduced. At times, improvement in other clinical parameters (eg, heart rate or PCV) is less than desired despite increased urine output. Rarely does maintenance of a high fluid administration rate correct these clinical abnormalities once urine output has increased. More often, patients with this response may need further supportive care such as treatments that increase oncotic pressure (eg, plasma or hetastarch) or that provide further analgesia for the underlying disease.

Observation of urine output is also warranted to assess for potential development of acute renal failure in moderately to severely dehydrated horses. Two signs that should increase suspicion for acute renal failure are a greater-than-expected degree of depression for the primary disease and oliguria (decreased urine output). The latter is most easily assessed by monitoring wetness of bedding in the stall rather than by continuous observation for urination. Next, horses in the incipient stage of acute renal failure will also gain excessive weight because of fluid retention. Serial weighing would likely detect fluid retention a day or two before it would be reflected by development of edema.

Discontinuation of fluid therapy

It is often easier to decide when a horse needs fluid therapy than to determine when this aspect of supportive care can safely be discontinued. In reality, fluid support is probably continued longer than necessary in many horses. Nevertheless, there are a couple of general rules that can be followed. First, the medical or surgical problem being treated should be stable or improving for 12 to 24 hours before discontinuation of fluid therapy is considered. This period would include correction of dehydration and at least 6 to 12 hours of fluid administration at a maintenance rate alone. Fluid therapy does not necessarily have to be continued until all laboratory data, including serum electrolyte concentrations and measures of renal function, have returned to the normal ranges, especially for horses that are improving in response to treatment. Second, when the medical or surgical disorder has been accompanied by partial or complete anorexia, a reasonable goal is for the horse to be eating at least 50% of a normal feed ration, preferably with an increasing appetite, before fluid therapy is discontinued. There are obvious exceptions to this rule; for example, a horse being treated for impaction colic with enteral fluids (through a nasogastric tube) usually will not be offered feed until after the last dose of enteral fluids has been given. When intravenous fluids have been employed either exclusively (eg, because of gastric reflux) or in conjunction with enteral fluids, intravenous fluids are often continued at a maintenance rate for 12 to 24 hours after feed is again offered. The main point is that fluids do not need to be continued until the patient is back on full feed. Third, a more cautious approach to discontinuing fluid therapy should be considered in horses receiving multiple potentially nephrotoxic medications (eg, gentamicin and flunixin meglumine or phenylbutazone), especially if indices of renal function are above the normal ranges. In addition, horses continuing to receive these medications may benefit from administration of oral electrolyte pastes, mostly NaCl given in an attempt to stimulate greater voluntary water intake and associated urine output, once enteral or intravenous fluids have been discontinued.

The decision to discontinue fluid therapy is more difficult in patients with long-standing ($>$ 5 days), ongoing fluid losses such as persistent gastric reflux with small intestinal disorders or persistent diarrhea with more severe cases of enterocolitis. Such cases are often receiving multiple intravenous infusions (eg, partial or total parenteral nutrition, lidocaine, and other therapies) in addition to maintenance fluid support. In fact, when all the fluids being administered are added up, these patients are often receiving fluid at a rate greater than maintenance needs. Further, they are often receiving excessive amounts of Na^+ and less-than-adequate amounts of K^+. Again, excess Na^+ replacement leads to greater urine output and exacerbates depletion of body K^+ stores. In addition to requiring more frequent assessment of acid–base status and serum electrolyte concentrations, such patients may be good candidates for using oral electrolyte pastes to correct replace K^+ deficits and provide further Na^+ when ongoing losses continue. At the same time, the approach should be to challenge these patients, once they are considered stable, by discontinuing fluid therapy for 12 to 24 hours. If their clinical condition deteriorates (eg, a decrease in appetite; greater depression; and increases in heart rate, PCV, and TS), fluid therapy can be started again. In these cases of more serious disease, affected horses may need to be challenged by discontinuation of fluid therapy several times before they can remain stable without this aspect of supportive care.

VETERINARY
CLINICS
Equine Practice

Vet Clin Equine 22 (2006) 15–35

Equine Fluid Therapy: Problem Set

Harold C. Schott II, DVM, PhD

Department of Large Animal Clinical Sciences, D-202 Veterinary Medical Center,
Michigan State University, East Lansing, MI 48824–1314, USA

Case 1

You are presented with an adult (assume 500-kg) horse that has been showing signs of mild abdominal pain for 12 hours. Examination reveals normal vital parameters and membrane color, but the membranes are slightly dry to the touch. A skin tent persists only momentarily, and you estimate dehydration at 5%. Intestinal sounds are decreased on auscultation of the abdomen, and rectal palpation reveals firm ingesta in the bowel in the left upper abdominal quadrant. Your tentative diagnosis is a pelvic flexure impaction as the cause of colic. Passage of a nasogastric tube yields no reflux. In addition to administration of an analgesic (eg, flunixin meglumine, 250 mg), you would like to pursue fluid therapy in an attempt to "overhydrate" the horse and soften the impaction. Typically, the approach to fluid therapy in this case would involve correction of dehydration and further administration of fluid at a rate of approximately twice the maintenance requirement. The volume of fluid required to correct dehydration is estimated by multiplying body mass in kilograms by the estimated percentage of dehydration. The result (in kilograms) is assumed to approximate the fluid deficit in liters. Maintenance requirements are 1 to 2 mL/kg/h or approximately 1 L/h for a 500-kg adult horse.

Your fluid therapy plan for the initial 12 hours is outlined as follows:

Fluid deficit from dehydration is 5%: 0.05×500 kg = 25 L
Maintenance requirement for 12 hours is 1 L/h = 12 L
Additional fluid requirement (to double maintenance) = 12 L
Total fluid volume for first 12 hours = 49 L
Rate of fluid administration is 49 L over 12 hours = 4 L/h[a]

E-mail address: schott@cvm.msu.edu

[a] Although this is the initial fluid rate selected, the rate is likely to be decreased within 4 to 6 hours after starting fluid therapy when frequent production of dilute urine is observed.

0749-0739/06/$ - see front matter
doi:10.1016/j.cveq.2005.12.001   *vetequine.theclinics.com*

Type of intravenous fluid selected: polyionic crystalloid fluid (eg, lactated Ringer's solution)

An alternate approach to fluid therapy in this patient would be to provide fluids enterally via a nasogastric tube. As long as small intestinal function is normal (which it likely is with an impaction), oral fluids are rapidly absorbed, often within the first hour after administration. Absorption is most rapid when the fluid administered is isotonic with body fluids (280–300 mOsm/kg), whereas administration of hypertonic fluids may transiently pull water into the bowel lumen before absorption ensues. Absorbed fluids are then secreted more distally in the colon to soften the impaction. An alternate approach to treat impaction colic is to administer a dose of an intestinal cathartic or laxative, such as a hypertonic fluid, that primarily contains a poorly absorbed ion (eg, magnesium). The cathartic agent acts to draw fluid into the bowel lumen, which can proceed distally to moisten the impaction. With the latter treatment, however, it is important to recognize that further dehydration of the horse may develop unless it starts to drink or other means of fluid support are provided. Gastric distention with either type of fluid administered via a nasogastric tube has the additional benefit of stimulating colonic motility.

To make an isotonic fluid, you need to know the following:

- Sodium chloride (NaCl; common table salt), 1 g, provides Na^+ and Cl^-, 17.1 mEq of each.
- Potassium chloride (KCl), 1 g, provides 13.4 mEq of K^+ and Cl^- each.
- "Lite" salt is 50% NaCl and 50% KCl, and 1 g provides 8.55 mEq of Na^+, 6.7 mEq of K^+, and 15.25 MEq of Cl^-.
- $NaHCO_3$ (baking soda), 1 g, provides 12 mEq of Na^+ and HCO_3^- each.
- For an anorectic horse, it is generally safe to provide a mix of NaCl and KCl (lite salt) as an oral fluid or a mix of table salt and lite salt.
- Adding NaCl, 30 g, or a mix of NaCl and KCl to each gallon (3.785 L) of drinking water makes a nearly isotonic solution. This is approximately 8 g/L.
- You can typically safely administer 8 L of fluid per hour to a horse via a nasogastric tube without distending the stomach enough to cause colic.

To replace the fluid deficits determined previously, you may need to pass a nasogastric tube four to six times over the first 12 hours. Alternately, you could leave it in place if it is well tolerated by the horse. It is important to check for reflux before administration of each successive dose of fluids to ensure that the previous dose has been absorbed. Assuming that absorption is adequate, an enteral fluid therapy plan for this horse using lite salt as the electrolyte source would be as follows:

Volume of fluid administered at a rate of 49 L over 6 doses = approximately 8 L per dose
Lite salt: 8 g/L × 49 L = 392 g
8 g/L × 8 L per dose = salt at a rate of 64 g per dose

Per liter of fluids: lite salt, 8 g/L, provides the following:
  68.4 mEq/L of $[Na^+]$
  53.6 mEq/L of $[K^+]$
  122 mEq/L of $[Cl^-]$
  Osmolality at the rate of 244 mOsm/kg

Case 2

You are presented with an adult (assume 500-kg) horse that has been off feed for 2 days and developed mild diarrhea on the morning of presentation. Examination reveals a rectal temperature of 39.2°C (102.5°F), a heart rate of 60 beats per minute, and a respiratory rate of 12 breaths per minute. The oral membranes are pale and tacky to the touch. A skin tent persists for a couple of seconds, and you estimate dehydration at 7%. Intestinal sounds are increased on auscultation of the abdomen, and fluid-like feces are passed during examination of the horse. Your tentative diagnosis is undifferentiated colitis. The approach to fluid therapy in this case would involve correction of dehydration and further administration of fluid at a rate to provide the maintenance requirement. In addition, fluids are administered to replace estimated losses in diarrhea (assume 1 L/h).

Your fluid therapy plan for the initial 12 hours is outlined below:

Fluid deficit from dehydration is 0.07×500 kg $= 35$ L
Maintenance requirement for 12 hours is 1 L/h $= 12$ L
Additional fluid requirement (for ongoing losses) is 1 L/h $\times$ 12 h $= 12$ L
Total fluid volume for first 12 hours $= 59$ L
Rate of fluid administration is 59 L over 12 hours $= 5$ L/h[b]
Type of intravenous fluid selected: polyionic crystalloid fluid (eg, lactated
   Ringer's solution)

After this plan has been initiated, you receive the following laboratory results (reference ranges):

Packed cell volume (PCV) $= 49\%$ (30%–45%)
Total solids (TS) $= 8.3$ g/dL (5.9–7.5 g/dL)
Fibrinogen $= 0.4$ g/dL (0.1–0.4 g/dL)
$Na^+ = 127$ mEq/L (128–158 mEq/L)
$K^+ = 2.7$ mEq/L (2.6–4.9 mEq/L)
$Cl^- = 85$ mEq/L (91–110 mEq/L)
Creatinine (Cr) $= 2.8$ mg/dL (0.8–1.8 mg/dL)
Venous blood gas:
   pH $= 7.357$ (7.377–7.423)
   $P_{CO_2} = 34.4$ mm Hg (36.9–54.4 mm Hg)

---

[b] Although this is the initial fluid rate selected, the rate is likely to be decreased within 4 to 6 hours after starting fluid therapy when frequent production of dilute urine is observed.

Po_2 43.1 mm Hg (27.9–46.2 mm Hg)
HCO_3^- = 18.7 mEq/L (24.5–30.4 mEq/L)
Base excess (BE) = −5.8 mEq/L (−2.8 to 3.1 mEq/L)

The Na^+ concentration in this horse's serum is low because the only replacement fluid it has had has been through drinking water, which is hypotonic. This horse would not have a normal stimulus to drink, because the primary stimulus for drinking is an increase in plasma tonicity, specifically Na^+ concentration.

In the euhydrated state, there is approximately 300 L of total body water in a 500-kg horse. Essentially two thirds of body fluid is intracellular fluid (ICF) and one third is extracellular fluid (ECF). Because K^+ is the primary intracellular cation and Na^+ is the primary extracellular cation, contents of these ions in body fluids are approximately 28,400 mEq for K^+ (100 L × 4 mEq/L in ECF + 200 L × 140 mEq/L in ICF) and approximately 16,000 mEq for Na^+ (100 L × 140 mEq/L in ECF + 200 L × 10 mEq/L in ICF). With the loss of total body water incurred during dehydration, it is important to recognize that there is also a loss of electrolytes, leading to concurrent cation and anion deficits. There are two components to the cation deficit that must be considered: the loss of cations in the deficit of total body water (this represents a loss of isotonic fluid) and a potential further cation deficit in the fluid remaining in the body when plasma tonicity is decreased (as in the horse in this example). Serum Na^+ concentration provides a reasonable measure of exchangeable cations (Na^+ in ECF and K^+ in ICF) in total body water, because the Na^+ concentration in ECF is comparable to the K^+ concentration in ICF. Thus, the exchangeable cation deficit can be estimated as follows: cation deficit = (pre-TBW × pre-Na^+ concentration) − (post-TBW × post-Na^+ concentration), where TBW is total body water.

We can calculate this horse's exchangeable cation deficit using a value of 140 mEq for the predehydration serum Na^+ concentration:

Predehydration TBW = 300 L
Water deficit (7% dehydration) = 35 L
Postdehydration TBW (300 L − 35 L) = 265 L
Exchangeable cation deficit: (300 L × 140 mEq/L) − (265 L × 127 mEq/L)
    = 8345 mEq cation deficit

An important concept to understand is that the nature of the fluid (and cation) deficit varies with the time course of dehydration. Although fluid is initially lost from the ECF, some of the ECF fluid deficit is replaced by fluid shifting from the ICF space to the ECF space. In general, the longer the time over which dehydration develops, the larger the ICF fluid deficit becomes in comparison to the ECF fluid deficit. For example, administration of furosemide causes a rapid fluid loss (10 L of urine produced within 60 minutes), and this fluid deficit is essentially all from the ECF. In contrast, when dehydration develops as a result of food and water deprivation, a larger fraction of the fluid deficit (up to 85%) may ultimately be incurred by the ICF space. Considering the time course over which dehydration develops allows the clinician to estimate the relative magnitude of cation (Na^+ and K^+) deficits more accurately.

In this case example, it is reasonable to assume that two thirds of the fluid loss is from ECF, whereas one third is from ICF. Thus, we can estimate the relative Na^+ and K^+ deficits as follows: Na^+ deficit: $2/3 \times 8345$ mEq = 5563 mEq and K^+ deficit: $1/3 \times 8345$ mEq = 2782 mEq.

Because most polyionic crystalloid fluid products have Na^+ concentration (range: 135–140 mEq/L) similar to that of serum, we can calculate the amount of Na^+ that should be administered with the fluid therapy plan outlined previously (first 12 hours) as follows: 140 mEq $\times$ 59 L = 8260 mEq.

Is this amount of Na^+ too little, adequate, or too much?

It is adequate. Although the amount administered is greater than the estimated ECF deficit (5563 mEq), we should anticipate ongoing losses attributable to diarrhea. Further, if excessive amounts are administered, urinary Na^+ excretion ensues. Hypernatremia is of essentially no concern as long as a source of fresh water is provided.

The K^+ concentration of most polyionic crystalloid fluid products is also similar to that of serum, typically around 5 mEq/L. Thus, we can also calculate the amount of K^+ that should be administered with the fluid therapy plan outlined previously (first 12 hours): 5 mEq $\times$ 59 l = 295 mEq.

Is this amount of K^+ too little, adequate, or too much?

It is too little; the amount administered would only be approximately 10% of the estimated K^+ deficit (2782 mEq). For this reason, it is common to add KCl at a rate of 20 to 40 mEq/L of fluids. For example, adding KCl at a rate of 20 mEq/L would provide an additional 1420 mEq of K^+ in the fluid therapy plan, but this would still not replace the estimated deficit of 2782 mEq. Thus, it is generally safe to supplement fluids with KCl in equine patients. The only exception would be in patients with severely compromised renal function, which may become hyperkalemic. For such reasons, it is always recommended to measure serum K^+ concentration before supplementing fluids with KCl. Because adding KCl to intravenous fluids is inconvenient and increases cost, alternate ways to provide KCl are to provide a second water bucket with KCl added (always continue to provide fresh nonsupplemented water as well) or to administer KCl via a nasogastric tube (ie, 8 L of water with KCl at a rate of 10 g/L would provide 80 g or 1072 mEq of K^+ with an osmolality of 268 mOsm/kg) or by oral dosing.

Estimate the bicarbonate deficit as follows: body mass in kilograms $\times$ 0.5 $\times$ base deficit = 500 kg $\times$ 0.5 $\times$ 5.8 mEq/L = 1450 mEq

Is specific correction of the acid-base status necessary?

No. As a general rule we do not worry about correcting acid-base status if the blood pH is normal and the HCO_3^- concentration exceeds 15 mEq/L. In this horse, volume expansion is most important, and mild acid-base disturbances generally resolve as dehydration is corrected and tissue perfusion improves.

Case 3

You are presented with an adult (assume 500-kg) horse that has had a decreased appetite for 5 days and has had watery diarrhea for the past 3 days. Little food was consumed over the last 3 days other than some grazing of the owner's lawn. The owner had been treating the horse with oral flunixin meglumine paste (250-kg dose) twice daily for the last 3 days. Examination reveals a rectal temperature of 37° (98.5°F), a heart rate of 88 beats per minute, and a respiratory rate of 16 breaths per minute with deep breaths. The oral membranes are dark red and dry to the touch. A skin tent persists for 10 seconds, and the ears and legs are cold. You estimate dehydration at 10%. Intestinal sounds are absent, and fluid-like feces are present in the rectum. Your tentative diagnosis is undifferentiated colitis.

The approach to fluid therapy in this case would involve correction of dehydration and further administration of fluid at a rate to provide the maintenance requirement. In addition, fluids need to be administered to replace estimated losses in diarrhea (assume a rate of 2 L/h).

Your fluid therapy plan for the initial 12 hours is outlined as follows:

Fluid deficit from dehydration is 0.10×500 kg = 50 L
Maintenance requirement for 12 hours is 1 L/h = 12 L
Additional fluid requirement (for ongoing losses) is 2 L/h $\times$ 12 hours = 24 L
Total fluid volume for first 12 hours = 86 L
Rate of fluid administration is 86 L over 12 hours = 7 L/h[c]
Type of intravenous fluid selected: polyionic crystalloid fluid (eg, lactated Ringer's solution)

After this plan has been initiated, you receive the following laboratory results (reference ranges):

PCV = 62% (30%–45%)
TS = 5.6 g/dL (5.9–7.5 g/dL)
Fibr = 0.6 g/dL (0.1–0.4 g/dL)
Na^+ = 99 mEq/L (128–158 mEq/L)
K^+ = 3.2 mEq/L (2.6–4.9 mEq/L)
Cl^- = 64 mEq/L (91–110 mEq/L)
Cr = 6.6 mg/dL (0.8–1.8 mg/dL)
Venous blood gas
    pH = 7.156 (7.377–7.423)
    PCO_2 = 37.1 mm Hg (36.9–54.4 mm Hg)

---

[c] Although this is the initial fluid rate selected, the rate is likely to be decreased within 4 to 6 hours after starting fluid therapy when frequent production of dilute urine is observed.

Po_2 = 40.2 mm Hg (27.9–46.2 mm Hg)
HCO_3^- = 12.1 mEq/L (24.5–30.4 mEq/L)
BE = −15.9 mEq/L (−2.8 to 3.1 mEq/L)

Because of the severity of dehydration and the 5-day course of the disease, you assume that there is likely a substantial K^+ deficit and decide to add KCl at a rate of 40 mEq/L of fluids.

This horse's exchangeable cation deficit can be calculated as follows:

Pre-TBW = 300 L
Water deficit = 50 L
Post-TBW = 250 L
Exchangeable cation deficit: (300 L × 140 mEq/L) − (250 × 99 mEq/L) = 17,250 mEq cation deficit

The relative Na^+ and K^+ losses (assume 60% from ICF and 40% from ECF because of longer duration of disease) can be calculated as follows:

Na^+ loss: 0.6 × 17,250 = 10,350 mEq
K^+ loss: 0.4 × 17,250 = 6900 mEq

How much Na^+ is to be administered with your plan during the first 12 hours? 140 mEq/L × 86 L = 12,040 mEq

How much K^+ is to be administered with your plan during the first 12 hours? 45 mEq/L × 86 L = 3870 mEq

Are the estimated cation deficits adequately replaced with this fluid therapy plan?

As in Case 2, the amount of Na^+ administered is greater than the estimated deficit, but we should again anticipate ongoing losses attributable to diarrhea. Further, if excessive amounts are administered, urinary Na^+ excretion ensues. If a similar rate of fluid administration is needed over a couple of days, the total Na^+ load administered becomes substantial—several times greater than the total amount of Na^+ in body fluids. Administration of excessive amounts of Na^+ in this manner usually leads to expansion of the ECF, primarily interstitial fluid volume, and development of edema. Obviously, development of edema is further compounded by decreased plasma oncotic pressure because of concurrent hypoalbuminemia. Again, hypernatremia should not develop as long as a source of fresh water is provided.

The amount of K^+ replaced is again too little, only a bit more than half of the estimated K^+ deficit, despite addition KCl at a rate of 40 mEq/L of fluids. Thus, as described previously, additional KCl should be administered via a nasogastric tube or by oral dosing. The clinical importance of total body depletion of K^+ in equine patients remains unclear, but severe hypokalemia can certainly lead to muscular weakness and cramping in other species.

The bicarbonate deficit can be calculated as follows: 500 kg × 0.5 × 15.9 mEq/L = 3975 mEq

Is specific correction of the acid-base status necessary? If so, how would you correct the bicarbonate deficit?

Yes, it would be helpful. Addition of $NaHCO_3$ at a rate of 50 mEq/L (50×86 L = 4300 mEq/L) would be a reasonable approach. $NaHCO_3$ cannot be added to calcium-containing fluids, however, because $CaCO_3$ precipitates may form. Thus, $NaHCO_3$ would need to be added to another base fluid, typically 0.9% NaCl. It is important to remember that when $NaHCO_3$ is added to a fluid in an attempt to correct a bicarbonate (base) deficit, Na^+ and HCO_3^- are being added, such that the final Na^+ concentration of the fluid would be greater than 200 mEq/L (154 mEq/L in 0.9% NaCl and 50 mEq from the added $NaHCO_3$). Although traditional teaching of the Henderson-Hasselbach approach to acid-base disorders would state that the bicarbonate deficit develops because of bicarbonate loss in diarrhea, proponents of the Stewart strong ion difference (SID) approach to understating acid-base disorders would argue that changes in concentrations of strong ions are more important. Thus, the benefit of adding $NaHCO_3$ to a base fluid may be more attributable to the additional Na^+ load administered than to the added bicarbonate. As with potassium supplementation, another means of providing $NaHCO_3$ would be administration of $NaHCO_3$ via a nasogastric tube (ie, 8 L of water with $NaHCO_3$ at a rate of 15 g/L would provide 120 g or 1440 mEq of HCO_3^-, with an osmolality of 360 mOsm/kg) or by oral dosing as a slurry (preferably in corn oil or another non–water-based liquid to limit fizzing).

Considering the expense of this fluid therapy plan, many owners may not be able to proceed with such treatment. Rather than giving up on such patients, an alternative can be to mix "homemade fluids" using distilled water, NaCl, KCl, and $NaHCO_3$. Given a fluid carboy that can hold 100 L of water, how many grams of each of these salts do you want to add to make an appropriate fluid? After preparing the fluid, calculate the concentrations of Na^+, K^+, Cl^-, and HCO_3^- as well as the estimated osmolality of the fluid.

A simple way to approach this problem is to start with a base fluid of 0.7% NaCl (7 g/L) and supplement this fluid with KCl at a rate of 60 mEq/L and $NaHCO_3$ at a rate of 50 mEq/L.

For each 100 L of carboy, we need:

NaCl: 100 L $\times$ 7 g/L = 700 g
KCl (1 g = K^+, 13.4 mEq): 60 mEq/L $\times$ 100 L = 6000 mEq/13.4 mEq per gram = approximately 450 g
$NaHCO_3$ (1 g = HCO_3^-, 12 mEq): 50 mEq/L $\times$ 100 L = 5000 mEq/12 mEq per gram = approximately 420 g

This mixture results in the following ion concentrations:

$[Na^+]$ = 120 mEq/L + 50 mEq/L = 170 mEq/L, or
(7 g/L as NaCl $\times$ 17.1 mEq/g) + (4.2 g/L as $NaHCO_3$ $\times$ 12 mEq/g) = 170 mEq/L

$[K^+] = 60$ mEq/L, or

(4.5 g/L as KCl $\times$ 13.4 mEq/g) = 60 mEq/L

$[Cl^-] = 120$ mEq/L + 60 mEq/L = 180 mEq/L, or

(7 g/L as NaCl $\times$ 17.1 mEq/g) + (4.5 g/L as KCl $\times$ 13.4 mEq/g) = 180 mEq/L

$[HCO_3^-] = 50$ mEq/L, or

(4.2 g as $NaHCO_3$ $\times$ 12 mEq/g) = 50.4 mEq/L

The osmolality of the fluid is as follows: 170 + 60 + 180 + 50 = 460 mOsm/kg.

This is only one example of a several possible fluid mixtures. In addition to the considerable cost savings, the homemade fluid recipe provided here allows more appropriate replacement of the estimated K^+ and HCO_3^- deficits in this case example. These fluids are not sterile or pyrogen-free, however, and it is not unusual for horses to develop unanticipated fevers when supported with homemade fluids. Thus, use of homemade fluids should only advocated as an alternative to euthanasia for owners who lack the financial resources to pursue treatment with commercially available sterile and pyrogen-free intravenous fluid products.

Case 4

A 19-year-old gelding in good body condition (assume 500 kg) is presented at noon with an acute onset of colic. The horse was reported to be normal at 10:00 PM the evening before. The referring veterinarian had seen the horse at 9:30 AM and administered flunixin meglumine, 500 mg, intravenously and xylazine, 250 mg, intravenously and promptly recommended referral. The horse is moderately painful, the heart rate is 72 beats per minute, the oral membranes are pale pink and capillary refill time is 3.5 seconds, intestinal sounds are absent, and distended loops of small bowel are detected on rectal palpation. Further examination reveals a mild persistence of a skin tent (3 seconds) and that the ears and extremities (from carpi and tarsi) are cool. Eight liters of reflux is obtained on passage of a nasogastric tube, and abdominocentesis yields serosanguinous fluid with TS of 3.5 g/dL (reference range: <2.5 g/dL). You recommend surgical exploration of the abdomen because you suspect a strangulating obstruction of the small bowel.

The owner authorizes the surgery, but the anesthesia service is concerned about anesthetizing the horse and asks you to provide initial therapy (30–60 minutes) to correct shock before general anesthesia is induced. You estimate dehydration at 7% because of shock secondary to fluid accumulation in the small intestine oral to the strangulating lesion and endotoxemia causing venous pooling of blood.

Shortly after this initial examination, you receive the following laboratory results (reference ranges):

PCV = 54% (30%–45%)
TS = 7.4 g/dL (5.9–7.5 g/dL)
Fibr = 0.4 g/dL (0.1–0.4 g/dL)
Na^+ = 133 mEq/L (128–158 mEq/L)
K^+ = 3.6 mEq/L (2.6–4.9 mEq/L)
Cl^- = 98 mEq/L (91–110 mEq/L)
Cr = 3.0 mg/dL (0.8–1.8 mg/dL)
Venous blood gas
    pH = 7.318 (7.377–7.423)
    P_{CO_2} = 35.1 mm Hg (36.9–54.4 mm Hg)
    P_{O_2} = 29.5 mm Hg (27.9–46.2 mm Hg)
    HCO_3^- = 24.0 mEq/L (24.5–30.4 mEq/L)
    BE = −1.9 mEq/L (−2.8 to 3.1 mEq/L)

Before surgery, you administer a 10-L bolus of a polyionic isotonic electrolyte solution and 7.5% NaCl (2 L). At surgery, a strangulating lipoma is found, and an intestinal resection is performed. During surgery, the horse received additional polyionic isotonic electrolyte solution (20 L), and the PCV was 42% and the TS were 5.8 g/dL at the end of surgery (after a total 30 L of the polyionic isotonic electrolyte solution had been given).

What was the reason for administering hypertonic saline?

Hypertonic saline (7.5% NaCl) can be administered in an attempt to rapidly yet transiently expand circulating volume and improve hemodynamics in patients that are showing signs of shock: tachycardia, weak peripheral pulses, and poor tissue perfusion. The large osmotic load administered intravenously draws water from interstitial and ICF fluid spaces into the vasculature to increase circulating volume. Administration of hypertonic saline also raises serum Na^+ and Cl^- concentrations and can stimulate thirst. In this case, drinking is not permitted and administration of hypertonic saline must be followed by continued administration of isotonic fluids.

Before surgery, the horse's fluid deficit was estimated at 35 L (500 kg × 0.07 = 35 L). Despite administration of nearly all this deficit by the end of surgery, endotoxemia is likely still contributing to poor tissue perfusion; thus, you elect to provide further intravenous fluid support at twice the maintenance rate (2 L/h) during the initial recovery period, starting when the horse returns to its stall at 8:00 PM. Ongoing losses should be negligible unless the horse begins to reflux after surgery. Therefore, the total volume for the next 12 hours should be 24 L. Because feed is being withheld from this horse, it should have an ongoing obligate K^+ loss in urine. Therefore, KCl (40 mEq/L) is added to the fluids.

On the morning after surgery, the gelding is more depressed and the heart rate has increased to 60 beats per minute (from a rate of 48 beats per minute at midnight). A regular "thumping," in synchrony with the heart rate is observed in the paralumbar fossa. Further examination reveals a lack of intestinal motility and cool lower limbs and ears. Overnight, one small pile of semiformed feces was passed, urine was passed two times (specific gravity of 1.028 on one sample), and the horse was intermittently observed to paw. At midnight, 8 L of reflux was obtained on passage of a nasogastric tube, prompting a decision to leave the tube in place. At that time, the fluid administration rate was also increased to 3 L/h. At 4:00 AM, 12 L of reflux was obtained, and 10 L was recovered at 8:00 AM. Thus, in the past 12 hours, 30 L of reflux was recovered and 32 L of fluid was administered (2 L/h for 4 hours, followed by 3 L/h for 8 hours). The following laboratory results are returned at 8:00 AM (reference ranges):

PCV = 44% (30%–45%)
TS = 7.2 g/dL (5.9–7.5 g/dL)
Fibr = 0.4 g/dL (0.1–0.4 g/dL)
Na^+ = 139 mEq/L (128–158 mEq/L)
K^+ = 2.8 mEq/L (2.6–4.9 mEq/L)
Cl^- = 95 mEq/L (91–110 mEq/L)
Cr = 2.9 mg/dL (0.8–1.8 mg/dL)
Ionized Ca^{++} = 4.6 mg/dL (5.4–6.8 mg/dL)
Venous blood gas
   pH = 7.466 (7.377–7.423)
   P_{CO_2} = 31.1 mm Hg (36.9–54.4 mm Hg)
   P_{O_2} = 44.5 mm Hg (27.9–46.2 mm Hg)
   HCO_3^- = 29.0 mEq/L (24.5–30.4 mEq/L)
   BE = 2.1 mEq/L (−2.8 to 3.1 mEq/L)

What is "thumps" and why did it develop in this horse?

Thumps, or synchronous diaphragmatic flutter, is a complication in horses with acid-base and electrolyte aberrations that results in neuromuscular excitability. It is most commonly associated with hypocalcemia, hypokalemia, and alkalosis. Thumps develops when the phrenic nerve, coursing over the right atria of the horse, fires with each depolarization of the atrial myocardium. The result is a weak to strong contraction of the diaphragm, causing an outward movement in the paralumbar fossa as abdominal contents are pushed caudally. It is of interest to note that in addition to a decrease in ionized Ca^{++}, the morning laboratory data also reveal alkalosis that is likely metabolic (further hypochloremia because of fluid loss into the upper gastrointestinal tract and an increase in HCO_3^- to the upper end of the reference range) and respiratory (hypocapnia, perhaps caused by hyperventilation in response to pain) in origin.

In this case, the volume of reflux recovered overnight was nearly the same as the amount of fluids administered and hydration and tissue perfusion needs have not been met. The patient is showing signs of poor perfusion and has mild tachycardia (a consequence of decreased circulating volume, hypocalcemia, or pain from upper intestinal and gastric distention). A decrease in circulating volume is further supported by the increase in TS since the end of surgery (from 5.8 to 7.2 g/dL). Immediate concerns are to improve circulating volume and correct hypocalcemia. The latter problem can also contribute to decreased intestinal motility and tachycardia (hypocalcemia can lead to decreased cardiac contractility and stroke volume). Thus, you start a 10-L fluid bolus over the next 2 hours and add 23% calcium borogluconate solution (125 mL) to each 5-L fluid bag.

What is the Ca^{++} deficit of this horse?

Determining the Ca^{++} deficit is not as straightforward as estimating the exchangeable cation (Na^+ and K^+) deficit, because only 0.1% of Ca^{++} in the body is in ECF and plasma. Further, only 45% to 55% of Ca^{++} in plasma is in the ionized (active) form, with the remainder bound to protein (primarily albumin) and a small amount complexed with other anions (citrate, phosphate, bicarbonate, and lactate). If we assume a normal total serum Ca^{++} concentration of 12 mg/dL and a normal ionized Ca^{++} concentration of 6 mg/dL, the following estimate of the ECF Ca^{++} deficit can be made (calcium is 40.1 g/mol and has 2 Eq/mol):

First, the total ECF Ca^{++} content is estimated in a normal horse as follows:

- Normal plasma and ECF = ionized calcium, 6.0 mg/dL
- 100 L of ECF × ionized Ca^{++} concentration of 6.0 mg/dL = 6000 mg or 6 g
- Plasma has a further 6.0 mg/dL of Ca^{++} bound to plasma protein
- Assuming that plasma volume is 30 L = 30 L × 6.0 mg/dL = 1800 mg or 1.8 g
- Thus, total ECF Ca^{++} concentration: 6 g + 1.8 g = 7.8 g
- 7.8 g per 40.1 g/mol = 0.20 mol × 2 Eq/mol = 0.40 Eq or 400 mEq

Second, the ECF Ca^{++} deficit can be estimated as follows:

- Measured ionized Ca^{++} concentration is 4.6 mg/dL versus a normal concentration of 6 mg/dL
- Therefore, measured ionized Ca^{++} concentration is decreased by approximately 25%: (6.0 − 4.6/6.0) × 100 = approximately 25%
- Deficit is 0.25 × 7.8 g = approximately 2 g or approximately 100 mEq (calcium is 40.1 g/mol and has 2 Eq/mol)

How much Ca^{++} is replaced by adding 23% calcium borogluconate (125 mL) per 5-L bag of fluids?

Calcium borogluconate, 500 mL, contains calcium in the amount of 10.7 g or 535 mEq (1069 mEq/L); thus, 125 mL provides approximately 2.7 g or 134 mEq, which equals one third of the ECF ionized Ca^{++} pool.

Supplementation with calcium borogluconate solution (125 mL) per 5-L bag actually more than adequately replaces the estimated deficit. In fact, in many equine hospitals, it is routine to add this amount of calcium borogluconate solution when horses are receiving intravenous fluids, especially when they are not eating. As an example, if a horse receives a maintenance rate of fluids (~20 L over 24 hours) with calcium borogluconate solution at a rate of 25 mL/L, a total of 500 mL of the calcium borogluconate solution is administered. This equates to 10.7 g or approximately 535 mEq of Ca^{++} over the course of a day.

Another way to look at Ca^{++} supplementation is to compare it with the suggested dietary Ca^{++} intake of 40 mg/kg/d, or 20 g for a 500-kg horse. Because only 50% to 60% of this ingested Ca^{++} is absorbed, the total daily uptake of Ca^{++} by an adult horse is approximately 10 to 12 g/d. Thus, this uptake is closely matched by addition of a 23% calcium borogluconate solution (25 mL/L) in 20 L of fluid. Even if intravenous fluids were to be administered at twice the maintenance rate ($\sim$40 L over 24 hours), it is considered safe to continue adding 25 mL of the calcium borogluconate solution to each liter, because any excess Ca^{++} administered is excreted in urine. Further, few clinical problems (and none in horses) have been associated with transient increases in total or ionized serum Ca^{++} concentrations. In fact, infusion of excessive amount of Ca^{++} resulting in ionized serum Ca^{++} concentrations of 10 to 12 mg/dL has not been observed to cause untoward effects. Thus, because clinical problems readily develop with hypocalcemia and are essentially nonexistent for hypercalcemia, somewhat overzealous Ca^{++} replacement therapy has become a standard therapeutic approach in equine practice.

Over the course of the day, the horse remains depressed and continues to produce reflux at a similar rate (2–3 L/h). You have already started a continuous-rate infusion (CRI) of lidocaine (0.05 mg/kg/min) for its prokinetic, antisecretory, and analgesic actions. The owners are quite concerned and ask if there is anything further that you can do to help the horse. You indicate that nutritional support could be useful. Energy expenditure at rest (basal metabolic rate) of a healthy anorectic horse in a thermoneutral environment (assuming a weight of 500 kg) ranges from 15 to 20 kcal/kg/d. For a 500-kg horse, that translates into 7500 to 10,000 kcal/d. Although your patient is anorectic, it is clearly not healthy. A reasonable estimate of the metabolic rate of your postoperative patient would be 1.0 to 1.5 times that of a normal horse. For the following calculations, we use a value of 12,500 kcal/d.

Glucose provides 4 kcal/g, and you want 12,500 kcal/d. Therefore, to provide for the horse's caloric needs completely, you would need to give glucose in the amount of 3125 g. A 500-mL bottle of 50% dextrose contains 50 g per 100 mL, or 250 g per 500-mL bottle. Thus, 12.5 bottles of 50% dextrose would be needed to supply the 3125 g required by this horse. This is a large amount of glucose, and if greater than 100 g/h is administered, hyperglycemia and glucosuria are likely to develop. A high rate of glucose administration also stimulates insulin release and inhibits fat mobilization. As a result, complete caloric support by administration of glucose alone should not be attempted in horses.

It is important to remember that approximately 50% of a horse's daily caloric needs are provided by volatile fatty acid absorption from the hindgut. Clearly, that energy source would be decreased in this horse, but additional calories can be derived from fat mobilized from tissues and, to a lesser extent, from ketone bodies. Thus, we would never really attempt to provide more than 60% to 70% of daily calories in the form of glucose.

Although not commonly pursued in most equine hospitals, addition of some glucose to intravenous fluids can have benefits, especially in patients that are at risk of developing hyperlipidemia. In this case, if the intravenous fluids were made into a typical approximately 5% glucose solution, 50% dextrose (500 mL) must to be added to each 5-L bag. Because the volume of the 5-L bag is now 5500 mL (or even more when the volume of KCl added is also taken into account), each liter actually contains dextrose in the amount of 45 g. If we administer fluids at 3 L/h (2.5 L/h of this fluid and 500 mL/h with the lidocaine CRI), the horse receives dextrose at a rate of approximately 112.5 g/h (or 2700 g/d). Although this would meet approximately 85% of the estimated energy requirement, it is an excessive rate of glucose administration. To avoid potential detrimental effects of excessive glucose administration, a more reasonable approach would be to prepare an approximately 2.5% glucose solution, which would provide glucose at the rate of approximately 62.5 g/h (or 1500 g/d) at a total fluid rate of 3 L/h (base fluid and lidocaine CRI). An approximately 2.5% glucose solution can be made by adding 50% dextrose, 50 mL/L (25 g/L), or 50% dextrose, 250 mL, to a 5-L bag. Again, because 50% dextrose (250 mL) is added to the 5-L bag, the final concentration of the solution is somewhat less than 2.5%.

When estimating daily caloric requirements, it is also of interest to consider the amount of energy expended to heat 72 L of fluids (3 L/h for 24 hours) from an ambient temperature of 20°C (68°F) to the horse's body temperature of 38° (100.4°F). If we assume that the specific heat capacity of fluid is similar to that of water (1 cal/g/°C = 1 kcal/kg/°C), dextrose, 1296 kcal or 324 g, ($\sim$10% of the daily caloric requirement) is needed to accomplish this.

For patients that remain off feed for more than 48 hours and are expected to remain off feed for 5 to 7 days because of persistent ileus or a severe diarrheal disease, nutritional support in the form of total parenteral nutrition (TPN) is worthy of consideration. The advantage of TPN over glucose alone is increased caloric density in the form of lipids, along with provision of amino acids. In addition, the insulin response is blunted, and catabolism of skeletal muscle is limited. The TPN formulations prepared for horses by the pharmacy at Michigan State University are detailed in Table 1.

In the author's experience, use of TPN for 3 to 5 days in the supportive treatment of critically ill patients with persistent reflux or other diseases that cause nearly complete inappetence has been of substantial benefit. Further, commercial products are now available that make mixing of TPN formulations rather simple in the hospital setting.

Table 1
Total parenteral nutrition formulations prepared for horses

	Adult horses			Foals[a]	
	Day 1	Day 2	Day 3+	Day 1	Day 2
50% dextrose (mL)	1000	1000	1000	1000	1000
20% lipid (mL)	500	500	500	500	500
10% amino acid (mL)	1000	1000	1000	1000	1000
Plasmalyte A (mL)	4000	4000	4000	4000	4000
Multivitamins (mL)	5	5	5	5	5
Volume per bag (mL)	6500	6500	6500	6500	6500
Rate (mL/hr)	500	750	1000	250	500
Bags per day	2	3	4	1	2
kcal/d	6600	9900	13,200	3300	6600

kcal calculations per bag (total = 3300 kcal/bag):
    50% dextrose = 1000 mL/bag = 500 g × 4 kcal/g = 2000 kcal/bag
    20% lipid = 500 mL/bag = 100 g × 9 kcal/g = 900 kcal/bag
    10% amino acid = 1000 mL/bag = 100 g × 4 kcal/g = 400 kcal/bag
    [a] Sick foals have a much higher metabolic rate: approximately 100 kcal/kg/d × 50 kg = 5000 kcal/d

A final consideration in cases with persistent inappetence is total body K^+ depletion. Remember that we added KCl at a rate of 40 mmol to each liter of a base fluid that already had 5 mEq/L. Despite the administration of K^+ at 3480 mEq/d, or approximately 12% of the total body content, to this horse (3 L/h × 45 mEq/L = 145 mEq/h × 24 hours = 3480 mEq), up to 50% of supplemented K^+ may be lost in urine. Further, if we add TPN to the treatment plan, the amount of KCl administered may decrease unless we remember to add additional KCl to the TPN formulation. To assess the adequacy of K^+ replacement further, the fractional urinary clearance of K^+ can be determined by measuring K^+ and Cr concentrations in serum and urine as follows: fractional K^+ clearance = {(urine [K^+]/serum [K^+]) × (serum [Cr]/urine [Cr])} × 100%.

Values in normal horses are typically in the range of 30% to 100%, and the author considers values less than 20% to be indicative of inadequate K^+ in horses receiving intravenous fluid support.

Case 5

A 1-year-old Miniature Horse gelding in fair body condition (weight = 60 kg) is presented for evaluation of a 4-day history of depression, decreased appetite for grain, and fever (40°C [104°F]) on day 1. Treatment with flunixin meglumine, an oral potentiated sulfonamide antibiotic, and oxytetracycline intravenously resulted in little improvement, and the Miniature Horse stopped eating altogether on the evening of day 3, prompting presentation for further evaluation the following afternoon. Feces passed had been scant but of normal consistency. No signs of colic had been observed, and there was no history of coughing or nasal discharge. The Miniature Horse was dewormed every 4 to 6 weeks, and its diet consisted of 1 cup of 12% sweet feed and a handful of hay twice daily. Examination reveals a moderately depressed Miniature Horse with a rectal temperature of 38°C (100.5°F), a heart rate of 84 beats per minute, and a respiratory rate of 42 breaths per minute. Intestinal sounds are present but decreased in all quadrants. The oral membranes are pink but tacky to the touch, and the capillary refill time is 2 seconds. Further examination reveals the mild persistence of a skin tent (3 seconds), and the ears and extremities (from carpi and tarsi) are cool. Edema is not apparent. Abdominocentesis yields a clear pale yellow fluid with TS of less than 2.5 g/dL. When walked to its hospital stall, the Miniature Horse was also noted to seem ataxic in the hind limbs.

The following data are returned (admission, day 1): white blood cell count (WBC) of 5500 cells/µL, 48% segmented neutrophils, 1% band neutrophils, 50% lymphocytes, and 1% monocytes, and few toxic changes in neutrophils; subjectively, platelets seem to be adequate. The following laboratory results are also received (reference ranges):

PCV = 52% (30%–45%)
TS = 2.9 g/dL (5.9–7.5 g/dL)
Fibr = 0.4 g/dL (0.1–0.4 g/dL)
Na^+ = 118 mEq/L (128–158 mEq/L)
K^+ = 3.1 mEq/L (2.6–4.9 mEq/L)
Cl^- = 93 mEq/L (91–110 mEq/L)
BUN = 35 mg/dL (11–25 mg/dL)
Cr = 1.9 mg/dL (0.8–1.8 mg/dL)
Total protein (TP) = 2.7 g/dL (5.9–7.8 g/dL)
Albumin = 0.6 g/dL (3.3–4.2 g/dL)
Total calcium = 7.9 mg/dL (0.2–12.8 mg/dL)
Ionized Ca^{++} = 4.4 mg/dL (5.4–6.8 mg/dL)
Venous blood gas
    pH = 7.433 (7.377–7.423)
    P_{CO_2} 34.6 mm Hg (36.9–54.4 mm Hg)
    P_{O_2} 28.6 mm Hg (27.9–46.2 mm Hg)
    HCO_3^- = 23.2 mEq/L (24.5–30.4 mEq/L)
    BE = −1.2 mEq/L (−2.8 to 3.1 mEq/L)

On further evaluation, the gait deficits are more consistent with weakness than ataxia. For the time being, you consider that the weakness observed could be attributable to the combined effects of poor perfusion and electrolyte alterations. You decide to initiate fluid therapy and re-evaluate for neurologic disease once the patient's perfusion is improved. In this patient, the elevated PCV, coupled with marked hypoproteinemia, indicates a substantially decreased effective circulating volume. In addition to this deficit in plasma volume, you further estimate the overall fluid deficit to be 7%. Therefore, the volume to be administered over the next 12 hours is as follows:

Correct dehydration (estimated deficit) is 0.07×60 kg $= 4.2$ L
Maintenance at 2 mL/kg/h: 132 mL/h $\times$ 12 hours $=$ approximately 1.4 L
Ongoing losses: none are apparent
Total volume $= 5.6$ L

This horse's exchangeable cation deficit can be calculated as follows:

Pre-TBW $= 40$ L
Water deficit $= 4$ L
Post-TBW $= 36$ L
Exchangeable cation deficit: $(40$ L $\times 140$ mEq/L$) - (36 \times 118$ mEq/L$) =$
    $5600 - 4248 = 1352$ mEq cation deficit

The relative Na^+ and K^+ losses can be estimated as follows (assume 60% from ICF and 40% from ECF because of longer duration of disease and lack of excessive ECF loss, as with diarrhea):

Na^+ loss: $0.4 \times 1352 = 541$ mEq
K^+ loss: $0.4 \times 1352 = 811$ mEq (KCl ~ 60 g)

What is the Ca^{++} deficit of this Miniature Horse?
First, the total ECF Ca^{++} content is estimated for a normal horse of this size:

- Normal plasma and ECF $=$ ionized calcium, 6.0 mg/dL
- Approximately 15 L of ECF $\times$ ionized Ca^{++} concentration of 6.0 mg/dL $= 900$ mg
- Plasma has a further 6.0 mg/dL bound to plasma proteins
- Assuming plasma volume is approximately 4 L $= 4$ L $\times 6.0$ mg/dL $=$ 240 mg
- Thus, the total ECF Ca^{++} concentration is 900 mg $+$ 240 mg $= 1140$ mg
- 1140 mg/40.1 mg/mmol $= 28$ mmol $\times 2$ mEq/mmol $= 56$ mEq

Second, the ECF Ca^{++} deficit can be estimated as follows:

- Measured ionized Ca^{++} concentration is decreased by approximately 25% from normal
- 0.25×1140 mg $=$ approximately 280 mg or approximately 14 mEq
- Replacement of this deficit requires administration of 23% calcium borogluconate solution, approximately 130 mL
- Note that the deficit in protein-bound Ca^{++} cannot be replaced until hypoproteinemia is corrected

The initial fluid therapy plan developed consists of a bolus (2 L) of a polyionic crystalloid solution, followed by 200 mL/h. To address the Ca^{++} deficit, you add a 23% calcium borogluconate solution (50 mL) to each of the first two fluid bags (1-L bags) and 25 mL to each of the subsequent fluid bags. This yields a total volume of 4150 mL of fluid with the first four bags of fluid administered. Because the Miniature Horse should be able to absorb electrolytes administered orally, you elect to correct the K^+ deficit as well as anticipated ongoing losses in urine by administering KCl, approximately 5 g (67 mEq of both K^+ and Cl^-), in corn oil (30–40 mL) orally every 6 hours over the initial day of hospitalization (for a total of 268 mEq of both K^+ and Cl^-). Because of the low TP concentration and clinical evidence of decreased perfusion, treatment with colloids is added to the fluid therapy plan: a bolus (500 mL) of 6% hydroxyethyl starch in a 0.9% NaCl solution, followed by an additional 500 mL at a rate of 100 mL/h for a total dose of approximately 17 mL/kg.

What is hydroxyethyl starch, and what advantages does it have over the use of plasma?

Hydroxyethyl starch, a substituted amylopectin, comprises a heterogeneous group of molecules (essentially substituted glucose polymers) ranging in molecular mass from 10,000 to greater than 100,000 d, with an average of 450,000 d. Commercially available hydroxyethyl starch consists of a 6% solution in 0.9% NaCl and comes in 500-mL units. A dose of 10 to 20 mL/kg has been recommended. It is designed to increase colloid oncotic pressure (COP) for resuscitation purposes, in comparison to crystalloid fluids, which more transiently expand plasma volume but lower COP. Hydroxyethyl starch administration should also lead to less interstitial tissue edema formation than with crystalloid fluid administration. The overall effects should be to administer a smaller volume of fluid for resuscitation and prolong the effect of the crystalloid fluids. The main benefit of using hydroxyethyl starch rather than plasma for colloid replacement is largely practical, because 500-mL bags of hydroxyethyl starch are commercially available and can be stored at room temperature. Thus, when colloid therapy is needed, there is no need to wait for plasma to thaw or to use a filtered fluid administration set (required for administration of blood or plasma). Potential adverse effects of hydroxyethyl starch include alterations in hemostasis with higher doses, but anaphylactic reactions are less common than with administration of plasma.

Overnight, the Miniature Horse's attitude improved, but it remained inappetent. One small pile of formed feces was passed, and urine was voided several times (specific gravity of 1.006 on most recent sample). At 8:00 AM, the rectal temperature is 38.4°C (101.1°F), the heart rate is 66 beats per minute, and the respiratory rate is 32 breaths per minute. The horse weighs 62 kg. No edema is detected.

The following data are returned at 8:00 AM on day 2 (reference ranges):

PCV = 38% (30%–45%)
TS < 2.5 g/dL (5.9–7.5 g/dL)
Na^+ = 126 mEq/L (128–158 mEq/L)
K^+ = 3.0 mEq/L (2.6–4.9 mEq/L)
Cl^- = 102 mEq/L (91–110 mEq/L)
BUN = 25 mg/dL (11–25 mg/dL)

Cr = 1.6 mg/dL (0.8–1.8 mg/dL)
TP = 1.8 g/dL (5.9–7.8 g/dL)
Albumin = 0.4 g/dL (3.3–4.2 g/dL)
Total calcium = 8.1 mg/dL (10.2–12.8 mg/dL)
Ionized Ca^{++} = 5.1 mg/dL (5.4–6.8 mg/dL)
Venous blood gas
   pH = 7.470 (7.377–7.423)
   P_{CO_2} 40.4 mm Hg (36.9–54.4 mm Hg)
   P_{O_2} 34.1 mm Hg (27.9–46.2 mm Hg)
   HCO_3^- = 29.5 mEq/L (24.5–30.4 mEq/L)
   BE = 5.7 mEq/L (−2.8 to 3.1 mEq/L)

The initial fluid plan included crystalloids at a rate of approximately 70 mL/kg (4.15 L) and hydroxyethyl starch at a rate of approximately 17 mL/kg (1 L). Fluid therapy seems to have partially corrected electrolyte abnormalities and resulted in improved perfusion and circulatory status. The decrease in PCV is consistent with expansion of plasma and effective circulating volumes, but administration of crystalloid and colloid fluids (along with the underlying disease) has caused a further decline in TP and albumin concentrations.

You decide to discontinue further intravenous fluid therapy, but oral KCl slurries are continued (KCl, 5 g, in corn oil administered every 6 hours). The patient is taken outside several times to graze grass but has little interest and remains weak in the hind limbs. Abdominal ultrasonography reveals no evidence of abdominal effusion, and the right dorsal colon measures within normal ranges. The small intestine is not dilated or thickened but has less than desired motility. Mild gastric ulceration of the squamous epithelium just above the margo plicatus is detected on endoscopic examination of the stomach. Later that afternoon, the Miniature Horse seems more depressed, the rectal temperature is 38°C (100.3°F), the heart rate is 72 beats per minute, and the respiratory rate is 24 breaths per minute. The PCV is 42%, and the TS are less than 2.5 g/dL.

In the absence of obvious pain, the heart rate is a reasonably good measure of effective circulating volume. During the course of the day, a portion of the fluids (especially the crystalloids) has been eliminated through urine or extravasation into the interstitium, and this is reflected by the increases in heart rate and PCV. On the following morning (day 3), the patient is more depressed. The heart rate is 76 beats per minute, the PCV is 45%, the TS are less than 2.5 g/dL, and the horse's weight is 61 kg. The Miniature Horse has been noted to pass clear urine frequently, and an occasional formed fecal ball has been passed. A urine sample is collected and has a specific gravity of 1.006 and a pH of 6.5. Dilute urine is attributed to ongoing elimination of crystalloid fluids. Urine Cr and electrolyte concentrations are as follows:

Na^+ = 54.6 mEq/L

$K^+ = 13.6$ mEq/L
$Cl^- = 57.2$ mEq/L
$Cr = 41.4$ mg/dL

These urine measurements can be used to calculate fractional electrolyte clearance values (using day 2 serum chemistry values). As provided in case 4, the formula for determining fractional electrolyte clearances is as follows: fractional electrolyte clearance = {(urine [electrolyte]/serum [electrolyte]) × (serum [Cr]/urine [Cr])} × 100%.

The fractional electrolyte clearance (FCl) values can be calculated (with percent reference ranges) as follows:

FCl Na = (54.6/126) × (1.6/41.4) × 100% = 1.67% (<1.0%)
FCl K = (13.6/3.0) × (1.6/41.4) × 100% = 17.5% (30%–100%)
FCl Cl = (57.2/102) × (1.6/41.4) × 100% = 2.17% (<1.0%)

The elevated values for FCl Na and FCl Cl are consistent with elimination of the excess amounts administered with the initial fluid therapy (eg, Na^+ replacement was {[140 mEq × 4L] + [154 mEq × 1L of hydroxyethyl starch]} = 714 mEq in the face of an estimated deficit of 541 mEq, and Cl^- replacement would have been even more excessive with the additional Cl^- as oral KCl). The low value for FCl K, despite oral supplementation, reflects renal K^+ conservation attributable to total body K^+ depletion and ongoing losses in urine. Paradoxic aciduria likely reflects renal potassium conservation via exchange with H^+ in the distal tubule and collecting duct.

Further diagnostic evaluation for a protein-losing enteropathy on day 3 includes the result of a xylose absorption test, which reveals a blunted curve (flatter than normal) with a delayed peak (3 hours). A fecal flotation test has negative results, and no *Salmonella* spp were detected on the initial sample submitted for culture. After these tests, the patient is again taken out to graze but has little interest and still seems to be weak in the hind limbs when walked. You decide to measure indirect blood pressure with a tail cuff, and the values recorded are 95/45 (systolic/diastolic), with a mean of 60 mm Hg. Because of the persistent and marked hypoproteinemia and limited improvement with the initial fluid therapy, omeprazole, and KCl supplementation, you recommend a plasma transfusion.

The owner authorizes a plasma transfusion, and 1.5 L is administered over a period of 3 hours. What is the expected increase in plasma TP concentration with the plasma transfusion (assume a TP concentration of 6.5 g/dL in administered plasma)?

Plasma volume (4 L) × TP concentration of 1.8 g/dL (day 2) = 72 g
Protein in administered plasma: 1.5 L × 6.5 g/dL = 97.5 g
TP concentration immediately after plasma transfusion (169.5 g/5.5 L) = 3.1 g/dL
After the excess fluid is eliminated (169.5 g/4 L) = 4.2 g/dL

By that evening, the Miniature Horse seems brighter and is more interested in grazing. At 8:00 PM, the heart rate is 60 beats per minute, the PCV is 26%, and the TS are 3.4 g/dL. At 8:00 AM on day 4, the patient continues to be brighter, the PCV is 27%, the TS are 4.3 g/dL, and the horse's weight is 62 kg. Indirect blood pressure values have increased to 128/92 (systolic/diastolic), with a mean of 105 mm Hg.

The changes in body weight observed since admission suggest that the magnitude of body fluid loss (dehydration) estimated at admission was likely inaccurate (too high), because only a 1-kg increase in body weight persisted by the morning of day 3. It warrants mention that recent studies in human and small animal patients have revealed that the clinical (eg, moisture of oral membranes, skin tenting, temperature of extremities) and laboratory (eg, PCV, TS) measures used to estimate hydration status are actually rather poor indicators of hydration status. Serial measurement of body weight is a more accurate measure. Unfortunately, because euhydrated body weight is not known when patients are admitted, these less accurate measures are still used in clinical practice. When available, however, serial determination of body weight at 12- to 24-hour intervals after hospitalization is a more useful monitor of hydration and response to fluid therapy.

The following data are also returned at 8:00 AM on day 4 (reference ranges):

Na^+ = 132 mEq/L (128–158 mEq/L)
K^+ = 3.3 mEq/L (2.6–4.9 mEq/L)
Cl^- = 105 mEq/L (91–110 mEq/L)
Total Ca^{++} = 8.8 mg/dL (10.2–12.8 mg/dL)
BUN = 11 mg/dL (11–25 mg/dL)
Cr = 1.4 mg/dL (0.8–1.8 mg/dL)
TP = 4.0 g/dL (5.9–7.8 g/dL)
Albumin = 1.4 g/dL (3.3–4.2 g/dL)

The Miniature Horse's appetite continues to improve, omeprazole is continued, and KCl in corn oil is decreased to every 12 hours. The working diagnosis is diffuse ulceration of the intestinal tract because of excessive concentrate feeding. The patient is discharged 2 days later with instructions to continue omeprazole paste for a total of 2 weeks and that feeding should consist of hay only, along with grazing ad libitum. A re-examination 2 weeks later reveals continued improvement, and the TP and albumin concentrations have increased to 5.1 g/dL and 2.2 g/dL, respectively.

VETERINARY
CLINICS
Equine Practice

ELSEVIER
SAUNDERS

Vet Clin Equine 22 (2006) 37–42

Duodenal Stricture in a Foal

Bonnie S. Barr, VMD

Rood and Riddle Equine Hospital, 2150 Georgetown Road Lexington, KY 40580, USA

History

A 3-month-old Thoroughbred filly was evaluated for colic, bruxism, ptyalism, hypersalivation, and depression. The filly had a history of hospitalization for enteritis. The initial visit to the hospital was 3 weeks earlier, and the clinical signs resolved with medical management, including fluids and muzzling. The most recent hospitalization was 5 days before this visit, and treatment was instituted as for the initial visit. The filly had been dewormed every 30 days and had not yet received her first set of vaccinations.

Physical examination

On physical examination the filly was quiet, grinding her teeth, and hypersalivating. Vital signs were as follows: temperature 38.3°C (101.4°F), pulse 52 beats/minute, and respiratory rate 36 breaths/minute. Auscultation of the heart and lungs did not detect any abnormalities. Borborygmi were quiet and decreased. There was minimal abdominal distension, and fecal consistency was soft. There was no evidence of lameness or joint effusion.

Case assessment

Causes for colic in a 3-month-old foal include enteritis, enterocolitis, colitis, gastric ulcers, intussusception, a strangulating lesion, or ruptured viscous. Bruxism usually indicates pain, most likely associated with the gastrointestinal tract. Ptyalism can occur with oral ulcers, oral foreign body, esophageal ulceration, slaframine toxicity, or gastric ulcers. Occasionally ptyalism is noted in the case of enteritis or enterocolitis. Oral examination did not identify any oral ulcers or foreign bodies, so these could be ruled out as a cause of the clinical signs noted in this foal. Additionally, slaframine toxicity is uncommon in young foals. To differentiate further

E-mail address: bbarr@roodandriddle.com

0749-0739/06/$ - see front matter © 2006 Elsevier Inc. All rights reserved.
doi:10.1016/j.cveq.2005.12.015

the cause of the colic, bruxism, and ptyalism in this foal, further diagnostics were necessary.

Procedures

Laboratory work included complete blood chemistry and a master panel. No significant abnormalities were noted on laboratory work. A nasogastric tube was passed, and 2 L of foul-smelling reflux was obtained. After gastric decompression the foal's heart rate improved. Gastroscopy was performed with a 3-m endoscope, and severe gastric ulceration and distal (reflux) esophagitis with linear erosions were noted (Figs. 1, 2). A transabdominal ultrasound was performed with a 7.5-MHz transducer; there was no excessive peritoneal effusion, but there were several loops of mildly distended fluid-filled small intestine. After the results of the abdominal ultrasound were available, peritonitis and ruptured viscous were less likely. An abdominocentesis was not performed because there was not an excessive amount of peritoneal fluid, and the risk of inadvertent bowel wall perforation is higher in foals. Because of the concern of a potential gastric outflow obstruction, contrast gastrointestinal radiography was performed. Once the stomach was completely empty, barium (10 mL/kg) was administered through a nasogastric tube. Serial standing lateral radiographs of the abdomen were taken before administration of the barium, immediately after barium administration, and at 5, 10, 15, 20, 30, and 60 minutes after barium administration [1]. A normal foal should have evidence of barium in the duodenum by 5 to 10 minutes after barium administration. In this case the barium did not empty out of the stomach, even after 1 hour; therefore the diagnosis was delayed gastric emptying (Fig. 3).

Differential diagnosis

Delayed gastric emptying in a foal could result from a functional outflow disorder or a mechanical outflow disorder. A functional outflow disorder

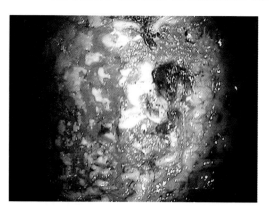

Fig. 1. Severe, diffuse gastric ulceration.

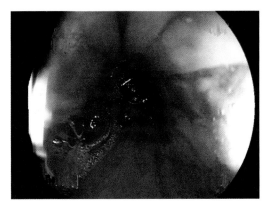

Fig. 2. Distal (reflux) esophagitis. Note linear ulcerative lesions.

could result from inflammation, erosion, or ulceration causing impairment of gastric emptying by affecting the myoelectric activity of the gastrointestinal tract [2]. Diseases such as gastric/duodenal ulceration, anterior enteritis, peritonitis, endotoxemia, and enterocolitis could result in a functional outflow problem. On the other hand, disorders that result in a mechanical obstruction include pyloric/duodenal stricture, small intestinal volvulus, small intestinal intussusception, or large colon displacement [2]. A small intestinal volvulus and large colon displacement were ruled out because the foal's pain level could be controlled with frequent gastric decompression; in this author's experience, foals with a small intestinal volvulus or large colon displacement do not stay comfortable even with frequent gastric decompression. Enterocolitis could be ruled out because the foal had normal feces. The gastroscopy identified severe gastric ulceration and distal (reflux) esophagitis. In this author's experience, the presence of distal esophagitis (along with

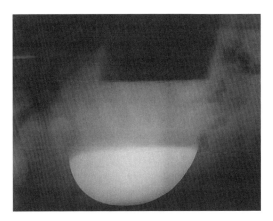

Fig. 3. Barium that has not emptied out of the stomach 60 minutes after administration.

the gastric ulcers) and the lack of emptying of barium from the stomach suggest inflammation or stricture of the pylorus or proximal duodenum. Often it is difficult to differentiate between inflammation without stricture and duodenal stricture. If the foal's comfort level can be maintained with gastric decompression and other medical therapies, medical management is the initial treatment in the hope that there is no stricture.

Treatment

Medical management included frequent decompression of the stomach, antiulcer medications, and intravenous fluids. Treatment with intravenous potassium penicillin (20,000–40,000 IU/kg every 6 hours) and gentamicin (6.6 mg/kg every 24 hours) was started. Because the foal initially was refluxing, intravenous antiulcer medication (ranitidine) was administered (Table 1). Often these foals have mild electrolyte abnormalities; thus balanced polyionic fluids with appropriate supplementation are administered. This author's rule of thumb for fluid management is

Fluid rate for 1 hour = maintenance requirement (2.2 – 4.4mL/kg/hour)
+ fluid deficit (% dehydratyion × body weight in kg/24 hours)
+anticipated hourly losses (caused by refluxing or diarrhea)

A constant-rate infusion is best, but if it is not practical, fluids can be administered every 4 to 6 hours. Typically medical management is tried for 2 to 3 days. Signs of improvement include a decrease or resolution of gastric reflux, a decrease or resolution of bruxism and ptyalism, and the ability to nurse or eat without pain. If the ulceration has progressed to fibrosis, and medical management does not result in improvement, surgical intervention is needed [3,4]. After 3 days of medical management, this filly showed no signs of improvement. An exploratory celiotomy identified a duodenal stricture. A gastrojejunostomy was performed to bypass the duodenal stricture. Postoperative care typically includes allowing nothing by mouth for 2 days, appropriate fluid therapy, antimicrobials, antiulcer medication, and nutritional support if needed. The nutritional support can range from

Table 1
Typical anti-ulcer medications for use in foals

Drug	Dose	Route	Frequency
Sucralfate	10–20 mg/kg	po	Q 6 hr
Cimetadine	10–20 mg/kg	po	Q 4 hr
Cimetadine	6.6 mg/kg	iv	Q 4 hr
Ranitidine	5–10 mg/kg	po	Q 6–12 hr
Ranitidine	0.8–2.2 mg/kg	iv	Q 6 hr
Omeprazole	4 mg/kg	po	Q 24 hr

intravenous dextrose (5% solution) as an additive to fluids to partial or total parenteral nutrition (TPN). The need for intravenous nutritional support is based on the debilitation or body condition of the foal. The author has had best success with a TPN formula of dextrose (10 g/kg/day), amino acids (2 g/kg/day), and lipids (1 g/kg/day). The rate of administration varies according to the foal's caloric needs, weight, and ability to tolerate the TPN. Usually the TPN is started at one fourth the foal's caloric needs and then increased over a 12- to 24-hour period depending on the foal's ability to tolerate the TPN, primarily the dextrose. The blood glucose level is initially monitored every 2 to 4 hours and then every 6 hours, depending on the patient. A dextrometer purchased from a human pharmacy is a cheap and accurate assessment of the blood glucose. Postoperatively, antiulcer medication should be switched to an oral medication (omeprazole or ranitidine) once the foal is no longer refluxing. Antimicrobial therapy should be continued for 7 days postoperatively. Foals that have undergone surgical correction have a fair long-term prognosis [5]. Immediate postoperative complications include ileus, colitis, incisional infection, or possible strangulation of the intestine. If surgery is not an option, medical management can be continued longer, and motility-enhancing drugs can be considered. In this situation one of the most commonly used prokinetic drugs used is bethanecol (Table 2). If the foal is to continue on medical therapy, intravenous nutrition such as 5% dextrose or TPN may be required. Response to continued medical treatment will be noted by the decrease/resolution of reflux, decrease/resolution of bruxism and ptyalism, and the foal's ability to nurse without any signs of abdominal discomfort. In the author's experience, medical management carries a poor prognosis unless the foal receives treatment early in the course of the disease, before stricture formation. Often, however, the problem is not diagnosed until the lesion is extensive.

The exact cause of duodenal strictures is unknown. Probably the lesion begins as inflammation or ulceration of the proximal duodenum that progresses to fibrosis and stricture. Factors predisposing foals to gastroduodenal ulcers include use of nonsteroidal anti-inflammatory drugs, stress, or a disease process that results in an imbalance between the protective and aggressive factors of the gastric mucosa [6–8]. There have been a few reports of several foals on one farm being affected, leading to the belief that an

Table 2
Common prokinetic agents for use in foals

Drug	Dose	Route	Frequency
Bethanecol	0.02 mg/kg followed by	sc	Q 4–6 hr
	0.35 mg/kg	po	Q 8 hr
Lidocaine 2%	1.3 mg/kg followed by	iv	Bolus in 1 L
	0.05 mg/kg/min	iv	CRI
Metaclopramide	0.1 mg/kg	iv	Q 6 hr (in 1 L saline over 1 hr)
Erythromycin	0.5–2 mg/kg	iv	Q 6 hr (in 1 L saline over 45 min)

infectious agent may be involved, although one has not definitively been identified [3,4].

Because the exact cause of duodenal strictures is unknown, effective preventative measures can be hard to define. Minimal usage of nonsteroidal anti-inflammatory agents is recommended. If they are used, antiulcer medication can be administered at the same time. In addition, good management practices are avoiding overcrowding, reducing stress, and limiting exposure to possible infectious diseases [8]. A 12-month follow-up has shown this foal/yearling to be doing well.

Overall the best treatment for a foal with delayed gastric emptying is surgical exploration. Unfortunately, the exact cause of this disease is unknown, but common clinical signs are bruxism, ptyalism, and colic

References

[1] Campbell ML, Ackerman N, Peyton LC, et al. Radiographic gastrointestinal anatomy of the foal. Vet Radiol Ultrasound 1984;25(5):194–204.
[2] Murray MJ. Stomach disease of the foal. In: Mair T, Divers T, Ducharme N, editors. Equine gastroenterology: gastrointestinal disease in the foal. London: W.B. Saunders; 2002. p. 469–76.
[3] Campbell-Thompson ML, Brown MP, Slone DE, et al. Gastroenterostomy for treatment of gastroduodenal ulcer disease in 14 foals. J Am Vet Med Assoc 1985;188(8):840–4.
[4] Orsini JA, Donawick WJ. Surgical treatment of gastroduodenal obstructions in foals. Vet Surg 1986;15(2):205–13.
[5] Zedler ST, Embertson RM. Surgical resolution of gastric outflow obstruction in the horse. In: Programs and abstracts of the 8th International Equine Colic Research Symposium. 2005.
[6] Borrow HA. Duodenal perforations and gastric ulcers in foals. Vet Rec 1993;(March):297–9.
[7] Murray MJ. Gastroduodenal ulceration in foals: a tutorial article. Equine Vet Educ 1999; 11(4):199–207.
[8] Barr BS. Gastric ulcer prophylaxis in the critically ill equine neonate. In: Wilkins PA, Palmer JE, editors. Recent advances in equine neonatal care. International Veterinary Information Service; 2001.

ELSEVIER
SAUNDERS

VETERINARY
CLINICS
Equine Practice

Vet Clin Equine 22 (2006) 43–51

Neonatal Diarrhea and Septicemia in an American Miniature Horse

Jonathan H. Magid, DVM, MS

Dr. T's Equine Clinic, 586 Lonesome Dove Lane, Salado, TX 76571, USA

History

A 30-hour-old American Miniature Horse colt weighing 10.9 kg was presented for evaluation of a possible scrotal hernia and mild dehydration. The foal was born without apparent difficulty, stood within 30 minutes of birth, and nursed normally. The foal passed normal meconium, followed by normal foal feces. The umbilicus had been dipped in iodine several times. The 8-year-old dam was not current on vaccinations. The mare was dewormed 1 month before foaling with fenbendazole and was regularly dewormed at 2-month intervals. This was the dam's fourth foal. The mare passed fetal membranes shortly after parturition. This horse had never received a blood transfusion and had belonged to the present owner for 7 years. The dam developed signs of colic and anorexia 6 hours after foaling. The foal developed diarrhea at the same time. The referring veterinarian examined the mare and foal. The foal was diagnosed with a bilateral scrotal hernia. The foal received intramuscular injections of tetanus toxoid and vitamin E–selenium. The mare was treated with mineral oil and intravenous fluids with dextrose because her liver enzymes were elevated. There is a strong association between anorexia and hyperlipidemia or fatty liver syndrome in periparturient Miniature Horse mares. The foal was treated for diarrhea with kaolin and pectin as well as probiotic paste, and manual reduction of the scrotal contents into the abdomen was performed at 3-hour intervals. The owner described the appearance of the testes and scrotum as unchanged since birth. On the morning of presentation, the foal had a temperature of 38.3°C (101.0°F) and continued to have diarrhea. He was active and nursing well.

E-mail address: jmagid@twoalpha.net

doi:10.1016/j.cveq.2005.12.013
vetequine.theclinics.com

Physical examination

The foal's temperature was 38.5°C (101.4°F), the heart rate was 112 beats per minute with strong synchronous pulses, and the respiration rate was 60 breathes per minute. The foal was bright, alert, and responsive. He was in good flesh, had a good appetite, and nursed strongly from his dam. The mare's udder and milk production seemed to be normal. Thoracic auscultation of the foal revealed no cardiac abnormalities or abnormal lung sounds. The gums were pink, moist, and slightly hyperemic, with a capillary refill time of 2 seconds. The conjunctiva and sclera were hyperemic. No other ocular abnormalities were detected. Dehydration was estimated to be 5% by skin tenting. The umbilicus was dry and normal and stained with iodine. Palpation of musculoskeletal structures was normal. The palate seemed to be complete based on digital examination. Gut sounds were normal, but defecation of small amounts of pasty yellow feces was frequent. A digital rectal examination revealed no abnormalities. Gentle palpation of the abdomen did not seem to cause discomfort, and ballottement of the abdomen did not produce a fluid wave. Urination was normal. The testes seemed to be large for the foal's body size but of normal shape and consistency. No gut was palpable in the scrotum or inguinal area. The skin, ears, and hair coat were normal for full-term gestation, age, and breed.

Case assessment

The primary problems identified in the foal were (1) diarrhea; (2) dehydration; and (3) hyperemic gums, conjunctiva, and sclera.

Diarrhea in foals is associated with bacterial, viral, and protozoal enteritis; septicemia; nutritional causes; obstruction of the gut; ingestion of irritants; antibiotic administration; parasitism; and foal heat in the mare. The role of *Escherichia coli* as a pathogen in foal diarrhea is controversial [1]. *E coli* is a well-documented pathogen in other species, however, and is the bacterium most commonly isolated from blood cultures of neonatal foals with diarrhea and septicemia [2]. The presence of *E coli* in blood cultures in foals with diarrhea may be attributable to bacteria crossing an already damaged intestinal barrier rather than primary invasion from the intestine. Proven causes of bacterial diarrhea in the neonatal foal include *Salmonella* and *Clostridium* species. *Salmonella* species cause disease by invading the mucosa, multiplying in macrophages, and then potentially spreading throughout the body. *Clostridium* species multiply in the bowel lumen and then produce toxins that damage the mucosa, resulting in diarrhea, toxemia, and possible septicemic spread of other bacteria. *Rhodococcus equi* can cause diarrhea in older foals by infecting the intestinal lymph nodes, but *Rhodococcus* septicemia has been seen in extremely young foals. Other bacterial causes of diarrhea considered were *Actinobacillus*, *Bacteroides fragilis*, *Klebsiella* and other coliforms, and *Streptococcus*. Viral diarrhea was considered less likely because of the early onset. The most likely viral cause for neonatal foal diarrhea is rotavirus, which has been documented to occur as early as 2 days of age. Other viral causes (coronavirus, adenovirus, and parvovirus) are less strongly associated with foal diarrhea. Rotavirus causes diarrhea by invading the epithelium of the small intestine and causing villus atrophy, malabsorption, and maldigestion. This allows lactose and fatty acid fermentation in the large intestine, which then leads to osmotic diarrhea. Protozoa, notably *Cryptosporidium*, have been associated with diarrhea in neonatal foals. This was ruled out in the current case, because protozoal diarrhea has a 3- to 7-day prepatent period. Nutritional diarrhea can occur in the foal of a heavily milking mare. The foal's small intestine can be overwhelmed, allowing undigested milk to ferment in the large intestine, which causes osmotic diarrhea. This could not be ruled out. Partial blockage of the intestine was unlikely, because colic was absent. Irritant ingestion and antibiotic use were ruled out by the history. Parasitism attributable to transmammary infection with *Strongyloides westeri* was possible, but its role in clinical disease is questionable, especially at this foal's age. Other types of parasitism were ruled out by the foal's age, as was foal-heat diarrhea. Foal-heat diarrhea is probably related to diet rather than to changes in the dam's milk or udder contamination, because orphan foals frequently have diarrhea at the same age.

Dehydration occurs because of abnormal fluid losses (attributable to the environment or to internal pooling) or inadequate intake of fluids. Inadequate intake of fluid could be ruled out because of the foal's normal appetite and the mare's apparently normal milk production. Diarrhea seemed the most obvious route of fluid loss to the environment, but endotoxemia can cause pooling of fluid by damaging the cardiovascular system. Renal water loss was unlikely, because neonatal foals with renal disease are usually oliguric. Bladder rupture can result in apparent dehydration by anorexia and osmotic means, because the hypertonic urine in the abdomen can cause fluid to move from the tissues into the abdominal cavity. Bladder rupture was considered unlikely in this case, however, because urination behavior and ballottement of the abdomen were observed to be normal at physical examination. Had this foal's scrotum actually been enlarged, bladder rupture and scrotal hernia would have been included in the differential diagnosis.

Hyperemic gums, sclera, and conjunctiva are associated with septicemia. Septicemia can only be definitively diagnosed by blood culture; however, neutropenia, neutrophilia, increased numbers of bands (immature neutrophils), hyperfibrinogenemia, toxic cell changes, and hypoglycemia are all suggestive of sepsis.

Case management

A CITE test (Idexx, Portland, Maine), complete blood cell count (CBC), fibrinogen value, serum chemistries, and urinalysis were run on day 1

(Table 1). It should be noted that normal hematologic and serum chemistry values vary with the age of the foal [3,4]. Blood was drawn using aseptic technique and submitted for aerobic and anaerobic blood cultures. The CITE test showed an IgG value greater than 800 mg/dL. Leukopenia (4170 cells/μL) and toxic granulocytes were noted on the CBC. The hematocrit (Hct) was 39%, whereas total hemoglobin (Hgb) was 13.7 g/dL. Serum chemistry showed hypocalcemia (8.5 mg/dL) and a slight hypokalemia (3.4 mEq/L). The results of the urinalysis were unremarkable (Table 2). The characteristic changes in serum chemistry that occur because of a ruptured bladder, including azotemia, hypochloremia, hyponatremia, and hyperkalemia, were not present (Table 3). Serum bicarbonate was within normal limits, and respiratory disease was absent; therefore, measurement of blood gases was not indicated. The CITE test indicated normal passive transfer of maternal antibodies. In calves and kids, gamma-glutamyltransferase (GGT) elevations are a marker of colostrum ingestion [5]. If this were the case in foals, the low normal GGT in this foal might indicate failure of passive transfer. Significant serum GGT elevation from ingestion of colostrum does not seem to occur in foals, however [6,7].

Table 1
Hematology report

Date/hospital day (%)	Normal values	8/7/98 Day 1	8/8/98 Day 2	8/10/98 Day 4
PCV	28–46	39	36.8	30.0
RBC × 10⁶/μL	8.2–11.0	7.22	6.88	6.67
MCV (fL)	30–50	54	53.4	52.8
MCH (pg)	10–19	18.9	18.8	20.3
MCHC (%)	31–38	35	35.3	38.4
Reticulocytes/μL		0	0	0
Hemoglobin (Hb) g/dL	11–16.6	13.7	13	11.5
RBC morphology		Normal	Normal	1 + anisocytosis
Nucleated RBCs/μL	0	0	0	0
White blood cells/μL	5010–12,600	4170	4120	4760
Metamyelocytes/μL				
Band neutrophils/μL	0–150	0	0	0
Semented neutrophils/μL	2000–10,200	2627	2431	2190
Lymphocytes/μL	600–5000	1543	1607	2047
Monocytes/μL	20–390		41	524
Eosinophils/μL	0–70		41	
Leukocyte morphology		Rare toxic granulocytes	Rare toxic granulocytes	Normal
Platelets/μL	100–500	292	273	139
Coomb's test (direct/indirect)		Direct +		
Fibrinogen mg/dL	100–400	300	500	

Abbreviations: MCH, mean corpuscular hemoglobin; MCHC, mean corpuscular hemoglobin concentration; MCV, mean corpuscular volume; PCV, packed cell volume; RBC, red blood cell.

Table 2
Urinalysis report

Date/hospital day	Normal values	8/7/98/Day 1
Source (eg, catheter/void/cystocentesis)		Free catch
Color		Pale yellow
Appearance		Clear
Specific gravity	1.001–1.027	1.012
pH	5.5–8.0	5.0
Protein	Negative to + 30	Trace
Glucose	Negative	Negative
Acetone	Negative	Negative
Bilirubin	Negative	
Blood	Negative	Negative

The low white blood cell (WBC) count and toxic granulocytes (see Table 1) suggested bacterial septicemia. An Hct/Hgb ratio that is less than 3 (Hct/ Hgb = 2.85 in this case) suggests hemolysis or laboratory error. The most likely cause of hemolysis in this foal was neonatal isoerythrolysis (NI). Serum bilirubin, although normal, was higher than usually seen from our laboratory, supporting the suspicion of hemolysis. The increase in bilirubin could also have been physiologic or caused by endotoxemia or hepatic disease, however. Other causes of increased bilirubin in a neonate could be septicemia, congenital defects of the liver, fatty liver in the foal or the dam, or

Table 3
Chemistry report

Date/hospital day		Normal values	8/7/98 Day 1	8/8/98 Day 2	8/11/98 Day 5
BUN	(mg/dL)	0–29.4	8.2	9.0	
Creatinine	(mg/dL)	0.4–3.6	0.9	0.8	
Alk phos	(IU/L)	530–2700	2209	1824	
SGOT (AST)	(IU/L)	85–460	122	125	
SDH	(IU/L)	0.6–4.6	5.4	8.3	
CPK	(IU/L)	25–350	201	156	
GGT	(IU/L)	10–38	10	12	
Total bilirubin	(mg/dL)	0.5–4.3	4.0	2.5	1.9
Glucose	(mg/dL)	108–223	201	141	
Na	(mEq/L)	123–159	137	136	
K	(mEq/L)	3.6–5.6	3.4	4.5	
Cl	(mEq/L)	90–114	106	106	
Ca	(mg/dL)	9.7–13.7	8.5	9.6	
P	(mg/dL)	3.4–7.4	5.2	6.5	
Total protein	(m/dL)	4.4–7.6	4.8	4.6	
Albumin	(m/dL)	2.3–3.4	2.4	2.4	
Cholesterol	(mg/dL)	100–478	139	134	
HCO₃	(mEq/L)	19–27.4	21.9	21.9	

Abbreviations: Alk phos, alkaline phosphatase; BUN, blood urea nitrogen; CPK, creatine kinuse; GGT, gamma glutamyltransferase; SDH, sorbitol dehydrogenase; SGOT, serum glutamic-oxaloacetic transaminase.

equine herpesvirus type 1 (EHV-1) infection in utero. Toxic causes, such as iron supplementation and drug (eg, corticosteroids, gas anesthesia, antiseizure medications) administration, were ruled out by the history. Physiologic hyperbilirubinemia is probably caused by a proportionally larger volume of blood in the neonate, shorter red blood cell (RBC) life, low volume of feed leading to increased absorption of bilirubin from the gut, insufficient ability to conjugate bilirubin, and lessened ability to excrete bilirubin. In physiologic hyperbilirubinemia, most of the bilirubin is unconjugated. Hemolytic disease also results in elevated unconjugated bilirubin, although endotoxin may decrease the ability of the bile canaliculi to excrete bilirubin, leading to increased conjugated bilirubin. Our laboratory did not differentiate between conjugated and unconjugated bilirubin.

Despite the elevated bilirubin concentration, hepatic disease was considered unlikely, because liver enzymes were normal, except for an unremarkable increase in sorbitol dehydrogenase (SDH) (5.4 IU/L, normal range: 0.6–4.6 IU/L). Hypokalemia was unremarkable (3.4 mEq/L, normal range: 3.6–5.6 mEq/L). Hypocalcemia (8.5 mEq/L, normal range: 9.7–13.7 mEq/L) was probably caused by a decrease in the protein-bound calcium, with normal ionized calcium because of low normal serum albumin. Because hemolytic disease was suspected, a direct Coomb's test was run. The direct Coomb's test was positive, which means that the foal's RBCs were coated with immunoglobulin or complement. This was suggestive of NI.

When sepsis was scored [8], the foal received 2 points for having a neutrophil count between 2000 and 4000 cells/μL, 0 points for having less than 50 bands/μL, 2 points for having toxic granulocyte changes, 0 points for having a fibrinogen level less than 400 mg/dL, 0 points for having a blood glucose level greater than 80 mg/dL, 0 points for having an IgG value greater than 800 mg/dL, 3 points for marked scleral injection, 0 points for having a normal temperature, 0 points for having a normal mental state, 3 points for having diarrhea, and 3 points for having a sick dam (colic). The total sepsis score was 13. Scores greater than 11 on this scale indicate sepsis. Because of these findings, diagnoses of diarrhea, probable septicemia, and possible NI were made.

Treatment and outcome

Treatment on day 1 included aseptic intravenous catheter placement, intravenous fluid supplementation with 0.45% sodium chloride (NaCl)/2.5% dextrose (100 mL) with 20% calcium dextrose (1 mL) added every 2 hours, potassium penicillin (22,000 IU/kg) administered intravenously every 6 hours, and amikacin (6.6 mg/kg) administered every 8 hours. The fluids were administered as supportive care for diarrhea and septicemia at a rate of approximately 90 mL/kg/d. This is a maintenance fluid rate for a foal, because a foal has proportionally more water than an adult. A maintenance rate was chosen because the foal was nursing well; therefore, this fluid rate and the foal's nursing would compensate for excess fecal fluid losses. Antimicrobials were chosen for broad-spectrum activity. Amikacin was chosen over gentamicin because it is less nephrotoxic. The dosing of amikacin was controversial. Dosing regimens ranging from 4 to 8 mg/kg every 8 to 12 hours to 20 to 25 mg/kg every 24 hours have been recommended. Monitoring of blood levels of aminoglycosides is recommended but was not possible in our clinic. Recently, once-daily dosing has been reported to be efficacious because of high blood levels and prolonged postantibiotic effect as well as safer because of lessened nephrotoxicity. In this case, at the time the foal was treated, dosing three times per day was deemed most legally defensible, and with the supplementation of fluid therapy so as to protect the foal's kidneys, safe and efficacious. The current recommendation for dosing of amikacin is 25 mg/kg administered once daily [9]. No corticosteroids were given for treatment of possible NI because of lack of symptoms and the contraindication of suspected septicemia. The foal's vital signs and membrane color were monitored closely.

On day 2 of treatment, the foal's temperature was 38.2°C (100.8°F), the heart rate was 100 beats per minute, and the respiration rate was 56 breathes per minute. The mucous membranes were normal, without signs of jaundice. The foal was bright, alert, difficult to catch, and nursing well. Defecation and urination were normal. A CBC and serum chemistry (see Tables 1 and 3) revealed that the Hct had decreased to 36.8%, Hgb to 13 g/dL, and Hct/Hgb ratio to 2.83 and that there was leukopenia (4120 cells/µL) with toxic granulocytes, increased fibrinogen (500 mg/dL), reduced total bilirubin, unremarkable serum calcium, and mild elevation in SDH. Laboratory findings were still suggestive of septicemia. Blood from the mare and foal was cross-matched to pursue the possibility of NI further. The mare's serum and the foal's RBCs were incompatible. This demonstrated that the previous finding of a positive Coomb's test was not spurious. NI was suspected. Treatment was unchanged, because the Hct was not so low as to warrant transfusion. On day 3, the foal's temperature was 38.6°C (101.5°F), the heart rate was 104 beats per minute, and the respiration rate was 36 breathes per minute. The Hct was further decreased to 33%, and plasma total solids were 4.9 g/dL. Blood culture confirmed septicemia with *E coli*, which was sensitive to aminoglycosides. Treatment was unchanged, because gram-positive or anaerobic pathogens were still possible. On day 4, the foal's temperature was 38.6°C (101.6°F), the heart rate was 116 beats per minute, and the respiration rate was 52 breathes per minute. A CBC was performed, and leukopenia was still present (4760 WBCs/ µL), but to a lesser extent and without toxic changes. The Hct was 30%, Hgb was 11.5 g/dL, and Hct/Hgb ratio was 2.61; yet, no signs of jaundice were present, and urine was observed to be of normal straw color. Fluids were discontinued. On day 5, the foal put up a remarkable struggle during the examination, which probably accounted for the elevated temperature of 39°C (102.2°F), pulse rate of 132 beats per minute, and respiratory rate of 52 breathes per minute. A final serum total bilirubin measurement was normal. This, combined with normal-colored urine and lack of jaundice, suggested that marked hemolysis was not occurring. On day 6, the physical examination was unremarkable, with a temperature of $38.7°C$ ($101.8°F$), pulse rate of 132 beats per minute, and respiratory rate of 32 breathes per minute. The foal was discharged. Because the owner's work schedule would not allow dosing three times daily, the foal was switched to once-daily intramuscular dosing of amikacin, 20 mg/kg, and twice-daily dosing of procaine penicillin G, 20,000 IU. This antibiotic regimen was to be continued for 5 additional days. The owner was advised to watch the foal for signs of jaundice or weakness. Careful observation for signs of NI was recommended for the mare's next foal. Blood typing the foal, the mare, and any stallion to which the mare might be bred was recommended. The foal and dam were reported to be in excellent health 22 days after admission. No anaerobic or gram-positive bacteria were isolated from the blood.

Possible reasons for the foal's failure to develop clinical NI despite being having a positive result on a Coomb's test and his dam's serum (and presumably colostrum) containing antibodies to his erythrocytes include the following:

1. The mare had antibodies to Ca antigen on the foal's erythrocytes without sensitization. This does not result in hemolysis. Anti-Ca alloantibodies may, in fact, be protective against NI caused by alloantibodies to other blood groups [10].
2. The mare was previously sensitized to a less antigenic blood antigen than the Qa or Aa antigens most commonly associated with clinical NI. Several other antigens have also been implicated in NI [11,12].
3. The mare had previous exposure to Qa, Aa, or other blood group antigens on the foal's cells but produced a weak antibody response.
4. The CITE test was in error, and the foal had partial failure of passive transfer and only a weak response to erythrocyte antigens. The CITE ELISA test has been found to have poor sensitivity and high specificity [13]. The poor sensitivity makes it more likely that the foal would have an unidentified false-negative test result for failure of passive transfer. It should be duly noted that the company has discontinued this test, replacing it with the SNAP ELISA (Idexx) test, which has higher sensitivity, although lower specificity.

References

[1] Wilson JH, Cudd T. Common gastrointestinal diseases. In: Koterba AM, Drummond WH, Kosch PC, editors. Equine clinical neonatology. Philadelphia: Lea & Febiger; 1990. p. 412–29.
[2] Marsh PS, Palmer JE. Bacterial isolates from blood and their susceptibility patterns in critically ill foals: 543 cases (1991–1998). J Am Vet Med Assoc 2001;218(10):1608–10.

[3] Bauer JE. Normal blood chemistry. In: Koterba AM, Drummond WH, Kosch PC, editors. Equine clinical neonatology. Philadelphia: Lea & Febiger; 1990. p. 602–14.

[4] Harvey JW. Normal hematologic values. In: Koterba AM, Drummond WH, Kosch PC, editors. Equine clinical neonatology. Philadelphia: Lea & Febiger; 1990. p. 561–70.

[5] Perino LJ, Sutherland RL, Woollen NE. Serum gamma-glutamyltransferase activity and protein concentration at birth and after suckling in calves with adequate and inadequate passive transfer of immunoglobulin G. Am J Vet Res 1993;54(1):56–9.

[6] Patterson WH, Brown CM. Increase of serum gamma-glutamyltransferase in neonatal Standardbred foals. Am J Vet Res 1986;47(11):2461–3.

[7] Warko G, Bostedt H. GGT activity in the blood serum of newborn foals after the absorption of a non-species specific colostrum preparation. Berl Munch Tierarztl Wochenschr 1991; 104(7):221–3 [in German].

[8] Brewer BD, Koterba AM. The development of a scoring system for the early diagnosis of equine neonatal sepsis. Equine Vet J 1988;20(1):18–22.

[9] Bucki EP, Giguere S, Macpherson M, et al. Pharmacokinetics of once-daily amikacin in healthy foals and therapeutic drug monitoring in hospitalized equine neonates. J Vet Intern Med 2004;18(5):728–33.

[10] Bailey E, Albright DG, Henney PJ. Equine neonatal isoerythrolysis: evidence for prevention by maternal antibodies to the CA blood group antigen. Am J Vet Res 1988;49:1218–22.

[11] Bailey E, Conboy HS, McCarthy PF. Neonatal isoerythrolysis of foals; an update on testing. In: Proceedings of the 33rd Annual American Association of Equine Practitioners Convention, 1987. p. 341–9.

[12] Zaruby JF, Hearn P, Colling D. Neonatal isoerythrolysis in a foal involving anti-Pa alloantibody. Equine Vet J 1992;24:71–3.

[13] Vaala WE. Neonatal anemia. In: Koterba AM, Drummond W, Kosch PC, editors. Equine clinical neonatology. Philadelphia: Lea & Febiger; 1990. p. 571–88.

ELSEVIER
SAUNDERS

VETERINARY
CLINICS
Equine Practice

Vet Clin Equine 22 (2006) 53–60

Chronic Hyperproteinemia Associated with a Probable Abdominal Abscess in an Appaloosa Stallion

Jonathan H. Magid, DVM, MS

Dr. T's Equine Clinic, 586 Lonesome Dove Lane, Salado, TX 76571, USA

History

A 12-year-old Appaloosa stallion used for pleasure riding and at stud in a small breeding operation had a history of weight loss that started 93 days before presentation. Initial signs were refusal of food and reluctance to move. The horse was stretching its neck forward and exhibiting abdominal discomfort. When the referring veterinarian (RDVM) examined the horse, it was febrile, with pale mucous membranes and a tense abdomen. Rectal palpation was normal. Nasogastric intubation revealed no reflux. Laboratory tests submitted by the RDVM showed a low normal white blood cell count with a left shift, hypokalemia, hyperbilirubinemia, and normal total protein (Tables 1 and 2). The horse was treated with flunixin meglumine and started on a 2-week course of procaine penicillin G. A slight improvement in the horse's condition was noted on day −89. A complete blood cell count (CBC) and serum chemistry panel submitted by the RDVM 89 days before presentation showed a mild left shift and moderate hyperbilirubinemia (see Tables 1 and 2). Forty-three days before presentation, all four legs were swollen and the RDVM found the horse reluctant to move in tight circles and sore in the right paralumbar area. Laboratory test results (see Tables 1 and 2) showed slight anemia, hyponatremia, 9.7 g/dL serum total protein (normal range: 5.6–8.0 g/dL), 2.4 g/dL albumin (normal range: 2.6–4.1 g/ dL), and a positive serum titer for equine protozoal myelitis (EPM). The horse was treated with penicillin and trimethoprim sulfa from day −37 through day −29 without improvement. On day −35, the horse was evaluated by another veterinarian. A CBC, serum chemistry, cervical radiographs, and bilateral hock radiographs were done. The hocks were found to be arthritic

E-mail address: jmagid@twoalpha.net

doi:10.1016/j.cveq.2005.12.006

Table 1
Complete blood cell count values

Date/hospital day	Normal values	10/30/97 Day −93	11/04/97 Day −89	12/10/98 Day −43	1/1/98 Day −29	1/29/98 Day 1	2/23/98 Day 26	3/24/98 Day 55
PCV (%)	32–53	45.3	34.5	30.4	30.0	31.5	36.4	37.2
RBC × 10⁶/µL	7–13	8.69	6.49	6.00	5.97	6.46	7.00	7.3
MCV (fL)	37–59	52.1	53.2	50.6	50.2	48.8	52.0	50.9
MCH (pg)	12–20	18.1	18.0	17.5	18.9	18	17.0	17.4
MCHC (%)	31–38	34.7	33.9	34.6	37.6	36.9	32.7	34.2
RBC morphology				1 + anisocytosis		1 + anisocytosis		
Hemoglobin (g/dL)	11–19					11.7		
Nucleated cells/µL	5.5–12 k	650	680	930	630	971	108	650
Metamyelocytes/µL	0–100	104	204	0	0		108	0
Band neutrophils/µL	3–7 k	409	374	669	441	776	756	396
Segmented neutrophils/µL	1.5–5 k	110	238	213	151	155	864	201
Lymphocytes/µL	0–1 k	195	340	372	252	388	432	390
Monocytes/ul	0–1 k	65	136		126	0	0	65
Eosinophils/µL	0–1 k				0	0	0	65
Leukocyte morphology				93		Normal		
Platelets/µL	Adequate	Adequate	Adequate	Adequate	Adequate	267,000	Adequate	Adequate
Fibrinogen (mg/dL)	100–400					600		

Abbreviations: k, 1,000; MCH, mean corpuscular hemoglobin; MCHC, mean corpuscular hemoglobin conceatration; MCV, mean corpuscular volume; PCV, packed cell volume; RBC, red blood cells.

Table 2
Chemistry report

Date/hospital day	Normal values	10/30/97 Day−93	11/04/97 Day−89	12/10/98 Day−43	1/198 Day−29	1/29/98 Day 1	2/23/98 Day 26	3/24/98 Day 55
BUN (mg/dL)	5–27	21	17	19	25	13.6	18	
Creatinine (mg/dL)	0.6–2.0	2.1	1.3	1.3	1.7	1.3	1.5	
Alk phos (IU/L)	66–212	70	113	103	104	95	121	83
SGPT (ALT) (IU/L)	0–40	6	11	8	14		9	13
SGOT (AST) (IU/L)	90–400	277	282	144	142	135	169	
LDH (IU/L)	110–450		211	150	157		171	
SDH (IU/L)	0–9					2.4		
CPK (IU/L)	60–330	153	105	54	79	89	124	
GGT (IU/L)	0–40			34	31	17	27	
Total bilirubin (mg/dL)	0–2.0	3.9	2.6	0.7	0.7	1.0	0.7	1.0
Direct bilirubin (mg/dL)	0.0–0.3			0.1	0.1		0.1	0.1
Amylase (IU/L)	0–30	6		7	6		7	
Glucose (mg/dL)	60–110	106	110	72	85	103	95	
Na (mEq/L)	132–146	139	139	137	129	129	134	
K (mEq/L)	3.2–5.0	2.9	4.2	4.0	4.0	3.7	4.5	
Cl (mEq/L)	98–109	98	104	106	99	97	102	
Ca (mg/dL)	10.4–13.8	11.8	11.5	11.7	11.6	10.5	11.7	
P (mg/dL)	1.7–4.7	2.3	1.9	2.3	2.2	2.1	121	
Total protein (g/dL)	5.6–8.0	7.2	7.5	9.7	11.2	10.1	10.0	7.7
Albumin (g/dL)	2.6–4.1	3.6	3.7	2.4	2.5	2.5	2.9	3.2
Globulin (g/dL)	2.0–5.0					7.6		
Cholesterol (mg/dL)	60–200				53	58	59	
HCO₃ (mEq/L)	24–34					28.4		

Abbreviations: Alk phos, alkaline phosphatase; ALT, alanine aminotransferase; AST, aspartate aminotransferase; BUN, blood urea nitrogen; CPK, creatine kinase; GGT, gamma glutamyltransferase; LDH, lactate dehydrogenese; SDH, sorbitol dehydrogenase; SGOT, serum glutamic-oxaloacetic transaminase; SGPT, Serum glutamic-pyruvic transminase.

and injected with corticosteroids. The serum total protein was 10.8 g/dL. The horse was started on a 5-day course of phenylbutazone. By day −29, there was no perceived improvement. The RDVM observed that the horse continued to be resentful of palpation in the paralumbar fossae. Laboratory tests (see Tables 1 and 2) again showed mild anemia, hyponatremia, elevated serum total protein of 11.2 g/dL, and serum albumin of 2.5 g/dL. The horse was treated with phenylbutazone for 3 days without improvement. It was dewormed with ivermectin on day −6 and had been dewormed routinely every 4 months prior. It had been vaccinated for eastern equine encephalitis, western equine encephalitis, tetanus, influenza, and rhinopneumonitis 8 months before presentation. The horse's last negative Coggin's test for equine infectious anemia (EIA) was 2 years before presentation. The horse ate 3 lb of oats and three flakes of mixed grass/alfalfa hay twice daily. It was presented for weight loss, leg edema, distended flanks, pain in the paralumbar fossae, elevated serum total protein, apparent neck pain, and reluctance to move.

Physical examination

The horse's temperature was 37.4°C (99.3°F), its heart rate was 36 beats per minute with synchronous pulses, and its respiratory rate was 12 breaths per minute. Its body condition was good, and its weight was 531 kg. The horse moved stiffly, and its hind legs were edematous below the hocks. The skin, mucous membranes, eyes, peripheral lymph nodes, genitals, and urination were all normal. The heart and lungs were normal on auscultation. The teeth were normal. The abdomen seemed to be distended. Gut sounds and feces were normal. The results of a rectal examination were normal. The horse was able to turn its head and flex its neck swiftly to either side in attempts to bite when the paralumbar fossae were pressed. Its neck did not seem to be sore. The horse exhibited unpredictable aggressive stallion behavior.

Case assessment and management

The initial problem list included weight loss, abdominal distention and discomfort, historically elevated serum protein, historical reluctance to move, and peripheral edema. Differentials for weight loss included chronic infection, neoplasia, liver disease, renal disease, and infiltrative bowel disease. Starvation and parasitism could be ruled out from the history. Dental disease, heart disease, and generalized pulmonary or pleural disease could be ruled out by physical examination, although a pulmonary abscess could not. Differentials for abdominal distention and discomfort were peritonitis or abdominal abscess, abdominal neoplasia, intestinal adhesion, and partial bowel obstruction. Heart failure, which can cause ascites, was unlikely based on physical examination. Chronic liver failure can also cause ascites but rarely in horses. Historically elevated serum total protein with normal serum albumin was probably attributable to chronic inflammatory disease, neoplasia, or chronic liver disease. There are numerous differentials for the historical reluctance to move, but broad categories would be musculoskeletal disease, neurologic disease, and abdominal pain. Leg edema might be from prolonged inactivity, obstruction of venous drainage, an immune-mediated vasculitis, or heart failure.

Because of severe snowy weather, the owner limited the amount of time available for workup of this case because she wanted to drive home during the daylight hours. A telephone conversation with the RDVM confirmed that weight loss had indeed occurred. The initial workup included a neurologic examination, brief lameness examination, CBC, plasma total protein and fibrinogen measurements, serum chemistry, and urinalysis. Fecal examination for parasites was not done because the horse had just been dewormed. The neurologic examination was normal, so the positive serum test result for EPM probably indicated exposure rather than clinical disease [1]. The horse was grade 1/5 lame in its left foreleg and right hind leg. Reluctance to move did not seem to be related to any lameness. Edema lessened after exercise, indicating that it was not important clinically. The results of the urinalysis were normal. The CBC (see Table 1) revealed mild neutrophilia and anemia. The plasma total protein was 9.3 g/dL. Fibrinogen was elevated at 600 mg/dL using the heat precipitation technique. Serum chemistry (see Table 2) revealed low blood urea nitrogen (BUN), elevated serum total protein of 10.1 mg/dL, normal albumin, hyponatremia, hypochloremia, and low creatine kinase (CK) and aspartate aminotransferase (AST). The results of the urinalysis were normal (Table 3). The mild neutrophilia combined with the low normal lymphocyte count indicated chronic bacterial infection, although a stress response could not be ruled out. Elevated fibrinogen is a sign of inflammation and is found in infectious, suppurative, neoplastic, and traumatic disease. Plasma total protein includes clotting factors, fibrinogen, albumin, and globulins. Serum total protein contains only albumin and globulins. Therefore, it is not possible for the serum total protein to be higher than the plasma total protein. This laboratory error can be explained by differences in measurement technique. Serum total protein is measured with a handheld refractometer. Plasma total protein is measured by the Biuret method, a colorimetric test used in automated chemistry analyzers. Elevated serum and plasma total protein are associated with dehydration if serum albumin is also increased. In this horse, serum albumin was actually at the low end of the normal range and, together with the lack of clinical signs of dehydration, ruled out dehydration as a cause of hyperproteinemia. The elevation in plasma total protein was partly attributable to increased fibrinogen, but the bulk of the elevation in plasma total protein and all the elevation in serum total protein were attributable to elevated immunoglobulins. Hyperglobulinemia occurs in chronic infections, such as an abdominal or pulmonary abscess, pleuritis, peritonitis, EIA [2], strongylosis, and chronic hepatic disease. Hyperglobulinemia also occurs in immune-mediated diseases, such as purpura hemorrhagica and amyloidosis, and

Table 3
Urinalysis report

Date/hospital day	Normal values	1/29/98 Day 1
Source (eg, catheter void cystocentesis)		Free catch
Color	Yellow to brown	Yellow
Appearance	Slightly turbid	Cloudy
Specific gravity	1.006–1.050	1.015
pH	7.0–9.0	8
Protein	0–trace	0
Glucose	0	0
Acetone	0	0
Bilirubin	0	0
Blood	0	0
Casts	None	0
Leukocytes/HPF	0–8	Rare
Epithelial cells/HPF	0	0
Erythrocytes/HPF	0–8	0
Crystals	$CaCo_3$	$CaCO_3$
Bacteria	In free catch	0
Other	Sperm (stallion)	0

Abbreviation: HPF, high-power field.

with neoplasia, especially of lymphocytes. In this case, hyponatremia can be explained as a function of the hyperproteinemia. Hyperproteinemia takes up a significant portion of the volume of serum or plasma. Sodium is only present in the aqueous phase of the sample. Therefore, measurement of sodium from the combined proteinaceous and aqueous portions of the serum results in a dilution of the sodium concentration perceived by the chemistry machine. Serum chloride, BUN, CK, and AST are affected in the same way by hyperproteinemia [3]. The low values for these substances are therefore insignificant. The mild anemia in this horse could be attributable to relative plasma expansion by hyperproteinemia. Causes of true anemia are bleeding, hemolysis, and inadequate erythrocyte production. In blood loss (eg, from gastric squamous cell carcinoma), low total protein would occur. With hemolysis, total protein should not change, and icterus, hemoglobinemia, or hematuria might occur if destruction of red blood cells was rapid. Hemolysis can be caused by toxins or immune-mediated responses directed against parasites or the body's own cells. In anemia of chronic inflammation, red blood cells may be damaged by passage through inflamed tissue or an overactive mononuclear phagocyte system, but the main cause of the anemia is thought to be a derangement of iron metabolism. This leads to sequestration of iron in the liver and bone marrow. There is also depression of the bone marrow's response to anemia. This may be a mechanism by which the body denies iron for bacterial metabolism [4]. Lymphosarcoma may be associated with signs of chronic inflammation (neutrophilia, leukocytosis, hyperfibrinogenemia, anemia, and hyperproteinemia) and can be associated with monoclonal or polyclonal gammopathies [5]. Plasma cell myeloma, although rare in horses [6], can cause anemia by chronic inflammation and myelophthisis, and is associated with monoclonal gammopathy and, occasionally, Bence-Jones proteinuria [7]. Myeloid neoplasia of a bone marrow–derived cell line can cause anemia by myelophthisis but does not usually cause hyperglobulinemia [5]. Bone marrow cytology can be used to characterize anemia and diagnose neoplasia. Serum protein electrophoresis aids in evaluation of hyperglobulinemia.

Leading differentials to account for all serious clinical signs with one lesion were EIA; chronic localized infection in the abdomen; and neoplasia localized in the abdomen, bone marrow, or both. A pulmonic abscess was also possible. Chronic hepatic disease and immune-mediated hemolysis were unlikely, because neither hepatic enzyme elevations nor hyperbilirubinemia occurred. Strongylosis was also unlikely.

Further diagnostic steps discussed with the owner and the RDVM were a Coggin's test for EIA, abdominocentesis, thoracic radiographs to rule out thoracic disease, abdominal ultrasonography, serum protein electrophoresis, and bone marrow aspiration. A Coomb's test would have been useful in further ruling out immune-mediated anemia. The owner and the RDVM were concerned about the cost of the thoracic radiographs and about the low yield of abdominal ultrasonography. The owner had further concerns about the time required for these procedures. Ultrasonography was unavailable until the following day, and a 2-hour wait would be required for thorax radiographs. The owner declined radiography and ultrasonography. Blood was submitted for a Coggin's test, and serum was submitted for protein electrophoresis. The horse was sedated and twitched for abdominocentesis and bone marrow aspiration from his sternebrae. Bone marrow was submitted for cytologic examination. Abdominal fluid was submitted for cytologic examination and aerobic and anaerobic culture and sensitivity testing.

The horse was discharged with an open diagnosis pending laboratory results. In her haste to leave the clinic because of the stormy weather, the client neglected to fasten her trailer hitch properly. The stallion spent the night stuck in the trailer in a ditch but had no ill effects from this incident.

Cytologic examination of the bone marrow and abdominal fluid was completed on day 2. Bone marrow cytology was normal, but the abdominal fluid had an elevated total protein of 4.7 g/dL and an elevated white blood cell count of 14,100 cells/µL. These cells were 98% nondegenerate neutrophils, with the rest being macrophages and mesothelial cells, with no evidence of neoplasia. This seemed to be a suppurative process. Culture results from the abdominal fluid were obtained on day 3. α-*Streptococcus* and *Corynebacterium* species were grown. Both of these bacteria were sensitive to ceftiofur, chloramphenicol, erythromycin, and oxytetracycline. Because of bacterial growth and a relatively low cell count in the abdominal fluid, a walled-off infection or abscess was suspected and generalized peritonitis or neoplasia was considered less likely. Ultrasonography may have been useful in locating a mass if it was not too deep in the abdomen to detect. If it had been possible to detect an abscess, it could have been monitored or drained during treatment. The horse was started on ceftiofur administered once daily at a dose of 2 mg/kg because of availability and relative safety. Ceftiofur treatment was to be continued for 4 to 6 weeks and monitored by the RDVM by serial CBCs, abdominocentesis, and serum chemistries. The results of the Coggin's test and the protein electrophoresis came back on day 10. The Coggin's test was negative for EIA. EIA has a 30- to 60-day period from infection to seroconversion [8]; thus, a negative test result is not always diagnostic. The main route of EIA transmission is by insect bites, however, so it was highly unlikely that the horse had been infected during the preceding 60-day period of cold weather. Serum protein electrophoresis showed a polyclonal gammopathy that was consistent with chronic antigenic stimulation or lymphoid neoplasia. This was consistent with a diagnosis of an abdominal abscess. Monoclonal gammopathy would have strongly suggested neoplasia. On day 26, the RDVM performed abdominocentesis, a CBC, and serum chemistry. The stallion still had neutrophilia and elevated serum total protein. The abdominocentesis sample was contaminated with gut content. The RDVM refused to repeat the procedure because he did not wish to be kicked again. The horse remained on ceftiofur until day 55, when a CBC and partial serum chemistry were repeated. All values were within normal limits, and the horse was clinically normal; thus, medication was discontinued. Resolution of the anemia suggests anemia of chronic disease. The RDVM and the owner reported the stallion to have had no further signs of disease 8 months after examination. An important aspect of this case is the haste that was required in the workup. Had time been allowed to get the results of the abdominocentesis, much expense could have been avoided.

References

[1] Saville WJ, Reed SM, Granstrom DE, et al. Seroprevalence of antibodies to Sarcocystis neuroma in horses residing in Ohio. J Am Vet Med Assoc 1997;210(4):519–24.
[2] Russell KE, Walker KM, Miller RT, et al. Hyperglobulinemia and lymphocyte subset changes in naturally infected, inapparent carriers of equine infectious anemia virus. Am J Vet Res 1998;59(8):1009–15.
[3] Carlson GP. Clinical chemistry tests. In: Smith BP, editor. Large animal internal medicine. 3rd edition. St. Louis (MO): Mosby; 2002. p. 396.
[4] Carlson GP. Diseases of the hematopoietic and hemolymphatic systems. In: Smith BP, editor. Large animal internal medicine. 3rd edition. St. Louis (MO): Mosby; 2002. p. 1064–5.
[5] Savage CJ. Lymphoproliferative and myeloproliferative disorders. Vet Clin North Am Equine Pract 1998;14(3):563–78.
[6] Kent JE, Roberts CA. Serum protein changes in four horses with monoclonal gammopathy. Equine Vet J 1990;22(5):373–6.
[7] Tizard IR. Veterinary immunology; an introduction. 5th edition. Philadelphia: WB Saunders; 1996. p. 134–7.
[8] Sellon DC. Equine infectious anemia. Vet Clin North Am Equine Pract 1993;9(2):321–36.

ELSEVIER
SAUNDERS

VETERINARY
CLINICS
Equine Practice

Vet Clin Equine 22 (2006) 61–71

Postpartum Hemoperitoneum and Septic Peritonitis in a Thoroughbred Mare

Tony D. Mogg, BVSc(Hons), PhD*, James Hart, BVSc,
Jamie Wearn, BVSc(Hons)

*University Veterinary Centre Camden, Faculty of Veterinary Science,
University of Sydney, 410 Werombi Road, Camden, NSW 2570, Australia*

Periparturient hemorrhage and hemoperitoneum in mares has been described secondary to arterial rupture or rupture of the uterus. Septic peritonitis may occur concurrently with hemoperitoneum in cases of uterine rupture. The history, physical examination findings, case assessment, treatment, and outcome of a Thoroughbred mare with postparturient hemoperitoneum and septic peritonitis (suspected to be the result of a uterine tear) are described in this case report.

Case details

History

A 5-year-old Thoroughbred full-term multiparous mare foaled unobserved overnight within a 5-hour interval and when first discovered by her owners was noted to be showing signs of colic. An ambulatory veterinarian examined the mare approximately 1 hour later. Physical examination revealed normal vital signs (heart rate 40 beats/minute, respiratory rate 12 breaths/minute, and rectal temperature 37.3°C (99.1° F) but no detectable borborygmi. Rectal examination failed to reveal any abnormalities. Some hemorrhagic discharge was present on vaginal examination. A nasogastric tube was passed; no net reflux was obtained, and the mare was given 6 L of water. Repeated attempts at abdominocentesis revealed sanguineous peritoneal fluid, whose packed cell volume (PCV) and total protein (TP) concentration were 19% (normal, negligible) and 3.8 g/dL (normal, <2.0g/dL),

---

* Corresponding author.
 E-mail address: T.D.Mogg@camden.usyd.edu.au (T.D. Mogg).

respectively. Her PCV and total plasma protein (TPP) were within normal limits (Table 1). Examination of the placenta was unremarkable, except for a small tear at the tip of the nongravid horn. The foal was clinically normal. The mare was treated with flunixin meglumine and xylazine but showed signs of colic again 30 minutes later. Referral to the University Veterinary Centre for further investigation was recommended, but the owner declined at that time because of financial constraints.

Approximately 36 hours later the mare was examined by another ambulatory veterinarian and was referred to the University Veterinary Centre. The owners reported that since the initial veterinary visit the mare had been depressed, inappetent, and febrile but showed fewer signs of abdominal discomfort. The foal continued to be bright and alert. The mare had been treated by the referring veterinarian with procaine penicillin, gentamicin sulfate, flunixin meglumine, and mineral oil immediately before referral.

Physical examination

The mare was quiet but responsive and weighed 440 kg. She was tachycardic (heart rate 70 beats/minute) but afebrile (rectal temperature 38.2°C; 100.8°F). She had prolonged skin turgor and dry oral mucous membranes. Her oral mucous membranes and sclerae were slightly injected. Her heart and lung sounds were within normal limits. She had decreased borborygmi. Her udder contained normal milk, and there was evidence that the foal had been nursing. The remainder of her physical examination was unremarkable. The foal was bright and clinically normal.

Table 1
Selected hematology and biochemistry results

Test (reference range)	Days of Hospitalization							
	−1	1	2	3	4	6	7	18
PCV (32%–52%)	34	28	28	26	24	27	25	25
TPP (5.5–8.4 g/dL)	6.5	5.2	6.1	6.2	7.2	7.2	7.2	6.6
White blood cells (6.0–13.0 × 10^3/μL)	ND	2.92	ND	6.5	ND	ND	18.7	11.2
Band neutrophils (0–0.24 × 10^3/μL)	ND	ND	ND	0.33	ND	ND	0.37	0.0
Neutrophils (2.47–6.96 × 10^3/μL)	ND	2.4	ND	3.7	ND	ND	13.09	8.62
Neutrophil morphology	ND	ND	ND	moderate toxic changes	ND	ND	mild toxic changes	no toxic changes
Fibrinogen (200–400 mg/dL)	ND	ND	ND	1000	ND	ND	870	580
Serum creatinine (1.0–1.7 mg/dL)	ND	ND	ND	1.0	ND	ND	0.7	0.7

Abbreviations: ND, not done; PCV, packed cell volume; TPP, total plasma protein.

Case assessment

The following diagnostic procedures were performed on admission to the hospital:

- Rectal examination: No abnormalities were detected.
- Manual vaginal and uterine examination: A small volume of nonmalodorous brown lochia was present. There was no evidence of a uterine tear.
- Routine hematology: The mare was anemic, hypoproteinemic, leukopenic, and neutropenic (see Table 1). Biochemistry was not performed because of lack of after-hours laboratory facilities.
- Transabdominal ultrasonography: A large volume of hyperechoic "swirling" free peritoneal fluid was present, consistent with a hemoperitoneum (Figs. 1, 2). A loculated, irregularly shaped structure of mixed echogenicity was present in the ventral abdomen consistent with a hematoma secondary to hemoperitoneum (Fig. 3). No fibrin was detected within the abdominal cavity, and no other abnormalities were observed.
- Abdominocentesis: Copious amounts of sanguineous peritoneal fluid were obtained in which the PCV, TP, and nucleated cell count were 26%, 4.7 g/dL, and $60 \times 10^3/\mu L$ (normal $< 5 \times 10^3/\mu L$), respectively. Cytologic examination revealed 89% degenerative neutrophils and 11% activated mononuclear cells. Some cells contained coccobacilli. This sample was not submitted for culture and sensitivity because of the recent administration of broad-spectrum antimicrobials.
- Transrectal uterine ultrasonography: No evidence of a uterine tear or a hematoma in the uterus or broad ligament was detected.

A diagnosis of postpartum hemoperitoneum and septic peritonitis was made.

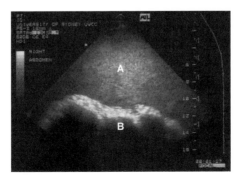

Fig. 1. Transverse sonogram of right ventral abdomen. (A) A large volume of hyperechoic "swirling" peritoneal fluid consistent with hemoperitoneum. (B) Normal large intestine. This sonogram was obtained using a 5-MHz sector-scanner transducer at a displayed depth of 16 cm.

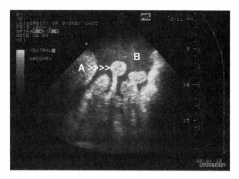

Fig. 2. Transverse sonogram of ventral abdomen. (A) Small intestine "floating" in hemoperitoneum. (B) Large volume of hyperechoic "swirling" peritoneal fluid consistent with hemoperitoneum. This sonogram was obtained using a 5-MHz sector-scanner transducer at a displayed depth of 20 cm.

Treatment and outcome

The mare and foal were admitted to the hospital for monitoring and conservative medical therapy. The mare was given water by nasogastric tube and no further medications overnight. The following morning she was depressed, tachycardic (heart rate 75 beats/minute), and febrile (40.0°C; 104.0°F). She was again given water by nasogastric tube, and abdominocentesis was repeated to obtain a sample of peritoneal fluid for culture and sensitivity. Treatment with procaine penicillin (22,000 IU/kg intramuscularly every 12 hours), gentamicin sulfate (6.6 mg/kg intravenously every 24 hours), and flunixin meglumine (0.5 mg/kg intravenously every 12 hours) was instituted, and the mare's clinical status was monitored closely. For the next 72 hours the mare continued to be depressed, inappetent, tachycardic

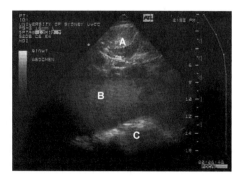

Fig. 3. Transverse sonogram of right ventral abdomen. (A) Loculated, irregularly shaped structure of mixed echogenicity consistent with an intra-abdominal hematoma. (B) Large volume of hyperechoic "swirling" peritoneal fluid consistent with hemoperitoneum. (C) Normal large intestine. This sonogram was obtained using a 5-MHz sector-scanner transducer at a displayed depth of 16 cm.

(heart rate 56–62 beats/minute), and febrile (rectal temperature 39.2–40.6°C, 102.6–105°F)). Her water intake improved, and enteral fluid therapy was discontinued. Because of her persistent fever, metronidazole (20 mg/kg by mouth every 8 hours) was added to her treatment regimen on day 3, but her clinical condition did not improve. Hematology performed on day 3 of hospitalization revealed normal white blood cell and neutrophil counts, a left shift, and hyperfibrinogenemia (see Table 1). Serum biochemistry was not performed (except for creatinine to assess renal function) because of financial constraints. Similarly, coagulation tests were not performed. Preliminary culture results from the peritoneal fluid revealed moderate growths of a *Streptococcus* and a gram-negative rod.

On day 4 transabdominal ultrasonography was repeated. Findings were similar to those on admission, with a large volume of hyperechoic "swirling" free fluid within the peritoneal cavity and no evidence of fibrin. Abdominal drainage and lavage were performed. The mare was sedated, and approximately 18 to 20 L of sanguineous fluid was drained from her ventral abdomen using a 28-French chest tube. Ultrasonography confirmed that the majority of the free peritoneal fluid within the ventral abdomen had been removed. Ten liters of warmed Hartmann's solution (similar to lactated Ringer's solution) was infused into the abdomen, drained, and the chest tube removed. Skin sutures were placed at the drainage site, but it continued to leak sanguineous fluid. A centrifuged sample of the peritoneal fluid revealed a port-wine supernatant, consistent with intra-abdominal hemolysis.

On day 5 the mare had developed a large plaque of warm, painful, pitting edema at the abdominal lavage site. Final results of the peritoneal fluid cultures were reported that day. Aerobic culture yielded growth of *Streptococcus equi ss zooepidemicus* and *Serratia liquefaciens/Citrobacter freundii* (organism not differentiated any further). Anaerobic culture yielded the same *Serratia liquefaciens/Citrobacter freundii* organism. Antimicrobial susceptibility testing was not initially performed on the *Streptococcus*. The *Serratia liquefaciens/Citrobacter freundii* was susceptible only to ciprofloxacin and tetracycline and was resistant to penicillin, ampicillin, ceftiofur, gentamicin, and trimethoprim/sulfonamide combinations. Subsequently the *Streptococcus equi ss zooepidemicus* was tested for susceptibility to tetracycline but was found to be resistant. Based on these results it was recommended that enrofloxacin be substituted for gentamicin in the mare's antimicrobial regimen, but the owners considered the cost to be prohibitive. The authors thus elected to treat the mare with oxytetracycline (6.6 mg/kg intravenously every 12 hours), beginning on the evening of day 5. Therapy with procaine penicillin and metronidazole was continued.

The mare's appetite and attitude improved rapidly. She was afebrile within 24 hours following the change in antimicrobial therapy, and her rectal temperature remained within normal limits (37.3–38.3°C; 99.1°–101.0°F) for the remainder of her hospitalization. Her anti-inflammatory therapy was changed to phenylbutazone (2.2 mg/kg by mouth every 12 hours) on day 6.

Hematology performed on day 7 revealed a leukocytosis, neutrophilia with a left shift, and decrease in plasma fibrinogen concentration (see Table 1). The mare's clinical condition continued to improve, and on day 12 she was turned out into a small paddock to graze. On day 13 therapy with phenylbutazone was changed to once daily, and on day 14 metronidazole therapy was discontinued. Neither of these changes resulted in deterioration of the mare's clinical status. Her ventral edema gradually resolved.

Because of financial constraints all antimicrobial therapy was discontinued on day 18, and the mare was discharged from the hospital. Hematology performed on that day revealed a mild neutrophilia and resolving hyperfibrinogenemia (see Table 1). Transabdominal ultrasonography revealed only a small volume of anechoic free peritoneal fluid, and the intra-abdominal hematoma was no longer visible. At the time of discharge the mare was bright and alert, afebrile, and weighed 434 kg. It was recommended that she be treated with phenylbutazone (2.2 mg/kg by mouth every 24 hours) for the next 5 days and monitored closely for signs of deterioration. It was also recommended that she not be rebred that season. Eight months after hospitalization the mare is reported to be clinically normal and has had no recurrence or complication of the hemoperitoneum and peritonitis. During the mare's hospitalization, the foal remained clinically normal, nursed vigorously, and gained body weight.

Discussion

The history of abdominal pain and the presence of sanguineous peritoneal fluid within hours of foaling were suggestive of a diagnosis of periparturient hemoperitoneum [1–3]. The initial diagnostic investigations performed on admission to the hospital also revealed abnormalities consistent with hemoperitoneum. The mare was anemic and hypoproteinemic, and a copious amount of frank blood was obtained on abdominocentesis. The PCV and TP of the peritoneal fluid were very similar to peripheral blood. The transabdominal ultrasonographic findings (large volume of hyperechoic "swirling" free peritoneal fluid and an intra-abdominal hematoma) were highly suggestive of hemoperitoneum [1,4,5]. Despite the diagnosis of periparturient hemoperitoneum, several observations were suggestive of a concurrent inflammatory or septic process. The mare had a history of fever before referral and remained febrile for the first 3 to 4 days of hospitalization (the mare was afebrile on admission, most probably as a result of the recent administration of flunixin meglumine by the referring veterinarian). Although mild fever has been reported in some horses with hemoperitoneum uncomplicated by sepsis [3], the magnitude of the mare's fever was more consistent with concurrent sepsis. The systemic leukopenia and neutropenia detected in this mare were also highly suggestive of acute inflammation or sepsis. In comparison, most horses with uncomplicated hemoperitoneum have either a normal leukogram or a stress response (neutrophilic leukocytosis) [3,5]. The peritoneal fluid cytology (and subsequent culture results) confirmed that the hemoperitoneum was complicated by septic peritonitis.

Internal hemorrhage and hemoperitoneum associated with parturition have been described as the result of arterial rupture or rupture of the uterus. Parturition-associated trauma to other intra-abdominal organs (eg, intestinal tract or spleen) could also result in hemorrhage and hemoperitoneum. Arterial rupture most frequently involves the middle uterine or utero-ovarian arteries and less commonly the external iliac artery [6,7]. Arterial rupture is most common in older mares and has been associated with age-related degenerative changes in the vessel walls [6–8]. Hemorrhage may be confined to tissues adjacent to the affected artery (ie, mesometrium) or enter the peritoneal cavity and result in hemoperitoneum [8]. Uterine rupture most commonly occurs during stage II of parturition [7]. It is most commonly reported to be associated with dystocia or postparturient uterine manipulation (eg, uterine lavage) [7,9]. It has also been reported in mares following uneventful parturition, most frequently occurring at the tip of the gravid uterine horn [7]. Unlike arterial rupture, rupture of the uterus is often complicated by the development of septic peritonitis [7,10]. Also, a hemorrhagic vaginal discharge may be present in cases of uterine rupture [1,3,7,10]. Other causes of hemoperitoneum (not directly associated with parturition) that were considered in this case included external trauma, vascular leakage from an intra-abdominal abscess or neoplasm, parasitic mesenteric artery rupture, hepatopathies, and coagulopathies [2,3]. Hemoperitoneum has also been described secondary to ovarian hemorrhage (eg, granulosa cell tumor or ovarian hematoma) [11–13], although such causes were considered unlikely in this mare given her reproductive status. Infection may have been introduced into the peritoneal cavity by hematogenous spread or, more likely, caused by direct bacterial contamination. Direct contamination could have been the result of trauma to the uterus or intestinal tract during parturition or of leakage from an intra-abdominal abscess.

Although the diagnostic tests confirmed that the mare had concurrent hemoperitoneum and septic peritonitis, a definitive cause was not identified. No evidence of artery rupture (eg, hematoma in the mesometrium), uterine rupture, trauma to the spleen or intestinal tract, intra-abdominal abscessation, or neoplasia was detected. Liver disease and coagulopathies could not be definitively excluded as a cause of the hemoperitoneum, because the appropriate diagnostic tests were not performed. Despite the lack of definitive findings, uterine rupture was considered the most likely cause of the hemoperitoneum and septic peritonitis in this case. The mare's clinical history and abdominocentesis abnormalities were typical of those described for mares with periparturient uterine rupture [7,10]. A diagnosis of uterine rupture can be made by either rectal examination or manual uterine examination, but the large size of the postpartum equine uterus may result in difficulty in making the diagnosis, especially if the rupture is a small tear at or near the tip of the gravid uterine horn [7,14]. Similarly, transrectal ultrasonography may not provide a definitive diagnosis [14]. Thus the inability to identify definitively a uterine tear in this mare is not inconsistent with this diagnosis. In one case hysteroscopy was used to confirm the diagnosis [14], and this procedure could have been considered in this mare. Hysteroscopy, however, requires air insufflation of the uterus, which could have resulted in pneumoperitoneum or disruption of a uterine hematoma and recurrence of hemorrhage.

Treatment for hemoperitoneum in horses is usually medical [2,5], although surgical intervention has been described in several cases [13,15]. Surgical intervention has been advocated in horses with hemoperitoneum (in the absence of septic peritonitis) when bleeding cannot be controlled within 12 hours or when hemorrhage occurs after previous surgery [3]. Surgery has also been advocated in horses with septic peritonitis to identify (and potentially correct) the source of the infection and to provide peritoneal drainage and lavage [16]. Both medical and surgical management of mares with uterine tears has been described [7,9,14]. Medical therapy is most likely to be successful with small dorsal uterine tears [7]. In this case, financial constraints precluded surgery.

The aims of medical management of hemoperitoneum are to stop continuing hemorrhage and provide supportive therapy (eg, fluid therapy, whole-blood transfusions, and analgesia) [2,5]. Medical therapies suggested in the literature for controlling on-going hemorrhage include antifibrinolytics (eg, aminocaproic acid), intravenous formalin, and naloxone [1,2,7]. The administration of oxytocin or ergonovine maleate has been suggested in cases of uterine rupture to decrease uterine hemorrhage [3,7,8,10].

The mare presented 36 hours after first showing signs consistent with hemoperitoneum and was not showing signs of hemorrhagic shock. It was thus decided to monitor her clinical condition and PCV/TPP closely to assess whether continuing hemorrhage was occurring [17] and thus to assess the need for hemostatic therapy or a whole-blood transfusion. Typically, changes in PCV/TPP do not reflect the severity of hemorrhage for 12 to 24 hours after bleeding begins [1]. Because the mare was admitted to the hospital more than 24 hours after the onset of hemorrhage, PCV/TPP measurements should have been representative of the severity of her anemia and a good indicator of on-going hemorrhage.

The mare was dehydrated, and fluid therapy was indicated, although financial constraints limited therapy to enteral fluids. The presence of concurrent septic peritonitis necessitated broad-spectrum antimicrobial therapy. Flunixin meglumine was administered for its anti-inflammatory, analgesic, and antiendotoxic properties. Nonsteroidal anti-inflammatory therapy was changed to phenylbutazone to decrease costs once the mare's condition was stable. Heparin has been advocated for the prevention of intra-abdominal adhesions in horses with peritonitis [18] but was considered contraindicated in this case because of the possibility of continuing hemorrhage. The administration of sedatives to horses with hemoperitoneum is controversial because of the potential for causing hypotension [1,3,17]. In cases of peripar-turient hemorrhage and hemoperitoneum, it is usually recommended not to separate the mare and foal, to avoid exciting the mare and potentially exac-erbating or reinitiating bleeding [7]. Similarly, it is recommended that horses with hemoperitoneum be confined to a box stall and that stress and agita-tion be minimized [3,5].

The antimicrobial regimen (penicillin and gentamicin) started by the re-ferring veterinarian was continued following admission to the hospital. This combination provided broad-spectrum antimicrobial coverage while awaiting peritoneal fluid culture and sensitivity results. Cultures from horses with septic peritonitis frequently yield multiple organisms, including obli-gate anaerobes (eg, *Bacteroides* spp.) [3]. Metronidazole therapy was with-held initially because of financial constraints but was included in the antimicrobial regimen on day 3 when the mare had failed to make significant clinical improvement. Culture and sensitivity results subsequently revealed that the *Serratia liquefaciens/Citrobacter freundii* was resistant to both pen-icillin and gentamicin. This resistance probably explains why the mare had not clinically improved. The *Serratia liquefaciens/Citrobacter freundii* was susceptible only to fluoroquinolones and tetracyclines. Ideally, the authors would have discontinued therapy with gentamicin and begun treatment with enrofloxacin, but cost precluded this approach, and the only option was oxytetracycline. The *Streptococcus* was resistant to tetracycline, necessi-tating continued penicillin therapy. Metronidazole therapy was continued because of the possibility that obligate anaerobes may have been present but not cultured. The combination of oxytetracycline and penicillin would normally be considered contraindicated because of concerns about the con-current administration of bactericidal and bacteriostatic antimicrobials [19]. In theory, the efficacy of bactericidal antimicrobial drugs (which are most effective against actively dividing bacteria) may be antagonized by the ac-tions of bacteriostatic antimicrobial drugs (which inhibit bacterial growth) [19,20]. For an antagonistic interaction to occur, however, the bacteria must be susceptible to both of the antimicrobial drugs [20]. In this case, in vitro susceptibility tests had shown that the *Streptococcus* was susceptible only to penicillin (and was resistant to oxytetracycline), whereas the *Serratia liquefaciens/Citrobacter freundii* was susceptible only to oxytetracycline (and was resistant to penicillin). Thus, if the in vitro results were representative of in vivo susceptibilities, no antimicrobial drug interactions should have oc-curred. The mare's rapid improvement following initiation of therapy with oxytetracycline suggests that if any interactions did occur, they were not clinically significant.

The decision to perform abdominal drainage and lavage was based on the failure of the mare to respond to more conservative medical therapy. Ultra-sonography was used to verify that the majority of the free peritoneal fluid in the ventral abdomen had been removed before lavage with a polyionic crystalloid solution. Drainage and lavage was performed only once because of the development of cellulitis at the drainage site and the mare's rapid clinical improvement following the introduction of oxytetracycline therapy. The aims of abdominal drainage and lavage are to reduce bacterial numbers and remove degenerate neutrophils, cellular debris, fibrin, bacterial toxins, and proinflammatory factors [21,22]. Abdominal drainage is usually not indicated in uncomplicated cases of hemoperitoneum because a large proportion of the red blood cells and protein will be reabsorbed into the systemic circulation. In this mare, however, the potential for the blood in the abdomen to enhance bacterial growth [1,3] was considered to be an indication for abdominal drainage (especially given her poor response to more conservative therapy). Several authors have questioned the efficacy of abdominal lavage in the standing horse [3,23]. It is likely that lavage is most efficacious if performed during surgical exploration of the abdomen [3,23]. Open peritoneal drainage and active intra-abdominal drains have also been described in the management of horses with septic peritonitis [24,25]. Consideration should be given to the type of lavage fluid chosen, because one study demonstrated that povidone-iodine solutions caused moderate-to-marked hemorrhagic peritonitis in normal ponies [26].

In this case the mare showed a rapid response to antimicrobial therapy based on the peritoneal fluid culture and sensitivity results. The case exemplifies the importance of submitting appropriate samples for bacteriologic culture and sensitivity rather than relying on empiric antimicrobial therapy. Sequential hematology revealed changes typical of a severe acute inflammatory process (leukopenia and neutropenia followed by rebound leukocytosis and neutrophilia, a left shift, and hyperfibrinogenemia). Ideally antimicrobial treatment would have continued until the mare's leukogram and plasma fibrinogen concentration were normal, but financial constraints did not allow continued therapy. Despite these financial limitations, which dictated many management decisions, the mare had a good outcome. The source of the hemoperitoneum and septic peritonitis remain unclear, although uterine rupture was considered most likely. Because of this possibility and the mare's poor body condition, it was recommended that the mare not be bred until the next breeding season.

References

[1] Jeffrey SC. Managing hemoperitoneum in horses. Vet Med 1996;91(9):850–6.
[2] Edens LM. Abdominal hemorrhage. In: Robinson NE, editor. Current therapy in equine medicine 4. Philadelphia: W.B. Saunders; 1997. p. 211–4.
[3] Semrad SD. Diseases of the peritoneum and mesentery. In: Colahan PT, Merritt AM, Moore JN, et al, editors. Equine medicine and surgery. 5th edition. St. Louis (MO): Mosby; 1999. p. 790–800.
[4] Reef VB. Adult abdominal ultrasonography. Diseases of the peritoneal cavity. In: Reef VB, editor. Equine diagnostic ultrasonography. Philadelphia: W.B. Saunders; 1998. p. 339–46.
[5] Pusterla N, Fecteau ME, Madigan JE, et al. Acute hemoperitoneum: a review of 19 cases (1992–2003). J Vet Intern Med 2005;19:344–7.

[6] Rooney JR. Internal hemorrhage related to gestation in the mare. Cornell Vet 1964;54:11–7.

[7] Blanchard TL, Varner DD, Schumacher J, et al. Dystocia and postparturient disease. In: Manual of equine reproduction. 2nd edition. St. Louis (MO): Mosby; 2002. p. 107–16.

[8] Lofstedt RM. Miscellaneous diseases of pregnancy and parturition. Hemorrhage associated with pregnancy and parturition. In: McKinnon AO, Voss JL, editors. Equine reproduction. Philadelphia: Lea & Febiger; 1993. p. 600–3.

[9] Fischer AT, Phillips TN. Surgical repair of a ruptured uterus in five mares. Equine Vet J 1986;18(2):153–5.

[10] Hooper RN, Carter GK, Varner DD, et al. Postparturient hemorrhage in the mare: managing lacerations of the birth canal and uterus. Vet Med 1994;89(1):57–63.

[11] Sedrish SA, Johnson PJ. Theriogenology question of the month. J Am Vet Med Assoc 1997; 210(2):179–80.

[12] Gatewood DM, Douglass JP, Cox JH, et al. Intra-abdominal hemorrhage associated with a granulosa-thecal cell neoplasm in a mare. J Am Vet Med Assoc 1990;196(11):1827–8.

[13] Alexander GR, Tweedie MA, Lescun TB, et al. Haemoperitoneum secondary to granulosa cell tumour in two mares. Aust Vet J 2004;82(8):481–4.

[14] van den Wollenburg L, van der Weijden GC, van Oldruitenborgh-Oosterbaan MMS. Uterine rupture as a cause of postpartum peritonitis in the horse. Pferdeheilkunde 2002;18(2): 141–6.

[15] Mitchell KJ, Dowling BA, Hughes KJ, et al. Unilateral nephrectomy as a treatment for renal trauma in a foal. Aust Vet J 2004;82(12):753–5.

[16] Hawkins JF. Peritonitis. In: Robinson NE, editor. Current therapy in equine medicine 5. Philadelphia: W.B. Saunders; 2003. p. 153–8.

[17] Boure L. Intra-abdominal hemorrhage. In: Brown CM, Bertone J, editors. The 5-minute veterinary consult—equine. Baltimore (MD): Lippincott Williams & Wilkins; 2002. p. 582–3.

[18] Parker JE, Fubini SL, Car BD, et al. Prevention of intraabdominal adhesions in ponies by low-dose heparin therapy. Vet Surg 1987;16(6):459–62.

[19] Dowling PM. Antimicrobial therapy. Combination antimicrobial therapy. In: Bertone JJ, Horspool LJI, editors. Equine clinical pharmacology. Edinburgh (UK): W.B. Saunders; 2004. p. 21–2.

[20] Chambers HF, Sande MA. Antimicrobial agents. General considerations. Therapy with combined antimicrobial agents. In: Hardman JG, Limbird LE, Molinoff PB, et al, editors. Goodman & Gilman's the pharmacological basis of therapeutics. 9th edition. New York: McGraw-Hill; 1996. p. 1046–9.

[21] Valdez H, Scrutchfield WL, Taylor TS. Peritoneal lavage in the horse. J Am Vet Med Assoc 1979;175(4):388–91.

[22] Davis JL. Treatment of peritonitis. Vet Clin North Am Equine Pract 2003;19(3):765–78.

[23] Hillyer MH, Wright CJ. Peritonitis in the horse. Equine Veterinary Education 1997;9(3): 136–42.

[24] Chase JP, Beard WL, Bertone AL, et al. Open peritoneal drainage in horses with experimentally induced peritonitis. Vet Surg 1996;25:189–94.

[25] Nieto JE, Snyder JR, Vatistas NJ, et al. Use of an active intra-abdominal drain in 67 horses. Vet Surg 2003;32:1–7.

[26] Schneider RK, Meyer DJ, Embertson RM, et al. Response of pony peritoneum to four peritoneal lavage solutions. Am J Vet Res 1988;49(6):889–94.

VETERINARY
CLINICS
Equine Practice

Vet Clin Equine 22 (2006) 73–84

Acute Diarrhea in the Adult Horse: Case Example and Review

Olimpo E. Oliver, DVM, MSc, DVSc[a],*,
Henry Stämpfli, DVM, Dr Med Vet[b]

[a]Clinica de Grandes Animales, Departamento de Salud Animal,
Facultad de Medicina Veterinaria y de Zootecnia,
Universidad Nacional de Bogota de Santa Fe, Bogota, Colombia
[b]Department of Clinical Studies, Ontario Veterinary College,
University of Guelph, Guelph, Ontario, Canada N1G 2W1

Acute diarrhea is a clinical sign of large intestinal (typhlocolic) disease in adult horses. Frequently, the major clinical signs also include colic, dehydration, and endotoxemia, which sometimes rapidly progress to shock and, occasionally, to death. Underlying pathologic causes are mostly colonic flora disturbances resulting in pathogen overgrowth and gastrointestinal motility alterations as well as intestinal fluid losses and electrolyte and acid-base imbalances. Diarrhea is defined as increased water content in the feces compared with homeostasis. Acute diarrhea may differ somewhat in foals and adult horses because of differences in causative infectious agents, the intestinal site affected, and different colonic absorptive capacity. The initiating cause of the problem of acute diarrhea is frequently (>60% of cases) not determined. Acute colitis also produces rapidly severe catabolic conditions with marked acute weight loss.

Acute undifferentiated diarrhea in a 4-year-old Thoroughbred stallion

A 4-year-old Thoroughbred stallion was presented with acute onset of severe diarrhea of 7 hours' duration. The pertinent history was unremarkable, and the horse had been in full training and racing at the local racetrack. On clinical examination, the horse was depressed, clinically estimated to be 10% dehydrated, mildly colicky, and mildly tachycardic, but the temperature was normal. Venous blood gases and electrolytes showed mild metabolic acidosis with hyponatremia, hypochloremia, absolute and relative

* Corresponding author.
E-mail address: ojoliver@cable.net.co (O.E. Oliver).

0749-0739/06/$ - see front matter © 2006 Elsevier Inc. All rights reserved.
doi:10.1016/j.cveq.2005.12.008   vetequine.theclinics.com

hypoproteinemia, an increased anion gap, a marked increase in the strong ion gap (lactate) compatible with the problems of fluid and electrolyte losses, inflammation of the colon, and general decreased tissue oxygenation as a result of severe dehydration (Table 1). A complete blood cell count (CBC) showed leukocytosis with a left shift and hyperfibrinogenemia, which were both compatible with severe toxic colitis (Table 2). The horse had received penicillin, gentamicin, and flunixin meglumine treatment by the referring veterinarian on the day of presentation.

Initial *Clostridium difficile* toxin A and B screening of feces was negative. Initial treatment consisted of parenteral fluid treatment using lactated Ringer's solution (LRS) spiked with one half of the deficit of sodium bicarbonate, calculated as 0.4 (sodium bicarbonate space) × body weight × negative base excess (as reported on blood gas results; note that the base excess is calculated from normal human bicarbonate concentrations and that the real base excess in this patient is higher at approximately 12 mmol/L; normal bicarbonate values of the horse are 28.3 ± 3.4; see Table 1). The rate of fluid administration in severely dehydrated animals may go up to 1 L/min for the first 30 minutes so as to improve hydration status. This can be accomplished with a fluid pump system. The remaining fluid deficit (% dehydration × body weight = fluid deficit in liters) should be corrected over 12 hours. The horse was also started on oral potassium supplementation using potassium chloride (KCl), 50 g, administered orally every 12 hours. As an adjunct treatment for undifferentiated diarrhea, the horse was also given oral zinc bacitracin (10 mg/kg) twice daily for the first 24 hours, followed by administration once daily until firm feces were observed. The horse was also treated flunixin meglumine at a rate of 0.25 mg/kg every 8 hours for its purported antiendotoxic effects.

The horse responded well to the supportive treatment in the first 24 hours, and vital signs were normal on day 2. Parenteral antibiotic

Table 1
Venous blood gases, total solids, and electrolytes at admission

	Case	Reference range
pH	7.20	7.4 ± 0.05
P_{CO_2}(mm Hg)	43.1	40 ± 2
P_{O_2}(mm Hg)	45.7	40 ± 4
HCO_3^- (mmol/L)	16	28.3 ± 3.4
Base Excess (mEq/L)	−8	0 ± (2–4)
Anion gap (AG; mmol/L)	20.4	12 ± 4
Strong ion gap (AG-A⁻) (mmol/L)	11.3	0 ± 2
Sodium (mmol/L)	125	139 ± 4.2
Potassium (mmol/L)	3.4	4.5 ± 0.04
Chloride (mmol/L)	92	101 ± 4
SID (Na^+ $K^-$$Cl^-$ HCO_3) (mmol/L)	36.4	40 ± 2
TP g/L	50	64 ± 10
A⁻ (TP × 0 .175) (mmol/L)	9.1	12 ± 4

Abbreviations: SID, strong ion difference; TP, total protein.

Table 2
Hemogram at admission

CBC	Case	Reference values
WBC (×10E9/L)	18.5	5.3–11.0
RBC (×10E12/L)	14.56	6.5–11.6
HGB (g/L)	190	109–188
HCT (L/L)	0.60	0.29–0.53
PLTS (×10E9/L)	100	80–397
Segmented	7.03	2.1–6.0
Bands	0.74	0.0–0.2
Lymphocytes	9.25	1.7–5.0
Monocytes	0.74	0.0–0.6
Fibrinogen (g/L)	5.0	<2.9
Rouleaux	+++	

Abbreviations: CBC, complete blood cell count; HCT, hematocrit; HGB, hemoglobin; PLTS, platelets; RBC, red blood cells; WBC, white blood cells.

treatment was not continued, and by day 3, there were firm feces present, parenteral fluid therapy was discontinued, and the horse recovered uneventfully. The main abnormalities noted on a biochemical profile were mild hypoalbuminemia (2.7 g/dL, normal range: 2.9–3.6 g/dL) and mild prerenal azotemia.

Bacteriologic culture of feces for *Salmonella* and *Clostridium* spp were repeatedly negative, as was a toxin assay testing for *C difficile* toxins A and B as well as for *C perfringens* enterotoxin (*C perfringens* Enterotoxin Test and *C difficile* tox A/B test; Techlab, Blacksburg, Virginia). The exact initiating cause of the diarrhea problem in this horse could not be established. The horse was not tested for Potomac horse fever (PHF). The final working diagnosis was acute undifferentiated diarrhea attributable to bacterial colonic overgrowth of unidentified pathogenic organism(s).

Pathophysiology of acute diarrhea

In approximately 40% of horses presented with the complaint of acute diarrhea, a causal association may be established, and in approximately 60% of cases, the originating cause is never found [1]. Diarrhea represents a disturbance of the normal fluid balance, including an imbalance of electrolyte secretion to absorption in the large intestine [2]. Because of the massive absorptive capacity of the large colon, small intestinal lesions do not usually cause diarrhea in adult horses as compared with other species. Small intestinal diarrhea may be seen in foals. Different mechanisms are involved in the development of diarrhea; these include hypersecretion, increased permeability (exudation), malabsorption, and abnormal motility [3,4]. Patients with severe acute diarrhea are usually also presented with signs of active inflammatory processes primarily localized in the large colon. Central to the problem of acute diarrhea is the cecocolic intestinal flora. Any "upsetter" of the flora may create a milieu that releases bacterial toxins (eg, lipopolysaccharide [LPS]) inducing inflammation (cytokines and other in-flammatory mediators), resulting in net fluid loss into the intestinal lumen and damage to the cell layers and vascular bed of the cecocolic mucosa as well as local edema formation, exudation, and toxin absorption into the bloodstream. The net result is massive fluid, electrolyte, anticoagulant, and procoagulant substances and protein losses with secondary signs, such as hypovolemia, acidemia, hypoalbuminemia, coagulation distur-bances, and cardiovascular and endotoxic shock [5].

Specific disease conditions associated with acute diarrhea include C difficile enterocolitis, C perfringens enterocolitis, antibiotic-associated diarrhea (AAD), salmonellosis, PHF, and nonsteroidal anti-inflammatory (NSAID)–associated diarrhea.

Clostridium difficile enterocolitis

C difficile enterocolitis is an inflammation of the colon caused by over-growth of toxigenic strains of C difficile, most commonly causing diarrhea and varying degrees of toxemia [6–9]. Proliferation of this organism occurs because of a disruption of the normal colonic flora. Two toxins are pro-duced, a cytotoxin and an enterotoxin, which work synergistically, with the net result of mucosal damage, local inflammation, and fluid secretion causing a vicious circle. Historically, there may be recent antibiotic use, which upsets the normal stable colonic bacterial milieu. Diagnosis is made by the presence of toxin in the feces using a commercial ELISA test [10,11]. A positive culture of C difficile in feces is not necessarily diag-nostic, because there are toxin-positive and toxin-negative strains of this organism present [11,12]. Viability of the organism in collected feces is poor even if kept refrigerated, whereas viability of the toxin is long term when feces are stored at 4°C [12,13]. The supportive treatment is identical to the case scenario. In addition, if feces are toxin-positive, a course with oral metronidazole at a rate of 15–25 mg/kg administered every 8 hours is in-dicated until feces are toxin-negative and are firming up [14]. Most of the isolates of C difficile at the Ontario Veterinary College clinic were sensitive to metronidazole but in vitro resistant to zinc-bacitracin [13]. The antibi-otic vancomycin (20–40 mg/kg administered two times daily to four times daily intravenously or orally) should be reserved for severe resistant infec-tions and should not be used in the horse if possible. Di-tri-octahedral smectite [15] has been shown in vitro to bind clostridial toxins and inhibit growth of C difficile but has not been critically evaluated as an adjunct treatment in horses with C difficile–induced colitis or in horses with undif-ferentiated acute colitis [16].

Clostridium perfringens enterocolitis

C perfringens has been associated with colitis in horses [9,17]. C perfrin-gens is classified based on the pattern of exotoxin production into five types:

A, B, C, D, and E (importance of type E in disease is questionable). *C perfringens* type A is the type most frequently associated with colitis in horses but is also isolated in normal horses. The main toxin that the virulent strains produces is the α toxin, which interferes with glucose uptake and energy production and triggers arachidonic acid metabolism and activation of secretion in enterocytes [10]. There is a novel toxin designed β_2 produced by *C perfringens* that could be described as similar to type A and has been found only in horses with colitis [18]. It biologic activity includes enterocyte necrosis, ulceration, intestinal hemorrhage, and inflammation. Virulent *C perfringens* also produces enterotoxin that alters permeability to water macromolecules, resulting in cell necrosis [10]. Diagnosis can be made by isolation of *C perfringens*, and demonstration of associated toxins in the absence of other pathogens is the strongest evidence of its causative role. The treatment approach is identical to *C difficile* therapeutic measures.

Antibiotic-associated diarrhea

Antibiotics that have been used experimentally to induce acute colitis in horses include lincomycin, clindamycin, oxytetracycline, and low-dose erythromycin ethylsuccinate [13,14,19,20].

Parenteral or oral antibiotics that have been temporally associated with the onset of acute diarrhea include tetracyclines, lincomycin, erythromycins, cephalosporins, trimethoprim-sulfas, and penicillins. Cases of colitis have also been associated with the administration of cloxacillin, florfenicol, ampicillin/sulbactam, chloramphenicol, and metronidazole as well as with ciprofloxacin more recently [21].

The core of the problem is the disruption of the normal cecocolic flora [22]. Theoretically, any broad-spectrum antibiotic has the potential to upset the local protective flora and to allow potential pathogens to "overgrow" and cause disease. In human beings, the main factors implicated in AAD are related to loss of colonization resistance through alterations in the gastrointestinal microflora, changes in fermentative conditions, and resulting increased toxin production by pathogenic organisms (eg, *C difficile* toxins) [23]. To date, only erythromycin ethylsuccinate has been implicated with *C difficile* as the specific pathogen causing acute colitis in the horse [6,19]. In many clinical cases, it is difficult to establish a pathogen and the antibiotic as the linked causative factors in disease. Most classes of antibiotics have been implicated in human AAD, but there is a greater association with cephalosporins, penicillins, and clindamycin [8,23].

Salmonellosis

Salmonellosis causes different clinical syndromes and is usually characterized by an acute septic colitis with profuse diarrhea [24]. Its incidence is low in nonhospital settings, but outbreaks occur occasionally on farms [25]. *Salmonella* species most frequently isolated from horses include *S typhimurium* (DT104), *S agona*, *S anatum*, and *S krefeld* [26,27]. *Salmonella* carrier horses have been reported with a frequency as high as 10% to 20%, but the frequency is thought to be between 1% and 2% in the general population [26]. The infection by *Salmonella* usually occurs orally and through the gastrointestinal tract. It can invade the pharyngeal, small intestinal, and colonic mucosa. It invades the intestinal M cells, is phagocytosed by macrophages and dendritic cells in the lamina propria and lymphoid tissue, and then passes into the bloodstream [24,25]. *Salmonella* causes diarrhea by different mechanisms involving virulent factors that promote infection. *Salmonella* produces a cytotoxin causing cell damage and altered permeability [28]. It also produces a thermolabile (LT) exotoxin similar to *Escherichia coli* that causes hypersecretion and may contribute to diarrhea [29], and the main cause of diarrhea is probably the ability of *Salmonella* to produce a severe intestinal inflammatory reaction [30]. The systemic effects caused by *Salmonella* can be attributed to LPS, often resulting in severe cardiovascular impairment and releasing factors triggering an inflammatory response of the host cumulating in further tissue damage and signs of endotoxemia [24,31]. Diagnosis of *Salmonella* is achieved by five serial fecal cultures that have a sensibility of 93% [32,33] or a positive fecal polymerase chain reaction (PCR) assay for *Salmonella* bacteria [34].

Potomac horse fever

PHF is an acute enterotyphlocolitis of horses caused by infection with the monocytotropic rickettsia, *Neorickettsia risticii* [35], formerly called *Ehrlichia risticii* [36]. The pathophysiology of PHF is poorly understood. *N risticii*, an obligate intracellular parasite, has a predilection for blood monocytes and tissue macrophages. Within days of infection, *N risticii* can be found in blood monocytes, and although readily phagocytosed by monocytes, *N risticii* survives within phagosomes in macrophages by inhibiting phagosome-lysosome fusion. The neorickettsemia persists throughout the clinical period [37].

The pathogen has a predilection for the cecum and large colon but is occasionally found in the jejunum and small colon. Colonic and small intestinal epithelial cells, colonic mast cells, and macrophages are the targets of infection. Even mild cases of PHF without diarrhea have evidence of colitis [38]. The major clinical signs observed resemble those of horses with salmonellosis or endotoxemia. It is possible that many pathophysiologic changes observed in horses affected with PHF are secondary to the effects of altered colonic flora (eg, diarrhea, endotoxemia).

Serology is the most commonly used method of diagnosing PHF. The indirect fluorescent antibody (IFA) test is the most widely used diagnostic test for PHF [37]. The interpretation of results can be challenging. PHF is diagnosed by demonstrating a fourfold or greater increase or decrease in IFA titers between acute and convalescent serum samples. The acute sample should be collected as soon as first clinical signs are observed, and the convalescent sample should be collected 5 to 7 days later. Failure to seroconvert does not rule out PHF. The expected antibody titer of naturally affected horses is greater than 1:80. Persistence of high antibody titers (eg, 1:2560) for more than a year has been noted in clinical and subclinical cases after natural infection [37]. An ELISA is also available [39]. A nested PCR technique has been developed [40]. This detects the partial 16S rRNA gene of *E risticii* and seems to be as sensitive as blood culture for detecting infection with *E risticii*. Isolation of *E risticii* by blood culture is the most definitive method of diagnosis of PHF. It requires collecting heparinized blood (100–400 mL) and harvesting buffy coat for culture [40]. Because conventional PCR assays are time-consuming and prone to contamination, a new real-time PCR assay has been developed and allows detection of *N risticii* in 2 hours [41].

Diarrhea associated with nonsteroidal anti-inflammatory drugs

Clinically, NSAID toxicity is described to cause two clinical syndromes: generalized NSAID toxicity and right dorsal colitis (RDC) [40,42]. All NSAIDs are potentially capable of causing toxicity. RDC is a localized ulcerative inflammation of the right dorsal colon that has been associated with NSAIDs given in excessive amounts in the presence of dehydration. The exact cause is not known, but there are associations with a history of phenylbutazone or flunixin meglumine treatments.

The most evident clinical signs of RDC are depression, anorexia, fever, colic, diarrhea, dehydration, and evidence of endotoxemia. Clinical signs of generalized NSAID toxicity may vary from no systemic signs to severe diarrhea along with the other sign of toxicity, such as anorexia, oral ulceration, fever, and peripheral edema [43]. NSAIDs inhibit cyclooxygenase activity (COX 1 and COX 2). It is believed that NSAIDs that are indiscriminately COX 1 and COX 2 inhibitors have a higher capacity to produce more toxicity (eg, phenylbutazone, aspirin). The gastrointestinal lesions caused by NSAIDs are manifested as mucosal ulceration, bleeding, protein-losing enteropathy, and a significant response to microbial products exposed to the lamina propria [43,44].

Therapeutic considerations in acute diarrhea cases

Because the net results of any case with severe acute diarrhea are massive fluid, electrolyte, and protein losses with secondary signs, such as hypovolemia, acidemia, and cardiovascular and endotoxic shock, the main goal of treatment is to re-establish homeostasis by supportive treatment. Based on the previous described alterations of homeostasis, the goals of colitis treatment, regardless of the cause, may involve fluid and electrolyte replacement, correcting acid-base disarrangements, circulatory support, treatment of hypoproteinemia, control of inflammation, endotoxin control, pain management, mucosal protection and repair, and the use of antibiotics and anticoagulants.

To correct fluid losses, the amount of fluid required to be replaced is calculated by the formula: BW × % DH, where BW is body weight and DH is dehydration. The calculated amount is administered at a speed based on cardiovascular status. Severely dehydrated animals may need rapid administration and require the use of peristaltic pumps to achieve it. The speed used can be between 10 and 40 mL/k/h. The use of 7.5% hypertonic saline (5–7 mL/kg in 20 minutes) is a resuscitation maneuver to reverse hypovolemia; however, in colitis cases with severe hyponatremia, it needs to be administered cautiously [45]. It needs to be always followed by the administration of isotonic solutions, with the amount compared with the total fluid loss plus the animal's daily maintenance requirement calculated. To restore and maintain fluid balance, LRS or acetated Ringer's solution and sodium chloride (0.9%) are commonly used [46]. Colloidal solutions (eg, whole blood, plasma, hetastarch, dextrans) can be used to maintain the fluid in the vascular space [46,47]. Colloids should be initiated when plasma proteins are less than 4 g/dL. Colloids should be from a commercial source or from appropriate donors (Aa and Qa isoantibody–negative).

Sodium bicarbonate is used to treat severe metabolic acidosis that does not correct with volume expansion. To calculate needs, use the following formula: 0.4 mEq × body weight (kg) × (base deficit). Give half the dose slowly intravenously over 20 minutes, and give the rest of the dose in crystalloid fluids over 4 hours. Hypokalemia can be treated by adding KCl to the hydration solution and can be administrated safely if the rate of administration does not exceed 0.5 mEq/kg/h. To correct body deficits, KCl should be administered orally at 50 g twice a day for several days.

Inotropic agents can be given to increase systemic blood pressure when it drops markedly. Dopamine hydrochloride, 1 to 5 µg/kg/min, is given by continuous intravenous administration

Dobutamine, 2 to 5 µg/kg/min, is given by continuous intravenous administration [48]. NSAIDS (eg, flunixin meglumine, ketoprofen, phenylbutazone, aspirin) are frequently used for attenuation of the inflammatory cascade. Flunixin meglumine seems to have the most potent antiendotoxic effects at a rate of 1.1 mg/kg administered every 8 to 12 hours or at 0.25 mg/kg administered every 6 to 8 hours, or ketoprofen can be administered at a rate of 0.5 mg/kg every 6 hours. Aspirin also prevents thrombus formation. NSAIDS inhibit vasodilator prostaglandins; therefore, care must be taken with regard to renal damage [49].

Hyperimmune antisera or plasma is used in endotoxemia. O-chain–specific antisera work well, but because of the antigenic diversity between gram-negative (GN0) bacteria in this region, they are not clinically useful. Different gram-negative bacteria share common core antigens; therefore, antibodies are aimed at the LPS core [50]. These antibodies may promote opsonization and reticuloendothelial clearance and inhibit the interactions of LPS. J5 hyperimmune plasma is used at a dose of 4.4 mL/kg initially. Some studies have failed to show positive results, however [51].

The use of antibiotics in treating acute enterocolitis is controversial [52]. Although bacterial seeding to other organ systems is rare, in severely neutropenic patients, the use of broad-spectrum antibiotics seems to be indicated. Oral antibiotics used as adjunct treatments to the supportive care are metronidazole (15–25 mg/kg administered every 8 hours) in cases with confirmed *C difficile* toxin-associated colitis and zinc bacitracin (10 mg/kg administered every 12 hours) in *C difficile* toxin-negative acute colitis with an open diagnosis for the cause of the diarrhea [1,14]. Improvement should normally be noted within 2 to 3 days. Metronidazole is potentially teratogenic and should not be used in pregnant mares. Both adjunct oral antibiotics are used in an extralabel form and have not been critically evaluated for efficacy in a controlled clinical trial.

In *Salmonella* cases, there are different opinions regarding the use of antibiotics in adult horses. Septicemic foals with salmonellosis are routinely treated with antimicrobial drugs, however. There are reasons for using antibiotics (may kill existing *Salmonella* bacteria, may prevent spread of *Salmonella* bacteria in the gastrointestinal tract to other organs, and may prevent spread of enteric bacteria through damaged intestinal mucosa to other organs), but there are also reasons for not using them (probably do not kill existing *Salmonella* bacteria, killing gram-negative bacteria may release additional LPS into the system, may prolong fecal shedding of *Salmonella* bacteria, may contribute to antibiotic resistance, and may further upset the colonic flora). The antimicrobials used in the treatment of salmonellosis include the combination of penicillin and gentamicin, the combination of ceftiofur and gentamicin, and fluoroquinolones (eg, enrofloxacin, orbifloxicin) [53].

Specific treatment for PHF includes oxytetracycline administered intravenously at a rate of 6.6 mg/kg every 24 hours for 3 to 5 days as the treatment of choice. A rapid recovery and dramatic decrease in fatality are observed when oxytetracycline therapy is commenced within 24 hours after the development of fever. A response to therapy (eg, decreased temperature, improved attitude, appetite, intestinal sounds) can be observed within 12 hours [39]. The combination of oral erythromycin estolate (25 mg/kg administered every 12 hours) and rifampin (10 mg/kg administered every 12 hour) is also effective when given early in the clinical course; however, the clinical response is not as rapid as when oxytetracycline is given intravenously. The risk of upsetting the colonic flora must be borne in mind, however [19,52].

During the acute phase, these animals demonstrate pronounced catabolism and lose condition quickly. Leukopenic and hypoproteinemic patients profit from hyperimmune serum and/or plasma transfusions as well as from broad-spectrum parenteral antibiotics to prevent seeding of infection peripherally. The energy requirement of a 500-kg horse at rest in a normal state is 33 kcal/kg/d; a horse with severe acute colitis needs approximately 50 kcal/kg/d. To counteract the severe catabolism with acute colitis, partial parenteral nutrition has also been reported. At this hospital, we use the following regimen: 50% dextrose (2 L) is combined with 8.5% amino acids (1.5 L) and LRS (1.5 L). This yields a hypertonic solution; therefore, the parenteral intravenous infusion has to evolve over time slowly and should be started at 140 mL/h and then gradually increased to 280 mL/h and then to 560 mL/h. In our clinical experience, this treatment approach has reduced the amount of plasma used, reduced mortality, shortened the hospitalization time, and reduced the total bill.

With regard to the prognosis of cases with acute colitis, there are limited numbers of studies in the literature. In a retrospective study at a veterinary teaching hospital, the case fatality rate was 42% [54], although in a more recent study, the case fatality rate was 25.4% [52]. Horses that were severely dehydrated were seven times more likely to die [53], and horses with a history of administration of an antimicrobial for a problem preceding diarrhea were 4.5 times more likely to fail to survive [55].

References

[1] Stämpfli HR, Prescott JF, Carman RJ. The etiology and treatment of idiopathic colitis—recent studies. Proc Am Assoc Equine Pract 1992;38:433–9.
[2] Cohen ND, Divers TJ. Acute colitis in horses. Part I. Assessment. Compend Contin Educ Pract Vet 1998;20:92–8.
[3] Schiller LR. Diarrhea. Med Clin North Am 2000;84:1259–74.
[4] Magdesian KG, Smith BP. Diarrhea. In: Smith BP, editor. Large animal internal medicine. 3rd edition. St. Louis (MO): Mosby; 2002. p. 102–8.
[5] Murray MJ. Digestive physiology of the large intestine in adult horses. Part II. Pathophysiology of colitis. Compend Contin Educ Pract Vet 1988;10:1309–16.
[6] Baverud V, Franklin A, Gunnarsson A, et al. Clostridium difficile associated with acute colitis in mares when their foals are treated with erythromycin and rifampicin for Rhodococcus equi pneumonia. Equine Vet J 1998;30:482–8.
[7] Donaldson MT, Palmer JE. Prevalence of Clostridium perfringens enterotoxin and Clostridium difficile toxin A in feces of horses with diarrhea and colic. J Am Vet Med Assoc 1999;215: 358–61.
[8] Fekety R, Shah AB. Diagnosis and treatment of Clostridium difficile colitis. JAMA 1993;269: 71–5.
[9] Weese JS, Staempfli HR, Prescott JF. A prospective study of the roles of Clostridium difficile and enterotoxigenic Clostridium perfringens in equine diarrhoea. Equine Vet J 2001;33(4): 403–9.
[10] Songer JG. Clostridial enteric disease of domestic animals. Clin Microbiol Rev 1996;9: 216–34.

[11] Arroyo LG, Weese JS, Staempfli HR. Experimental Clostridium difficile enterocolitis in foals. J Vet Intern Med 2004;18(5):734–8.

[12] Weese JS, Staempfli HR, Prescott JF. Survival of Clostridium difficile and its toxins in equine feces: implications for diagnostic test selection and interpretation. J Vet Diagn Invest 2000; 12(4):332–6.

[13] Weese JS, Staempfli HR, Prescott JF. Isolation of environmental Clostridium difficile from a veterinary teaching hospital. J Vet Diagn Invest 2000;12(5):449–52.

[14] McGorum BC, Dixon PM, Smith DGE. Use of metronidazole in equine acute idiopathic toxaemic colitis. Vet Rec 1998;142:635–8.

[15] Biosponge. Available at: http://platinumperformance.com/animal/equine/products/productcategories/product.cfm?category_id=458.

[16] Weese JS, Cote NM, deGannes RV. Evaluation of in vitro properties of di-tri-octahedral smectite on clostridial toxins and growth. Equine Vet J 2003;35(7):638–41.

[17] Wierup M. Equine intestinal clostridiosis. An acute disease in horses associated with high intestinal counts of Clostridium perfringens type A. Acta Vet Scand Suppl 1977;62:1–182.

[18] Herholz C, Miserz R, Nicolet J, et al. Prevalence of beta-2 toxigenic clostridium perfringens in horses with intestinal disorders. J Clin Microbiol 1999;37:358–61.

[19] Gustafsson A, Baverud V, Gunnarsson A, et al. The association of erythromycin ethylsuccinate with acute colitis in horses in Sweden. Equine Vet J 1997;29:314–8.

[20] Staempfli HR, Prescott JF, Brash ML. Lincomycin-induced severe colitis in ponies: association with Clostridium cadaveris. Can J Vet Res 1992;56:168–9.

[21] Weese JS, Kaese H, Baird JD, et al. Suspected ciprofloxacin-associated colitis in 4 horses. Equine Vet Educ 2002;4:232–7.

[22] White G, Prior SD. Comparative effects of oral administration of trimethoprim/sulphadiazine or oxytetracycline on fecal flora of horses. Vet Rec 1982;111:316–8.

[23] Hogenauer C, Hammer HF, Krejs GJ, et al. Mechanisms and management of antibiotic-associated diarrhea. Clin Infect Dis 1998;27:702–10.

[24] Smith BP. Salmonellosis infection in horses. Compend Contin Educ Pract Vet 1981; 3(Suppl):S4–13.

[25] Spier SJ. Salmonellosis. Vet Clin North Am Equine Pract 1993;9:385–97.

[26] Traub-Dargatz JL, Garber LP, Fedorka-Cray PJ, et al. Fecal shedding of Salmonella spp by horses in the United States during 1998 and 1999 and detection of Salmonella spp in grain and concentrate sources on equine operations. J Am Vet Med Assoc 2000;217:226–30.

[27] Weese JS, Baird JD, Poppe C, et al. Emergence of Salmonella typhimurium definitive type 104 (DT104) as an important cause of salmonellosis in horses in Ontario. Can Vet J 2001; 42(10):788–92.

[28] Koo FC, Peterson JW, Houston CW, et al. Pathogenesis of experimental salmonellosis: inhibition of protein synthesis by cytotoxin. Infect Immun 1984;43:93–100.

[29] Peterson JW, Molina NC, Houston CW, et al. Elevated cAMP in intestinal epithelial cells during experimental cholera and salmonellosis. Toxicon 1983;21:761–75.

[30] Ohl ME, Miller SI. Salmonella: a model for bacterial pathogenesis. Annu Rev Med 2001;52: 259–74.

[31] Clarke RC, Gyles CL. Salmonella. In: Gyles CL, Thoen CO, editors. Pathogenesis of bacterial infections in animals. 2nd edition. Ames (IA): Iowa State University Press; 1993. p. 133–53.

[32] van Duijkeren E, Flemming C, van Oldruitenborgh-Oosterbaan MS, et al. Diagnosis of salmonellosis in horses culturing multiple samples versus faecal samples. Vet Q 1995;17:63–6.

[33] Hyatt DR, Weese JS. Salmonella culture: sampling procedures and laboratory techniques. Vet Clin North Am Equine Pract 2004;20(3):577–85.

[34] Cohen ND, Martin JL, Simpson RB, et al. Comparison of polymerase chain reaction and microbiological culture for detection of salmonellae in equine feces and environmental. Am J Vet Res 1996;57:780–6.

[35] Dumler JS, Barbet AF, Bekker CPJ, et al. Reorganization of genera families *Rickettsiaceae* and *Anaplasmataceae* in the order *Rickettsiales*: unification of some species of *Ehrlichia* with *Anaplasma, Cowdria* with *Ehrlichia* and *Ehrlichia* with *Neorickettsia* description of six new species combination and designation of *Ehrlichia equi* and 'HE agent' as subjective synonyms of *Ehrlichia phagocytophila*. Int J Syst Evol Microbiol 2001;51:2145–65.

[36] Holland DH, Weiss E, Burgofer W, et al. *Ehrlichia risticii* sp nov.: etiological agent of equine monocytic ehrlichiosis (synonym. Potomac horse fever). Int J Syst Bacteriol 1985;35:524–6.

[37] Palmer JE. Potomac horse fever. Vet Clin North Am Equine Pract 1993;9:399–410.

[38] Wells MY, Rikisia Y. Lack of lysosomal fusion with phagosomes containing *Ehrlichia risticii* in P388D1cells: abrogation of inhibition with oxytetracycline. Infect Immun 1988;56: 3209–15.

[39] Baird. Potomac horse fever (PHF). In: Brown CM, Bertone JJ, editors. The 5-minute veterinary consult equine. Baltimore (MD): Lippincott Williams & Wilkins; 2002. p. 836–9.

[40] Mott J, Rikihisa Y, Palmer JE, et al. Comparison of PCR and culture to indirect fluorescent-antibody test for diagnosis of Potomac horse fever. J Clin Microbiol 1997;35:2215–9.

[41] Pusterla N, Leutenegger CM, Sigrist B, et al. Detection and quantitation of *Ehrlichia risticii* genomic DNA by real-time PCR in infected horses and snails. Vet Parasitol 2000;90:129–35.

[42] Karcher LF, Dill SG, Anderson WI, et al. Right dorsal colitis. J Vet Intern Med 1990;4: 347–53.

[43] Meschter Cl, Gilbert M, Krook L, et al. The effects of phenylbutazone on the intestinal mucosa of the horse: a morphological, ultrastructural and biochemical study. Equine Vet J 1990;22:255–63.

[44] Collins LG, Tyler DE. Phenylbutazone toxicosis in the horse: a clinical study. J Am Vet Med Assoc 1984;184:699–703.

[45] Sterns RH, Ocdol H, Schrier RW, et al. Hyponatremia pathophysiology, diagnosis and therapy. In: Narins RG, editor. Maxwell and Kleeman's clinical disorders of fluid and electrolyte metabolism. 5th edition. New York: McGraw-Hill; 1994. p. 583.

[46] Seahorn JL, Seahorn TL. Fluid therapy in horses with gastrointestinal disease. Vet Clin North Am Equine Pract 2003;19:665–79.

[47] Parsons D. Endotoxemia. In: The 5-minute veterinary consult equine. Baltimore (MD): Lippincott Williams & Wilkins; 2002. p. 380–1.

[48] Hosgood G. Pharmacologic features and physiologic effects of dopamine. J Am Vet Med Assoc 1990;197:1209–11.

[49] Moses VS, Bertone AL. Nonsteroidal anti-inflammatory drugs. Vet Clin North Am Equine Pract 2002;18:21–37.

[50] Spier SJ, Lavoie JP, Cullor JS, et al. Protection against clinical endotoxemia in horses by using plasma antibody to Rc mutant E. coli (J5). Circ Shock 1989;28:235–48.

[51] Morris DD, Whitlock RH, Corbeil LB. Endotoxemia in horses: protection provided by antiserum to core lipopolysaccharide. Am J Vet Res 1986;47:544–50.

[52] Papich MG. Antimicrobial therapy for gastrointestinal diseases. Vet Clin North Am Equine Pract 2003;19:645–63.

[53] Murray MJ. Salmonellosis. In: Brown CM, Bertone JJ, editors. The 5-minute veterinary consult equine. Baltimore (MD): Lippincott Williams & Wilkins; 2002. p. 940–1.

[54] Staempfli HR, Townsend JF, Prescott JF. Prognostic features and clinical presentation of acute idiopathic enterocolitis in horses. Can Vet J 1991;32:232–7.

[55] Cohen ND, Woods AM. Characteristics and risk factors for failure of horses with acute diarrhea to survive. J Am Vet Med Assoc 1999;214:382–90.

VETERINARY
CLINICS
Equine Practice

ELSEVIER
SAUNDERS

Vet Clin Equine 22 (2006) 85–94

Malabsorptive Maldigestive Disorder with Concurrent *Salmonella* in a 3-Year-Old Quarter Horse

Paul J. Plummer, DVM

Veterinary Microbiology and Preventative Medicine, Iowa State University,
Ames, IA 50011, USA

History

A 3-year-old Quarter Horse mare used for pleasure riding (340 kg) was treated 2 weeks before presentation for a small hind limb laceration by the local veterinarian. The mare was given a tetanus antitoxin booster, and hydrotherapy of the limb was initiated. No antibiotics or nonsteroidal anti-inflammatory drugs (NSAIDs) were prescribed or administered. The mare was pastured with one other gelding (no signs of illness) and fed 3 lb (1.4 kg) of 13% sweet feed twice daily. The mare was returned to the local veterinarian 1 day before referral for a history of anorexia of several days. Blood work demonstrated hypoproteinemia characterized by hypoalbuminemia. The horse was referred at this time for diagnostic evaluation. No fecal production had been observed for 2 days before referral. The horse had a current negative Coggin's test, had been wormed 2 weeks previously, and, with the exception of the tetanus toxoid booster, had not received any vaccinations during the previous year.

Physical examination

The mare was bright and alert but was underconditioned, with a body condition score of 3 on a scale of 9 (Appendix). While the horse was being unloaded, it passed a small volume of liquid feces and was admitted to the equine isolation unit. The mare's rectal temperature was 39.4°C (102.9°F), the heart rate was 60 beats per minute with a normal rhythm, and the respiratory rate was 40 breaths per minute. There was a plaque of pitting edema present on the pectoral region that extended caudally to the level

---

E-mail address: plummer@iastate.edu

doi:10.1016/j.cveq.2005.12.005
vetequine.theclinics.com

of the umbilicus. Thoracic auscultation aided by a rebreathing bag and thoracic percussion were unremarkable. Borborygmi were present in all quadrants of the abdomen. Oral mucous membranes were moist and pink and had a capillary refill time less then 2 seconds. Rectal palpation was within normal limits. There was a small healing laceration on the left hind metatarsus.

Initial diagnostics

Based on the history and physical examination, the following problems were identified: undercondition, anorexia, scant feces, diarrhea, pitting edema, hypoproteinemia, hypoalbuminemia, fever, and tachycardia. Initial diagnostics (Table 1) included a complete blood cell count, serum fibrinogen, serum chemistry, electrolytes, urinalysis, fecal flotation, fecal culture, fecal *Clostridium difficile* toxin assay, Potomac horse fever (PHF) titer, abdominal fluid analysis, and abdominal and thoracic ultrasound scans. Based on the ultrasound findings, small intestinal thickening was added to the problem list (thickness of 6–8 mm, normal is approximately 3–4 mm).

Case assessment

Based on the physical examination and initial diagnostics, the most prominent problems included the low body condition, hypoalbuminemia, pitting edema, diarrhea, and small intestinal wall thickening. Any animal with weight loss or low body condition should first be evaluated with respect to nutrition, parasites, and dentition. In this horse's case, the nutrition

Table 1
Laboratory results

	Results	Normal range
Complete blood cell count		
Total white blood cell count	6700	5400–14300
Neutrophils	4290	2700–8600
Lymphocytes	2080	1500–7700
Eosinophils	0	0–100
Monocyte	70	0–100
Total protein	4.0	5.7–7.8 g/dL
Packed cell volume	41.4	3%–53%
Chemistry profile		
BUN	18	9–20 mg/dL
Creatinine	1.1	0.9–1.8 mg/dL
Total protein	4.0	5.7–7.8 g/dL
Albumin	1.0	2.8–3.8 g/dL
Fibrinogen	300	<500 mg/dL

Abbreviation: BUN, blood urea nitrogen.

seemed to be adequate, a complete oral examination showed no abnormalities of the dentition, and the fecal floatation was negative for parasite ova. Poor body condition and weight loss can also be associated with changes in exercise level (none reported in this case) or systemic disease that affects absorption and digestion of nutrients.

Hypoproteinemia characterized by hypoalbuminemia was initially observed on the blood work before referral and was confirmed on the serum chemistry at the time of presentation. The pitting edema present on the pectoral region and abdomen suggested that the hypoalbuminemia was contributing to a low oncotic pressure with accumulation of interstitial fluid in a gravity-dependent fashion. Hypoproteinemia is primarily associated with three basic classes of abnormalities: (1) decreased production of albumin by the liver, (2) loss of albumin from the gastrointestinal (GI) system or the renal system or sequestration of albumin in a third space (pleuritis, ascites, or abscess), and (3) decreased absorption of nutrients from the diet. The lack of significant increases in gamma-glutamyltransferase (GGT), aspartate aminotransferase (AST), and bilirubin made liver disease unlikely, and a normal creatinine level and the absence of proteinuria ruled out significant losses of protein from the renal system. GI loss of albumin can be associated with gastric ulceration or right dorsal colitis and enterocolitis. Gastroscopy of the stomach and pylorus using a 3-m scope ruled out gastric ulcers. Abdominal ultrasound of the right dorsal colon was performed transabdominally. Although there was definite thickening of the mucosa, no evidence of local ulceration was present, and abdominocentesis did not show any abnormalities typically associated with right dorsal colitis. Additionally, the thickening was present diffusely throughout the small and large intestines, suggesting a more diffuse disease process than that typically seen with right dorsal colitis. Diffuse hypoechoic thickening of the GI mucosa can be observed with edema formation secondary to hypoproteinemia; however, in this case, there was definite hyperechogenicity, suggesting more of an infiltrative process than simple edema formation. The abdominal and thoracic ultrasound scans showed no evidence of abscessation or sequestration of significant volumes of fluid.

Procedures

To evaluate the diffuse intestinal thickening further, a D-xylose absorption curve (Table 2) and rectal biopsy were performed. Intestinal absorption of sugars can be measured over a time course and compared with published normal values in an attempt to document malabsorption or maldigestion by the intestine. It should be noted, however, that there is significant variation in published normal values and no standardized cutoff points have been determined. Glucose or D-xylose can be used for evaluation of proximal small intestinal absorptive capacity [1]. Glucose absorption curves have the advantages of ease of access to the test solution and the simplicity of

Table 2
Results of D-xylose absorption test

Time (min)	Xylose (mg/dL)
30	6
60	7
90	7
120	7
150	7
180	7
210	7
240	6

Interpretation: Because of the lack of the expected peak (ie, inverted V) at 1.5 to 2 hours and the flat line curve, the absorption curve is interpreted to be abnormal.

stall-side testing; however, the curve can be affected greatly by endogenous hormone release and mucosal metabolism. The use of D-xylose (not present in normal equine blood) to perform the absorption curve allows for more accurate assessments without the complications of endogenous processing of the sugar and effects of hormonal fluctuations. Variations in D-xylose levels can occur, however, as a result of differences in gastric emptying rate, renal clearance, and ileus. D-xylose was used at a dose of 0.5 g/kg administered as a 10% solution by nasogastric intubation after a 24-hour fast, and jugular blood samples were collected at different time points for D-xylose measurement. Although variations in normal curves do occur in different animals, the blood D-xylose level should not be a flat line as observed in this case, suggesting an abnormality of absorption or digestion. Normal curves would be expected to have an inverted "V" shape, with a maximum curve at 1.5 to 2 hours after administration. Abnormal D-xylose curves are most often associated with infiltrative disease of the jejunum.

Rectal biopsies can be performed with minimal risk if appropriate preparations are made [2]. They are limited purely because of the inability to sample further than one arm's length or so from the rectum. It should be remembered that the histopathologic findings at this level of the GI system may not be representative of the entire GI tract; however, they do at least provide some objective data. There are multiple means of collecting rectal biopsies, two of which are mentioned in this discussion. Endoscopic collection of biopsies has the advantage of visualization of the biopsy site; however, in the author's experience, the size and depth of the biopsy are often insufficient for achieving a diagnosis. Perhaps the preferred method for obtaining a diagnostic biopsy is the use of sterile uterine biopsy forceps guided by rectal palpation. The horse should be heavily sedated and restrained in stocks. The risk of rectal perforation should be discussed with the owner before the procedure, but this risk is minimized with appropriate restraint. Two percent lidocaine (60–120 mL) can be introduced into the rectum at the level of the biopsy using a 60-mL syringe and a 20-in intravenous extension set. Once the lidocaine is introduced, it should be given 10 minutes to take effect on the local mucosa. The biopsy may be easiest to obtain without the use of a rectal sleeve, because the dexterity and manipulation of the tissue are simplified. The forearm is thoroughly lubricated, and the rectal biopsy instrument is introduced into the distal rectum while being cupped in the hand to protect the end. Once a comfortable depth has been reached, the thumb and forefinger can be used to lift a piece of mucosa, with care being taken not to include the outer layers of the rectum. At no time should the biopsy be performed in a blind fashion or without placement under the guidance of a hand. One should also be especially careful to note the location of the biopsy so that if complications do occur, the site can be re-evaluated. Generally, two samples are collected, one for formalin fixation and histopathologic examination and the second for bacterial culture. After the procedure, the horse should be carefully monitored for complications associated with rectal perforation or bacterial translocation. In the case described here, histopathologic examination demonstrated significant infiltration of the lamina propria and submucosa with lymphocytes and lesser numbers of eosinophils. The bacterial culture also yielded a *Salmonella* species.

Discussion of differential diagnoses

A number of different causes can be associated with infiltration of the bowel wall and subsequent malabsorptive maldigestive disorders. As the names would imply, malabsorption refers to a decreased ability to absorb nutrients from the lumen into the enterocytes, whereas maldigestion refers to a decreased ability to digest the complex nutrients of the diet into fragments of appropriate size for subsequent absorption. Differentiating these two processes in the clinical patient is extremely difficult and often not done. One of the common causes of human maldigestive disorders is pancreatic insufficiency, a disease process not well described in the horse. As such, more equine cases likely arise from a malabsorptive situation interfering with the uptake of dietary carbohydrates, proteins, and fats by the enterocytes. Unless there is significant large intestinal involvement, electrolytes and water are absorbed normally. The clinical presentation of diarrhea in this case suggested large bowel involvement in addition to the small bowel thickening observed on ultrasound. Abnormal absorption of dietary carbohydrates by the small intestine increases the presentation of fermentable substrates to the microflora of the large bowel, which may induce bacterial population changes or overgrowth.

Classification of infiltrative bowel diseases with abnormal cellular infiltrates is most commonly made on the basis of the predominant cell type on histopathology [3]. In the case presented here, the predominant cell type was lymphocytes, with a lesser number of eosinophils and a few plasmocytes. Lymphocytic-plasmacytic enterocolitis is an uncommon disease process that is generally regarded as having a poor prognosis. In one study, 14 horses diagnosed with this condition were evaluated retrospectively for significant clinical features that would distinguish this process from other inflammatory diseases of the intestine [4]. The findings showed that the condition presented in adult horses of all ages (range: 3–26 years) with typical clinical signs of malabsorption and hypoproteinemia. Other organ systems were typically not involved, and 9 of 12 horses had an abnormal carbohydrate absorption curve. Rectal biopsies were performed on 7 of the horses, of which 3 showed abnormal histopathologic findings. Long-term treatment of all the cases was unsuccessful, and all the animals had the diagnosis confirmed at necropsy.

Other differentials that should be considered in diffuse infiltrative bowel disease include alimentary lymphosarcoma, proliferative enteropathy, multisystemic eosinophilic epitheliotropic disease (MEED), and granulomatous enteritis. Of these, the most common reported cause in foals is proliferative enteropathy associated with *Lawsonia intracellularis*, the cause of proliferative enteropathy in swine [5,6]. At this time, no epidemiologic link between affected foals and swine has been made. The foals are typically presented between 3 and 7 months of age for poor body condition, a rough coat, and a potbellied appearance. Abdominal ultrasound reveals diffuse thickening of the small intestinal wall, with a wall thickness between 6 and 10 mm. Antemortem diagnostics include a fecal polymerase chain reaction and *Lawsonia* serology. Many of these foals have a recent history of weaning, and the concurrent stress may be associated with the onset of disease. Treatment with erythromycin and rifampin for 2 to 4 weeks has been effective, and clinical improvement may be noted within 1 or 2 days after initiation of clinical therapy.

Granulomatous enteritis typically presents with similar clinical signs to all the previously mentioned disease processes and the absence of diarrhea. Most cases occur in young (generally less than 3 or 4 years of age) Standardbreds, although it has been reported to occur in other breeds, including Thoroughbreds. The overrepresentation of Standardbreds may suggest a genetic predisposition of the breed, although there is no formal evidence to confirm this at this time. Histopathologic examination of the small bowel reveals diffuse granulomatous inflammation with villus atrophy and abscesses, whereas the large colon is generally less affected. The exact etiologic cause of the syndrome is unknown; however, infectious (*Mycobacterium avium*), toxic, and immune-mediated hypersensitivity have all been suggested. The long-term prognosis is guarded, although some horses may respond to corticosteroids in the short term and one horse has been reported to have undergone clinical remission after a long-term course of treatment. In some cases, surgical resection of the affected bowel may be an option if the infiltration is confined to a specific portion of the jejunum.

MEED often has a slightly different presentation than the previously discussed syndromes [1]. These horses are more likely to have clinical diarrhea on presentation and frequently have severe exudative skin lesions of the coronary band. In many cases, the owner's initial complaint is the skin lesions as opposed to the weight loss or diarrhea. Age of onset is typically 2 to 4 years old, and there is an overrepresentation of Standardbreds and Thoroughbreds. Gross inspection of the large bowel reveals severe multifocal granulomatous lesions and bowel wall thickening. The gross lesions of the small intestine tend to be less obvious and tend to predominate in the proximal duodenum and distal ileum. Histopathologic examination of the lesions demonstrates a severe infiltration with eosinophils and lesser numbers of lymphocytes and extensive fibrosis. Notably, there is often eosinophil infiltration of other organs of the body, including the pancreas, liver, and mesenteric lymph nodes. Biopsies of the skin lesions reveal hyperkeratosis, acanthosis, and severe infiltration of eosinophils. The cause of the syndrome seems most likely to be chronic hypersensitivity to some unidentified antigen present in the lumen of the GI system. The prognosis is poor; however, when this syndrome is suspected, aggressive therapy with corticosteroids, antibiotics, and anthelmintics has been attempted with limited success. In part, involvement of other body systems, such as the liver and pancreas, may contribute to long-term treatment failure. It is noteworthy that although tissue infiltration with eosinophils is significant in these cases, most do not have systemic eosinophilia present on a complete blood cell count.

Alimentary lymphosarcoma is most commonly diagnosed in young horses 2 to 4 years of age of all breeds [7]. The onset may be rapid and progressive, and these animals can become quite ill acutely. The disease process is most commonly confined to the small intestine and associated mesenteric lymph nodes, which may be palpated on rectal examination. Although a rectal biopsy may be helpful in diagnosis, a surgical biopsy of the small intestine and lymph nodes should be considered if this disease is deemed likely. Systemically, the horses often demonstrate anemia and thrombocytopenia; however, systemic lymphocytosis is uncommon. Treatment includes chemotherapy and immunosuppression but is almost invariably unsuccessful. Short-term maintenance of these animals may be possible if it is justified by the benefit of such an endeavor.

The lack of skin lesions, systemic disease, and significant eosinophilia in the histopathologic findings of the case described here helped to rule out MEED as the primary cause. The predominance of lymphocytes on the biopsy and the diagnostic impression of the pathologist suggested that lymphocytic-plasmacytic enteritis was the best working diagnosis in this situation. Alimentary lymphosarcoma was deemed less likely, given the lack of pleomorphism in the observed lymphocytes and the more insidious onset of symptoms. Granulomatous enteritis could still be a consideration in this case and cannot be ruled out without a surgically obtained biopsy of the more anterior GI tract; however, if the rectal biopsy is representative of the entire tract, the predominance of lymphocytes would not be consistent with such a situation. A surgical biopsy was not obtained because of financial constraints and the lack of significant effect on treatment options.

The concurrent isolation of *Salmonella* from this patient is also worthy of discussion. Initially, bacterial cultures were submitted based on the clinical presence of significant diarrhea. Differentials that should be considered in acute diarrhea include infectious (eg, *Salmonella*, *Clostridium*, *Ehrlichia*, *Lawsonia*), parasitic, and toxic (eg, cantharidin, NSAID toxicity, heavy metal) causes. After the horse was admitted to the isolation facility, cultures for *Salmonella* were started as well as a *Clostridium difficile* toxin A assay and *Ehrlichia* serology. *Salmonella* shedding is transient in patients, and fecal culture should be performed daily for 5 days before ruling out salmonellosis. The diagnostic sensitivity can be improved with inclusion of a rectal biopsy bacterial culture or fecal polymerase chain reaction assay for *Salmonella*. In the case presented here, the clostridial toxin assay and *Ehrlichia* serology were negative and fecal flotation showed no signs of parasitism; however, the horse was found to be shedding *Salmonella*. Although the microbial pathogenesis of salmonellosis is not completely understood, a compromised host immune system and preexisting GI disease are considered predisposing factors in the development of clinical disease. Likely, the underlying malabsorptive maldigestive disease present in this case induced a change in the presentation of nutrients to the large colon and allowed for changes in colonic bacterial flora that may have predisposed the horse to salmonellosis. The diagnosis of *Salmonella* in an equine patient should be considered significant, and care should be taken to isolate that animal properly from other horses. The potentially zoonotic nature of the organism should also be discussed with the owner and all individuals in contact with the patient.

Treatment and outcome

Initial therapy of this case included fluid therapy and general supportive care until further diagnostics revealed the presence of infiltrative bowel disease and salmonellosis. The hypoproteinemia and hypoalbuminemia were addressed by administration of equine plasma at a dose of 10 mL/kg given slowly intravenously on day 1 and repeated on day 3. After the first dose of plasma, the horse was started on a constant-rate infusion of a commercially available balanced ionic solution at 60 mL/kg/d in anticipation of continued fluid loss via diarrhea. Care was taken to monitor the plasma total protein and packed cell volume (PCV) closely every 4 hours during the fluid therapy to make sure the hypoproteinemia was not exacerbated by the fluid therapy. A dose of flunixin meglumine was administered to control the fever and provide anti-inflammatory therapy during diagnostics. By day 2, the horse was nonfebrile, had normal feces, and the hypoproteinemia had not progressed. The fluid rate was decreased by half (30 mL/kg/d) for several hours and then discontinued. Fresh water and electrolytes were provided free choice at all times. After fasting for the D-xylose absorption curve on day 2, the horse was provided free-choice grass hay and limited sweet feed (1.5 lb [0.7 kg] every 12 hours) until the diagnostics were completed and the horse was discharged. The ventral edema accumulation was treated twice daily with hydrotherapy. Given the suspected presence of lymphocytic-plasmacytic enteritis, therapy with corticosteroids was initiated. The potential to exacerbate the salmonellosis by immunosuppression was weighed with the benefits of treatment of the infiltrative disease and discussed with the owner. Given the improvement in diarrhea and guarded prognosis, the owner elected to start therapy. In this case, prednisone was chosen for therapy, starting at a dose of 1 mg/kg administered orally every 24 hours and tapering over a 60-day period. Research on the absorption of oral prednisone published after this case was treated now suggests that the drug has a limited bioavailability after oral administration and suggests that prednisolone or dexamethasone may have been a better choice for oral administration [8]. The horse was discharged with instructions to keep it isolated from other horses until it was fecal- negative for *Salmonella*. The horse improved clinically, with resolution of the ventral edema, weight gain, and increased activity on pasture. At 40 days after discharge, the serum albumin level had doubled and was just slightly below normal. The steroids were continued for an additional month, after which they were discontinued. Eight months after discharge, the owners reported that the horse seemed to be normal and maintaining appropriate weight; however, contact with the owners was lost at this time, and no additional follow-up information was received.

Appendix

Equine body condition scores

1—Extreme emaciation; spinous processes, ribs, tuber coxae, and tuber ischia are extremely prominent. Bones of withers and neck are easily observed.

2—Emaciated, with slight fat covering the base of spinous processes. Spinous processes, ribs, tail head, and tuber ischia are prominent. Bones of neck and shoulder are fairly visible.

3—Thin, with fat build-up halfway up the spinous processes. Transverse processes of spine cannot be felt. Spine is prominent, but individual processes cannot be distinguished. Tuber coxae appear rounded, but the tuber ischia cannot be visualized.

4—Slight ridge along the back with ribs slightly visible. Tuber coxae are not discernible, and the neck does not appear thin.

5—Flat in the back, with ribs not visible from a distance. Tail head area starts to feel spongy. Shoulder and neck blend smoothly into the body.

6—May have a slight crease down the back line, and area over ribs feels spongy. Fat starts to be laid down around neck and withers.

7—May have a slight crease down the back. Ribs can be felt, but fat is laid down between ribs.

8—Crease down the back, ribs cannot be felt, and area around tail head is extremely soft. Neck appears thick, and fat is noticeable on inner thighs.

9—Obvious crease down the back and patchy appearance over ribs. Fat on inner thighs may rub together. Flank is filled with fat.

Adapted from Henneke DR, Potter GD, Kreider JL, et al. A scoring system for comparing body condition in horses. Equine Vet J 1983;15:371–2.

References

[1] Reed S, Bayly W, Sellon D. Equine internal medicine. 2nd edition. St. Louis: WB Saunders; 2004.

[2] Lindberg R, Nygren A, Persson SGB. Rectal biopsy diagnosis in horses with clinical signs of intestinal disorders: a retrospective study of 116 cases. Equine Vet J 1996;28:275–84.

[3] Scott EA, Heidel JR, Snyder SP, et al. Inflammatory bowel disease in horses: 11 cases (1988–1998). J Am Vet Med Assoc 1999;214:1527–30.

[4] Kemper DL, Perkins GA, Schumacher J, et al. Equine lymphocytic-plasmacytic enterocolitis: a retrospective study of 14 cases. Equine Vet J Suppl 2000;32:108–12.

[5] Lavoie JP, Drolet R, Parsons D, et al. Equine proliferative enteropathy: a cause of weight loss, colic, diarrhea and hypoproteinemia in foals on three breeding farms in Canada. Equine Vet J 2000;32:418–25.

[6] Williams NM, Harrison LR, Gebhart CJ. Proliferative enteropathy in a foal caused by Lawsonia intracellularis-like bacterium. J Vet Diagn Invest 1996;8:254–6.

[7] Van den Hoven R, Franken P. Clinical aspects of lymphosarcoma in the horse; a clinical report of 16 cases. Equine Vet J 1983;15:49–53.

[8] Peroni DL, Kollias-Baker C, Robinson NE. Prednisone per os is likely to have limited efficacy in horses. Equine Vet J 2002;34(3):283–7.

ELSEVIER
SAUNDERS

VETERINARY
CLINICS
Equine Practice

Vet Clin Equine 22 (2006) 95–106

Severe Metabolic Acidemia, Hypoglycemia, and Sepsis in a 3-week-old Quarter Horse Foal

Jonathan M. Naylor, BVSc, PhD*

*Department of Large Animal Clinical Sciences, Western College of Veterinary Medicine,
52 Campus Drive, University of Saskatchewan, Saskatoon,
Saskatchewan, SK 57N 5B4, Canada*

Signalment and presenting complaint

A 23-day-old female Quarter Horse foal was admitted (time = 0 hours) with a complaint of cloudy eye.

This was the mare's first foal. She was born without assistance but needed help to stand. At birth the foal was accepted by the mare and sucked from the udder. The navel was sprayed with iodine. No other assistance was given. Mare and foal were the kept at pasture. The day before admission the field was sprayed with an insecticide. Following the spraying, the foal was noted to have eyes that were dilated and runny. The foal spent an increased amount of time in recumbency. The foal was lethargic, ataxic, and sucked the mare with decreased frequency.

Initial examination

The standard work-up included a physical examination, blood gas analysis, hemogram, and chemistry panel (Tables 1–4).

Physical examination

The rectal temperature was 38.1°C (100.6°F), the heart rate was 84 beats/minute, the respiratory rate was 36 breaths/minute, and the weight was 60 kg.

---

* Current address: Ross University School of Veterinary Medicine, PO Box 334, Basseterre, St. Kitts, West Indies.
E-mail address: jnaylor@rossvet.edu.kn

0749-0739/06/$ - see front matter © 2006 Elsevier Inc. All rights reserved.
doi:10.1016/j.cveq.2005.12.016

Table 1
Venous blood gas values and heparinized plasma electrolyte and metabolite concentrations

Time (hours from admission)	pH	PCO₂ (mm Hg)	PO₂ (mm Hg)	Bicarbonate mmoles/L (1mmol = 1 mEq)	Base Excess (mmoles/L)	Sodium (mEq/L)	Potassium (mEq/L)	Chloride (mEq/L)	Ionized Calcium (mmoles/L) (mEq/L)[a]	Lactate (mmoles/L)[b]	Temperature (C)
0.63	6.944	30.9	53.7	6.5	−24.6	131.2	4.68	101	1.58	18.72	37.5
1.57	7.268	32.6	34.3	14.7	−11.3	132.6	4.11	96	1.24	19.59	36.1
5.50	7.091	35.1	37	10.1	−18	145.1	3.55	106	1.50	20.83	39.5
10.93	7.187	30.9	34.3	11.3	−15.3	144.2	4	109	1.59	19.67	38.2
12.75	7.447	40.5	35.6	27.3	3.1	140	3.28	96	1.23	18.79	37.3
20.37	7.292	39.3	37.5	18.2	−7.2	144.5	3.37	106	1.48	17.47	39.8
28.37	7.401	38.7	44.7	23.1	−0.8	144.3	2.74	113	1.41	8.72	38.8
33.17	7.398	42	46.3	24.9	0.5	146.4	2.73	114	1.4	5.2	38.7
37.08	7.374	39.9	53.7	22.4	−2.1	145.8	2.68	116	1.42	5.33	38.5
45.50	7.343	39.7	40.3	20.6	−4	144.9	2.61	114	1.47	5.16	39.1
69.75	7.247	48	23.4	19.8	−6.6	141.7	3.11	110	1.49	8.06	39.4

[a] To convert ionized calcium to mg/dL, divide value in mg/dL by 0.25. To calculate ionized calcium as mEq/L, divide mmol/L value in mmol/L by 0.25. To calculate ionized calcium as mEq/L, divide mmol/L value by 0.5.
[b] To convert lactate in mmoles/L to mg/dL, divide value by 0.111.

Table 2
Glucose administration rates during hospitalization*

Time from admission (hours)	Glucose administration rate (mg/kg/min)
0.63	0.00
1.57	6.94
2.25	0.06
5.50	0.06
6.25	1.54
10.93	1.54
12.75	41.67
20.37	0.00
28.37	0.00
33.17	0.00
37.08	0.00
45.50	0.00
69.75	0.00

* At a given time the rate of administration is calculated from the preceding time to the indicated time period. For example, between 0.63 and 1.57 hours from admission the mean glucose administration rate was 6.9 mg/kg/minute. Time periods correspond to points at which plasma glucose was measured in Fig. 1.

The foal was depressed, weak, and recumbent. The mucous membranes were light purple with a 5-second capillary refill time. There was bilateral corneal opacity with cloudy white material in the anterior chambers of both eyes. The right pupil was miotic. The lung sounds were increased in volume with an expiratory grunt that was sometimes louder following abdominal palpation. The foal had periods of bruxism.

The initial list of problems was rapid-onset weakness, depression, ataxia, corneal and anterior chamber opacities consistent with corneal edema and fibrin in the anterior chamber, a constricted right pupil, bruxism, and expiratory grunt.

The eye problems were diagnosed as uveitis, and an ophthalmology consult was requested. Shock was diagnosed on the basis of a prolonged capillary refill time, depression, weakness, and recumbency. A heart rate of 84 beats/minute is inappropriately slow for the foal's physical condition. Possible causes for bradycardia include hypothermia, which was not present, hyperkalemia, and hypoglycemia. The latter two possibilities were assessed using a blood gas analysis, which is the most rapidly completed laboratory test in the author's hospital. Based on the presence of shock and uveitis, septicemia was suspected. Leptospiral infection can cause uveitis in adult horses. Bruxism and an expiratory grunt aggravated by abdominal pressure indicate pain, likely of abdominal origin. Possible causes include gastric ulceration, enteritis, peritonitis, and acute hepatitis. Pleural pain was also possible but less likely.

The immediate concerns were to treat the presumed septic shock and to complete the standard work-up for a seriously sick foal.

Table 3
Hemogram findings*

Hours	White Blood Cell Count	Segmented Neutrophils	Band Neutrophils	Toxic Change	Lymphocytes	Monocytes	PVC (L/L)	Hemoglobin (g/L)	Fibrinogen (g/L)
0	8	2.56	**1.76[a]**	**3 +**	3.28	0.4	0.398	133	**6**
24	11.2	5.152	**1.68**	**2 +**	4.256	0.112	0.335	118	
70	17.4	9.918	**1.74**	**1 +**	5.394	0.348	0.303	105	3

* All cell counts are reported in units of 10^9/L, equivalent to thousands/mm^3.
[a] Abnormal values are in bold.

Table 4
Serum chemistry findings

Item	Units	Normal Range	Presentation	22.5 Hours	46 Hours
Urea	mmol/L	4.1–14.7	4.6	8.5	7.2
Creatinine	umol/L	52–126	123	**160**[a]	90
Total Bilirubin	umol/L	2–41	25	74	105
Gamma-glutamyltransferase	U/L	8–33	**71**	**71**	**67**
Sorbitol dehydrogenase	U/L	2–7	**249**	**38**	**17**
CK	U/L	88–439	369	555	171
AST	U/L	6–347	**2358**	**2382**	**1425**
Total Protein	g/L	60–74	58	48	42
Albumin	g/L	31–48	27	23	20
Globulin	g/L		31	25	22

[a] Abnormal values are in bold.

Initial therapy

A catheter was placed in a jugular vein using an aseptic procedure. Blood was collected anaerobically and aseptically and placed into the appropriate tubes for hemogram, chemistry, blood gas analysis, and blood culture.

Immediately following catheterization, sodium ampicillin (20 mg/kg every 8 hours) and gentamicin (6.6 mg/kg every 24 hours) were administered intravenously for suspected septicemia and septic uveitis. When the hemogram was completed 1 hour later, the sepsis score was 17, indicating a high likelihood of septicemia (Fig. 1). Gentamicin was chosen over amikacin because amikacin is less effective against gram-positive organisms. In the author's hospital, previous surveys have shown that gentamicin resistance is rare, even in gram-negative bacteria.

Lactated Ringers' solution, at an initial rate of 90 mL/kg/hour, was started as fluid therapy for shock. Within 30 minutes, 2.75 L of lactated Ringers solution had been administered, and its administration was stopped. The rate of fluid administration was reduced to less than 20 mL/kg/hour, and the type of fluid administered was re-evaluated in the light of the blood gas results, which showed severe metabolic acidosis, severe hypoglycemia, and severe L-lactic acidosis (see Table 1).

Intravenous 5% dextrose was infused either through a secondary line or as part of the saline-bicarbonate mixture. In this foal, the mean glucose infusion rate over the first 13 hours of therapy was 5.9 mg/kg/minute (see Table 2). Infusion rates were extremely variable, however, and in consequence plasma glucose varied between 0.7 and 33.5 mmol/L (13–600 mg/dL) (Fig. 2).

This foal had a severe metabolic acidosis and L-lactic acidosis (see Table 1). The bicarbonate deficit was calculated using the formula derived for calves [1–3]:

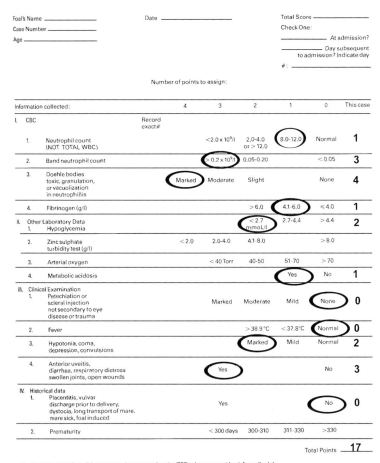

Fig. 1. Sepsis score for foal. (*Modified from* Brewer BD, Koterba AM. Development of a scoring system for the early diagnosis of equine neonatal sepsis. Equine Vet J 1988;20:19; with permission.)

Bicarbonate requirement in mmoles (1 mmol = 1 mEq)
= body weight in Kg × base deficit in mmoles/L × 0.5
= 60 × 24.6 × .5
= 738 mmol

After 1.57 hours of therapy, 300 mmoles of sodium bicarbonate (2 L of isotonic 1.3% sodium bicarbonate) had been administered, and blood pH was improved (Fig. 3). After infusion of a further 300 mmoles (2 L) of isotonic sodium bicarbonate by 10.93 hours, however, the foal was still severely acidotic (see Table 1), despite the restoration of urination. A urine sample

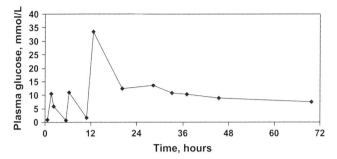

Fig. 2. Plasma glucose during therapy.

collected at 5 hours had a specific gravity of 1.012 and a pH of 5. An additional 600 mmoles (4 L) of isotonic sodium bicarbonate corrected acidemia at 12.57 hours, but another 300 mmoles were required between 20 and 28 hours of hospitalization to correct a minor recurrence (see Fig. 3).

The severity of acidemia in this foal was extreme. Calves generally die as venous pH falls below 7.00, and the foal's venous pH was below this critical point at presentation. The severity of L-lactic acidosis was also extreme. Muscular exertion from exercise and poor tissue perfusion from shock are the most common causes of L-lactic acidosis in large animals. In humans, in-shock L-lactate concentrations greater than 10 mmoles/L are associated with a very poor prognosis. The total amount of bicarbonate required to correct acidemia was 1200 mmoles, which is greater than predicted, perhaps because of individual variation in the degree of intracellular acidosis and bicarbonate space. The large bicarbonate requirement may also have reflected ongoing production of acids within the foal.

During hospitalization, therapy was further refined. The systemic antibiotic regimen was left unaltered, except for a switch to the intramuscular route following development of mild thrombophlebitis and removal of the

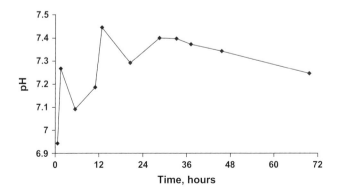

Fig. 3. Venous blood pH versus time from admission.

intravenous catheter at 48 hours. A half-dose of flunixin meglumine was given once a day for 3 days for its anti-inflammatory properties. An ophthalmologist examined the foal's eyes and agreed with the diagnosis of uveitis. Atropine drops were placed in the eyes every 6 hours until the pupils dilated, a topical nonsteroidal anti-inflammatory, fluribprofen, was administered every 6 hours, and a topical antibiotic combination of bacitracin, neomycin sulfate, and polymixin was administered every 8 hours.

Sequential hemograms showed steady improvement during hospitalization. The number of mature neutrophils increased, and the degree of inflammation as judged by degree of toxic change and fibrinogen concentration improved. The hematocrit and packed cell volume fell, indicating improvement in hydration with fluid therapy and resumption of nursing (see Table 3).

Serum chemistry initially showed evidence of hepatocellular damage with marked elevations of the liver-specific serum enzyme concentrations of sorbitol dehydrogenase (SDH) and gamma-glutamyltransferase and elevations of serum aspartate aminotransferase, which can be released by a variety of damaged tissues including liver (see Table 4). Liver damage may have been secondary to shock. Other possible causes of liver damage are Tyzzer's disease from *Bacillus piliformis* infection [4], leptospirosis, and idiopathic liver disease. Serum concentrations of SDH, which has a short half-life, declined steadily with therapy (see Table 4). Liver disease/damage may have contributed to abdominal pain in this foal.

The foal made a continuous and steady improvement in condition from the initiation of therapy. By 4 hours she had regained the ability to suck; by 12 hours she could stand without assistance and nurse. Bruxism was not observed after the first hour. The foal was comfortable between hours 1 and 30. Between hours 30 and 32, the foal had an episode of discomfort with signs of shifting weight on her hind legs and tail swishing. Around hour 57 there was transient diarrhea. Two separate blood cultures collected at admission yielded an alpha streptococcus species sensitive to ceftiofur, gentamicin, and ampicillin and resistant to amikacin. The tip of the intravenous catheter was cultured following its removal, and no bacteria were cultured.

The foal was discharged 72 hours following admission. At this time she could nurse and had normal feces but was judged to be slightly depressed. Following discharge she was given ceftiofur, 2.2 mg/kg intramuscularly every 12 hours for 4 days, and the nonsteroidal anti-inflammatory eye drops were continued every 8 hours for the next 4 days. The foal continued to improve, did not require further veterinary attention, and is currently a healthy 2-year-old being prepared for use as a riding horse.

Discussion

This case illustrates the complexity of managing acidemia and hypoglycemia in a neonatal foal.

The recommended rate for administering dextrose to correct hypoglycemia in foals varies, depending on the attending veterinarian, and none have been critically evaluated. Some recommend a separate infusion of 5% or 10% dextrose at a rate of 4 to 8 mg/kg/minute (0.8–0.16 mL/kg/minute of 5% dextrose). In this foal dextrose administration at a rate 6.94 mg/kg/minute between hours 0.4 and 2 successfully corrected the initial severe hypoglycemia (see Fig 2). To maintain these infusion rates, it would have been better to administer glucose continuously through a separate line, preferably with the rate of infusion controlled with a fluid pump. Other authors recommend adding dextrose to the replacement intravenous fluids to a final concentration of 5% [5]. If this solution is administered at a rate of 80 to 100 mL/kg/day, as recommended, then the glucose infusion rate could approach 3.5 mg/kg/minute. More rapid administration occurs with greater fluid rates. In this foal, adding dextrose to the saline-sodium bicarbonate mixture to a final concentration of 5% resulted in dextrose being administered at approximately 42 mg/kg/minute between hours 11 and 13, and the foal became severely hyperglycemic (see Fig. 2).

With the restoration of euglycemia at 2 hours, glucose administration, was decreased to below 4 mg/kg/minute, and hypoglycemia recurred by about 6 hours. A second sample about 0.5 hours later had a blood glucose concentration of 10.9 mmol/L (196 mg/dL), however. At the time this rapid fluctuation was attributed to changes in the rate of fluid administration depending on the position of the foal's neck. In retrospect this 10.9 mmol/L (196 mg/dL) value seems suspect. It is one of two measured with a patient side glucometer. The values on either side were 0.7 and 1.7 mmol/L (13–31 mg/dL), respectively, and were measured as part of the automated blood gas analysis. The 10.9 mmol/L value could have been high because of contamination (eg, if the sample was collected from the same vein through which glucose was infused) or because of technical error.

This case illustrates the importance of maintaining glucose infusion even though euglycemia had been attained, and the foal had started to drink. The foal sucked from the mare, with assistance, for the first time at 4 hours from admission. By 7.5 hours she could get up and nurse with encouragement, and by 10.5 hours she was standing and sucking without assistance. The foal was still hypoglycemic at hours 6 and 12, however (see Fig. 2).

The degree of lactic acidosis experienced by this foal was extreme. Several causes were considered, including the possibility of poisoning from aerial spraying. No documented case of L-lactic acidemia induced by poisoning in farm animals could be found, however. Respiratory chain poisons, such as cyanide derivatives, induce liver damage [6] and L-lactic acidosis [7], but these poisons prevent the use of oxygen and should be accompanied by bright red mucous membranes, not the cyanosis seen in this foal. Given the presence of a severely inflammatory hemogram, positive sepsis score, and cyanosis, a combination of poor tissue perfusion and sepsis were the likely causes of L-lactic acidosis [8–12]. Inflammatory factors released during endotoxemia promote glucose use [13] and increase L-lactic acid production [8,9]. L-lactic acid removal by the liver can also be deranged in shock [14], and liver disease predisposes to lactic acidosis [7–9,11,15]. This foal had evidence of hepatocellular damage. Survival of foals with this degree of L-lactic acidosis may be unusual. In humans and colicky horses, L-lactate concentrations above 4 mmol/L are associated with reduced survival, and prognosis becomes very poor when lactate concentrations are in the teens [8,9,16–19]. The amount of sodium bicarbonate needed to correct L-lactic acid in this foal was more than twice that calculated using the standard calf formula. This increased need may be partly related to the degree of intracellular acidosis, which is difficult to measure. Another important reason is likely to be continuing L-lactic acid production. In some cases, sodium bicarbonate administration can increase peripheral production of lactic acid because the increase in pH removes an inhibitory influence on phosphofructokinase activity, a key enzyme controlling the breakdown of glucose to pyruvate and hence to lactate [20].

Severe hypoglycemia in this foal likely contributed to mental depression and bradycardia [21]. Severe hypoglycemia (< 1 mmol/L; < 18 mg/L) can be seen in the terminal stages of starvation when body reserves are exhausted. Although this foal was unable to suck at presentation, the reported period of illness was short, and the foal was in normal body condition. Absence of intake of food would deplete glycogen stores and produce a mild hypoglycemia. The major reasons for hypoglycemia may be increased glucose use secondary to shock [14], partly because of the release of mediators that promote glucose use and partly because anaerobic metabolism is less efficient, and more glucose must be used to produce ATP.

The initiating causes of this foal's problems were never completely explained. Although it had a positive sepsis score, bilateral uveitis, and two positive blood cultures, the cultured streptococcus did not belong to a species commonly recognized as being a primary pathogen. This case may represent an unusual case of primary septicemia, or septicemia may have been secondary to some other problem. In dogs, shock and poor intestinal perfusion can lead to mucosal sloughing, facilitating the entry of microorganisms [22]. Shock may also facilitate entry of endotoxins and possibly bacteria in horses [23].

The only organs that were severely affected were the eyes and liver. In humans, liver disease can be secondary to shock [24]. The laboratory findings of severe inflammation, hypoglycemia, and elevated serum concentrations of liver-specific enzymes are similar to those reported in two foals that later died of Tyzzer's disease [25]. It is difficult to diagnose this condition if the foal survives, however. Uveitis in adult horses can be caused by leptospiral infection [26–29]. Leptospiral infection was not implicated as a cause of liver failure in one study in adult horses [30], but in the equine fetus leptospiral infection can cause abortion and hepatitis [31,32]. Experimental infection of adult horses with *Leptospira interogans* produced fever, anorexia, icterus, petechiation, and recurrent uveitis [28].

In conclusion, this foal survived severe hypoglycemia and L-lactic acidosis following aggressive antibiotic and fluid therapy. The case illustrates the difficulty of correcting severe acidemia and hypoglycemia in foals and emphasizes the need for monitoring blood glucose and pH until these items are stable and within their normal ranges.

References

[1] Kasari TR, Naylor JM. Clinical evaluation of sodium bicarbonate, sodium l–lactate and sodium acetate for the treatment of acidosis in diarrheic calves. J Am Vet Med Assoc 1986;187: 392–7.

[2] Naylor JM, Forysth GW. The alkalizing effects of metabolizable bases in the healthy calf. Can J Vet Res 1986;50:509–16.

[3] Vaala W. Neonatology; foal cardiopulmonary resuscitation. In: Orsini JA, Divers TJ, editors. Manual of equine emergencies: treatment and procedures. Philadelphia: W.B. Saunders; 1998. p. 473–503.

[4] Whitwell KE. Four cases of Tyzzer's disease in foals in England. Equine Vet J 1976;8:118–22.

[5] Brown CM, Bertone JJ. The 5-minute veterinary consult. Equine. Baltimore (MD): Lippincott Williams & Wilkins; 2002.

[6] Shaw IC, Harwood DG, Malone FE. Foxoil—a toxic experience in lambs. Vet Rec 1992; 131:268.

[7] Luft FC. Lactic acidosis update for critical care clinicians. J Am Soc Nephrol 2001; 12(Suppl 17):S15–9.

[8] Astiz M, Rackow EC, Weil MH, et al. Early impairment of oxidative metabolism and energy production in severe sepsis. Circ Shock 1988;26:311–20.

[9] De Backer D. Lactic acidosis. Intensive Care Med 2003;29:699–702.

[10] Lang CH, Bagby GJ, Blakesley HL, et al. Fever is not responsible for the elevated glucose kinetics in sepsis. Proc Soc Exp Biol Med 1987;185:455–61.

[11] Stacpoole PW, Wright EC, Baumgartner TG, et al. Natural history and course of acquired lactic acidosis in adults. DCA-Lactic Acidosis Study Group. Am J Med 1994;97:47–54.

[12] Vary TC, Murphy JM. Role of extra-splanchnic organs in the metabolic response to sepsis. Effect of insulin. Circ Shock 1989;28:41–57.

[13] Lang CH, Bagby GJ, Blakesley HL, et al. Glucose kinetics and pyruvate dehydrogenase actvity in septic rats treated with dichloroacetate. Circ Shock 1987;23:131–41.

[14] Naylor JM, Kronfeld DS. In vivo studies of hypoglycemia and lactic acidosis in endotoxic shock. Am J Physiol 1985;248:E309–16.

[15] Casaburi R, Oi S. Effect of liver disease on the kinetics of lactate removal after heavy exercise. Eur J Appl Physiol Occup Physiol 1989;59:89–97.

[16] Aslar AK, Kuzu MA, Elhan AH, et al. Admission lactate level and the APACHE II score are the most useful predictors of prognosis following torso trauma. Injury 2004;35:746–52.

[17] Husain FA, Martin MJ, Mullenix PS, et al. Serum lactate and base deficit as predictors of mortality and morbidity. Am J Surg 2003;185:485–91.

[18] Moore JN, Owen R, Lumsden JH. Clinical evaluation of blood lactate levels in equine colic. Equine Vet J 1976;8:49–54.

[19] Parry BW, Anderson GA, Gay CC. Prognosis in equine colic: a comparative study of variables used to assess individual cases. Equine Vet J 1983;15:211–5.

[20] Kreisberg RA. Lactate homeostasis and lactic acidosis. Ann Intern Med 1980;92:227–37.

[21] Pollock G, Brady WJ Jr, Hargarten S, et al. Hypoglycemia manifested by sinus bradycardia: a report of three cases. Acad Emerg Med 1996;3:700–7.

[22] Hardie EM, Kruse-Elliot K. Endotoxic shock. Part I: a review of causes. J Vet Intern Med 1990;4:258–66.

[23] Morris DD. Endotoxemia in horses: a review of cellular and humoral mediators involved in its pathogenesis. J Vet Intern Med 1991;5:167–81.

[24] Nordstrom G, Saljo A, Hasselgren P. Studies on the possible role of oxygen-derived free radicals for impairment of protein and energy metabolism in liver ischemia. Circ Shock 1988;26: 115–26.

[25] Brown CM, Ainsworth DM, Personett LA, et al. Serum biochemical and hematological findings in two foals with focal bacterial hepatitis (Tyzzer's disease). Equine Vet J 1983;15:375–6.

[26] Brem S, Gerhards H, Wollanke B, et al. 35 intraocular leptospira isolations in 32 horses suffering from equine recurrent uveitis (ERU). Berl Munch Tierarztl Wochenschr 1999;112: 390–3.

[27] Dwyer AE, Crockett RS, Kalsow CM. Association of leptospiral seroreactivity and breed with uveitis and blindness in horses: 372 cases (1986–1993). J Am Vet Med Assoc 1995; 207:1327–31.

[28] Girio RJS, Mathias LA, Lacerda Neto JC, et al. Experimental leptospirosis in horses infected with *Leptospira interrogans serovar copenhageni*: clinical and serological aspects. Arq Inst Biol (Sao Paulo) 1999;66:21–6.

[29] Wada S, Yoshinari M, Katayama Y, et al. Nonulcerative keratouveitis as a manifestation of Leptospiral infection in a horse. Vet Ophthalmol 2003;6:191–5.

[30] Zientara S, Trap D, Fontaine JJ, et al. Survey of equine hepatic encephalopathy in France in 1992. Vet Rec 1994;134:18–9.

[31] Poonacha KB, Donahue JM, Giles RC, et al. Leptospirosis in equine fetuses, stillborn foals, and placentas. Vet Pathol 1993;30:362–9.

[32] Wilkie IW, Prescott JF, Hazlett MJ, et al. Giant cell hepatitis in four aborted foals: a possible leptospiral infection. Can Vet J 1988;29:1003–4.

ELSEVIER
SAUNDERS

VETERINARY
CLINICS
Equine Practice

Vet Clin Equine 22 (2006) 107–116

Cholelithiasis and Hepatic Fibrosis in a Standardbred Mare

Emily A. Graves, VMD, MS

Equine Consulting of the Rockies, PO Box 27–1760, Fort Collins, CO 80527–1760, USA

Signalment and history

The mare was presented with a 1-week history of mild depression, decreased appetite, weight loss, and intermittent fevers. Six weeks previously, the horse exhibited non–weight-bearing lameness of the left forelimb; a nail puncture injury into the frog was discovered. The mare was hospitalized for treatment of sepsis of the left front distal interphalangeal joint and navicular bursa. A decreasing dose of phenylbutazone had been administered since that time. Mild left forelimb lameness at a walk persisted. Three weeks before presentation, the mare delivered a full-term colt. During the week in which signs developed, phenylbutazone, 1 g, had been administered orally every 12 hours.

Approximately 4 weeks before the foaling date, the mare was vaccinated for influenza, rhinopneumonitis, tetanus, eastern and western equine encephalitis, and West Nile virus. On an alternating schedule, deworming was performed every 2 months with ivermectin or pyrantel pamoate; double-dose pyrantel was administered each fall. This was the mare's ninth foal, and no other horses on the breeding farm were showing similar clinical signs.

Physical examination

At admission, the mare was depressed and had mildly icteric oral membranes that were slightly tacky. The body condition score was 4/9 (Henneke scale [1]), with visible ribs. The rectal temperature was 100°F (37.7°C), the pulse was 52 beats per minute (bpm), and the respiratory rate was 20 breaths per minute (brpm). The sclerae were also mildly icteric. Normal

E-mail address: dr.egraves@gmail.com

bronchovesicular sounds were auscultated in all lung fields. Peripheral pulse quality was good, and no heart murmurs were auscultated. Gastrointestinal (GI) sounds were reduced, but feces passed were normal in consistency. Mild dehydration was estimated at 5%. Transrectal palpation revealed a prominent left kidney and well-involuted uterus. No other significant findings were palpated. Mild distal limb edema was present in the left forelimb, and mildly increased digital pulses were palpated in both forelimbs. The packed cell volume (PCV) was 32% and total solids (TS) were 9.0 g/dL.

Case assessment

At admission, the problem list consisted of intermittent fever (historical), depression, weight loss, poor appetite, icterus, mild tachycardia, mild dehydration, increased digital pulses, and elevated plasma TS. Rule-outs for intermittent fever, in conjunction with depression, poor appetite, and weight loss, included infection of any body system or local site. In light of the history of nonsteroidal anti-inflammatory drug (NSAID) use, right dorsal colitis (RDC) and associated peritonitis was a suspected diagnosis. Infectious colitis, antimicrobial-induced colitis, hepatobiliary disease, genitourinary tract infection, and persistent septic navicular bursitis and/or arthritis and subsequent systemic illness were other possible infections. Although the mare was not passing loose feces, GI-related disorders were considered nonetheless because of the potential for altered GI flora.

Icterus could have been associated with a decreased appetite or caused by altered bilirubin metabolism or cholestatic disease. With the mare's history of not eating well for several days, fasting hyperbilirubinemia was considered the most likely cause. It is theorized that anorexia leads to depletion of ligandin from hepatocyte stores. This common cytosolic protein is critical for the transfer of bilirubin from albumin into hepatocytes [2]. Other differential diagnoses were cholangitis, cholelithiasis, or hepatitis as well as plant alkaloid-induced hepatotoxicity. The mild dehydration and tachycardia were consistent with the patient's history of poor food intake. An increased heart rate may also result from anxiety, hypovolemia, shock, pain, endotoxemia, cardiovascular disease, and fever. Of these, anxiety and low-level pain may have been contributory.

The dehydration was most likely caused by inadequate food and water intake, because the mare exhibited no signs of increased fluid losses, such as diarrhea, gastric reflux, cavity effusion, or excessive sweating. The increased TS value was markedly elevated and not consistent with dehydration alone. Additional sources of elevated plasma proteins include increased globulin or fibrinogen production, and both occur with ongoing inflammatory states. B lymphocytes produce globulins in response to more chronic antigenic stimulation; fibrinogen is an acute-phase protein that increases in concentration as part of the inflammatory cascade. Active inflammation typically leads to a febrile state as well as to increased fibrinogen and globulin production over time. The associated mental depression often limits appetite and then results in a slow decline in body weight. Based on the presence of high TS, history, and other clinical findings, an established inflammatory or infectious disease process was considered the most likely root of the mare's signs. RDC was thought to be a less likely primary disease, because TS values typically drop as a result of gradual albumin loss into the GI tract. The elevated forelimb digital pulses suggested the presence of pain or inflammation within the hoof capsule. With the previous septic synovial disease, the pulse changes were most likely attributable to persistent pain and inflammation in the left foot as well as to early stages of contralateral limb laminitis.

Diagnostic procedures

A complete blood cell count (CBC) on day 1 showed a mildly elevated mean corpuscular hemoglobin concentration (MCHC), mature neutrophilia, and monocytosis with mild toxic changes and reactive lymphocytes (Table 1). All abnormalities were consistent with a stress leukogram and immune response to a bacterial infection. Primary GI disease was considered less likely, because neutropenia is more typical. Low neutrophil counts result from endotoxemia and induced neutrophil margination and migration into GI tissues. As expected, the fibrinogen concentration was elevated, indicating active inflammation. Increased TS concentration, in light of a normal PCV, may have been caused by long-term infection and subsequent increased globulin production or dehydration in an anemic patient. Based on the mare's mildly dehydrated status, the former was considered most likely. An MCHC increase typically accompanies intra- or extravascular hemolysis. Subclinical extravascular hemolysis was considered as an explanation because of the patient's systemic inflammatory state. Because the mare had no signs of active hemolysis, however, the mild MCHC increase was considered clinically insignificant.

Chemistry profile results revealed mild hypoalbuminemia, hyperglobulinemia, hyperbilirubinemia, elevated gamma-glutamyltransferase (GGT), hypoglycemia, and low creatine kinase (CK) activity (Table 2). Albumin was slightly decreased, consistent with protein-losing enteropathy (PLE) and chronic NSAID use. In addition, the minor loss could be explained by cholangitis or hepatitis and local protein loss attributable to vascular leakage or protein-losing nephropathy. No evidence of renal dysfunction was found, and a dipstick urinalysis revealed no protein. The increased globulin value supported a diagnosis of chronic infection. With icterus and elevated GGT also present, primary cholestatic disease became the top differential diagnosis. The bilirubin rise was small and primarily attributable to an increased unconjugated fraction, which typically reflects acute hepatocyte injury more than cholestasis. A rise in the conjugated bilirubin more reliably signifies primary liver dysfunction [2]. With this mare's mild elevation,

Table 1
Complete blood cell count results

Date/hospital day	Day 1	Day 2	Day 4	Day 8	Day 37	Normal values
PCV (%)	34		25	27	26	30–45
RBC × 10^6/µL	7.93		5.96	6.38	5.40	6.91–10.36
MCV (fL)	41.9		41.3	41.6	45.8	38.1–52.7
MCH (pg)	16.5		16.1	16.3	16.3	12.7–18.8
MCHC (%)	39.3		39.0	39.2	35.5	32.6–37.2
RBC morphology	Normal; rouleaux formation		Normal; rouleaux formation	Normal	2 + echinocytes	
Nucleated cells/uL	0		0	0	0	
Nucleated RBC/uL	0		0	0	0	
White blood cells/uL	20,860		7340	8820	9680	5100–13,120
Metamyelocytes/uL	0		0	0	0	
Band neutrophils/uL	0		0	0	0	
Segmented neutrophils/uL	16,900		4550	5410	6940	1940–7400
Lymphocytes/uL	3340		2820	2770	2350	960–5740
Monocytes/uL	630		310	360	250	10–350
Eosinophils/uL	0		80	170	60	0–1070
Basophils/uL	0		80	50	30	30–260
Leukocyte morphology	Few reactive lymphocytes		Normal	Normal	Few reactive lymphocytes	
Platelets/uL	245,000		224,000	248,000	172,000	97,000–309,000
Fibrinogen (g/dL)	0.6		0.6	0.6	0.5	0–0.4
PT (seconds)		14.5				10.0–12.3
APTT (seconds)		44.2				23–43

Abbreviations: APPT, activated partial thromboplastin time; MCH, mean corpuscular hemoglobin; MCHC, mean corpuscular hemoglobin concentration; MCV, mean corpuscular volume; PCV, packed cell volume; PT, prothrombin time; RBC, red blood cell.

bilirubin concentration did not help to discern if or what type of liver disease was present. The concurrent rise in the GGT concentration with a normal aspartate aminotransferase (AST) concentration made cholestatic disease more likely [2]. Hypoglycemia was mild and consistent with a poor appetite. The low CK value fit with depression and decreased physical activity. Possible hepatic disorder rule-outs were bacterial cholangitis or hepatitis, cholelithiasis, megalocytic hepatopathy (ie, pyrrolizidine alkaloid toxicity), and chronic active hepatitis.

A venous blood gas (VBG) analysis showed elevated lactate and decreased magnesium concentrations (see Table 2). Mild dehydration and hypovolemia explained the increased lactate, which is a sign of poor tissue perfusion. Low magnesium is a consequence of inadequate intake, which was supported by the mare's partial anorexia.

A peritoneal fluid analysis showed an increased white blood cell (WBC) count and total protein concentration and was interpreted as a nonseptic exudate. The lack of bacteria and toxic WBC changes supported a diagnosis of a primary intra-abdominal inflammatory process, such as RDC and cholangitis or cholelithiasis. The brief initial ultrasound examination on day 1 focused on intestinal wall thickness because of the mare's long-term phenylbutazone treatment. The overall impression was mildly thickened large colon walls measuring from 0.3 to 0.6 cm [3]. On day 2, a complete abdominal ultrasound examination was performed and showed marked hepatomegaly, similar gut wall thickness as measured on day 1, and no other abnormal findings. The liver extended well past the costochondral junctions and had generally rounded edges. In the most cranial images, repeatable acoustic shadows were seen within the parenchyma. Based on the history, elevated cholestatic enzymes, and these findings, a working diagnosis of cholelithiasis and possible ascending cholangiohepatitis was made [4–7].

Differential diagnosis

In addition to cholelithiasis, other differential or concurrent diagnoses included bacterial cholangitis or hepatitis, cholelithiasis, megalocytic hepatopathy (ie, pyrrolizidine alkaloid toxicity), other hepatotoxic insults, and chronic active hepatitis. Bacterial cholangitis or cholangiohepatitis can be associated with ascending infection of enteric organisms from the GI tract. This condition may also be seen concurrently with cholestasis and the formation of choleliths [2,5–11]. Common clinical signs in cases of cholangitis or cholelithiasis are intermittent fever and mild to moderate colic [10]. Rarely, formation of choleliths has been related to the presence of a foreign body in the common bile duct and subsequent cholangitis [12].

Pyrrolizidine alkaloid toxicity results after long-term or a large ingestion of various alkaloid-containing plants (eg, *Senecio* spp, *Crotalaria* spp, *Amsinckia* spp, *Heliotropium* spp). Multiple toxic principles have been isolated and can vary with the season. The toxins are metabolized by the liver to

Table 2
Chemistry profile results

Date/hospital day	Normal values	Day 1	Day 2	Day 3	Day 4	Day 8	Day 37	Day 57	Day 59	Day 151
BUN (mg/dL)	11–31	12			11		17	13	11	
Creatinine (mg/dL)	0.8–1.8	0.6			0.6		0.9	0.7	0.7	
Alk phos (IU/L)	90–295	196			277		176	252	381	
SGOT (AST) (IU/L)	210–380	267			410		169	251	451	
ID (IU/L)	No reference range		18.9		19.2		4.6	10.7	28.3	
CK (IU/L)	156–417	112			91		129	90	87	
GGT (IU/L)	6–17	50			100		51	105	161	21
Total bilirubin (mg/dL)	0.1–2.1	5.4			1.4		1.2	4.3	3.8	
Direct bilirubin (mg/dL)	No reference range	1.0			0.4		0.3	1.0	1.4	
Triglyceride (mg/dL)	9–71					42				
Glucose (mg/dL)	75–119	60			88		65	76	85	
Na (mEq/L)	128–158	130			137		135	128	132	
K (mEq/L)	2.6–4.9	2.9			3.4		4.3	4.2	3.3	
Cl (mEq/L)	91–110	92			99		100	97	94	
Ca, total (mg/dL)	10.1–13.7	10.5			11.9		12.0	10.8	11.8	
P (mg/dL)	1.2–4.6	2.2			1.8		3.1	2.6	2.8	
Mg (mmol/L; from venous blood gas, not serum chemistry)	No reference range	0.3								

	No reference range							
Osmolarity (calculated) (mOsm/L)	No reference range	267.6			282.8	279.7	264.6	272.8
Total protein (g/dL)	6.1–8.9	8.5			8.7	9.5	8.9	8.7
Albumin (g/dL)	3.5–4.7	2.8			2.8	3.1	3.1	3.0
Globulin (g/dL)	2.4–4.2	5.7			5.9	6.4	5.8	5.7
Cholesterol (mg/dL)	51–117	40			54	63	68	74
Ammonia (µmol/L)	Control 62.9		1.7					
Bile acid (pre) (µmol/L)	0–7		15.5					
Bile acid (post)								
pH		7.421	7.381	7.434				
Po_2 venous (mm Hg)		27.8	38.4	42.8				
Pco_2 venous (mm Hg)		40.7	39.9	40.0				
HCO_3 (mmol/L)		26.6	24.4	26.7				
Total CO_2 (mmol/L)	22–30	27.8	25.6	27.9			24	27
Lactate (mmol/L)		4.6	0.8	1.2				
Base excess (mmol/L)		2.6	0.2	3.2				

Abbreviations: Alk phos, alkaline phosphatase; AST, aspartate aminotransferase; BUN, blood urea nitrogen; CK, creatine kinase; GGT, gamma-glutamyltransferase; ID, inositol dehydrogenase; SGOT, serum glutamic-oxaloacetic transaminase.

toxic pyrrole compounds that interfere with nucleic acid and protein synthesis. This results in altered cellular division and megalocyte formation. Once these abnormal megalocytes die, fibrosis follows [2,8,9]. Another hepatotoxic plant to consider was alsike clover. Although the toxin itself has not been elucidated, the risk of exposure seems to be greatest at times of clover bloom. The characteristic histologic changes are biliary hyperplasia and periportal or bridging fibrosis, thus making the distinction from pyrrolizidine alkaloid toxicity difficult [2,8,9].

Finally, the insidious onset of liver disease may be caused by an idiopathic disease called chronic active hepatitis. Horses can exhibit a range of signs, including fever, depression, encephalopathy, icterus, and weight loss. The diagnosis is confirmed by histopathologic findings of biliary inflammation and hyperplasia as well as periportal inflammation and fibrosis [2].

Treatment and clinical outcome

Initial supportive care consisted of intravenous fluid therapy with isotonic crystalloid fluids containing 23% calcium (Ca^{++}) borogluconate (25 mL/L), potassium (K^+) chloride (20 mEq/L), and magnesium sulfate (1 g/L). Because the mare's appetite was poor and most of these electrolytes come from the diet, Ca^{++} and K^+ were supplemented; magnesium was given to replace the deficit (varied from 20–40 mg/kg/day of magnesium sulfate). To replace the mare's fluid deficit, fluids were given as a bolus (20 L) and then maintained at a rate of 1 to 2 mL/kg/h. Other prescribed medications included potassium penicillin (22,000 IU/kg administered intravenously every 6 hours) and gentamicin (6.6 mg/kg administered intravenously every 24 hours) for broad-spectrum antimicrobial coverage because of the potential diagnosis of bacterial cholangiohepatitis, as well as omeprazole (4 mg/kg administered orally every 24 hours) for inhibition of gastric acid production. Gastric ulceration risk factors were numerous, including the stress of illness and lactation, poor appetite, and long-term NSAID use. The mare was offered timothy-grass mixed hay and water ad libitum plus Purina Horse Chow (5 kg; Purina Mills, LLC, St. Louis, Missouri) daily.

On day 2, medical therapy continued, including intravenous fluids (1–2 mL/kg/h), and the mare's attitude improved slightly. VBG analysis was normal, indicating that tissue perfusion was adequate. To describe the mare's disease better, a liver biopsy was indicated. Before collection, other diagnostic modalities were completed to assess liver function, including a coagulation profile and blood ammonia, bile acid, and inositol dehydrogenase (ID) measurements. A coagulation profile was performed because of the potential association between liver disease and decreased clotting factor production and subsequent bleeding tendencies. Findings included a slightly elevated prothrombin and activated partial thromboplastin times relative to the control patient (see Table 1). These may have suggested hepatic insufficiency (decreased clotting factor production), although the differences from the control patient were quite small and may have only reflected patient variability [2,8].

The ammonia concentration was normal; however, bile acids and ID values were moderately increased (see Table 2). The bile acid concentration strongly supported the presence of liver disease, because bile acids are removed from enterohepatic circulation by the liver [2]. Bile acids are not specific for the actual disease process, however. Because ID is a cytosolic enzyme, the ID rise confirmed acute liver damage and some degree of cellular injury.

A liver biopsy was performed because of the prognostic value of histopathologic information as well as the low incidence of bleeding complications in horses with confirmed liver disease [2]. On day 3, using a Tru-Cut biopsy needle (Baxter International, Inc., Deerfield, Illinois), three liver samples were collected through the right thirteenth intercostal space. One sample was macerated and submitted for bacterial tissue culture and sensitivity testing; the other two samples were sent for histopathologic examination. No bacterial agents were isolated. Endoscopy was performed to evaluate gastric mucosa as well as to visualize the proximal duodenum. No gastric mucosal lesions were observed. In some reported cases, choleliths present in the distal common bile duct are visible via endoscopy. Unfortunately, with several attempts, duodenoscopy was not successful. Ensuing ultrasound examinations showed consistent images.

The final histopathologic interpretation described severe cholangiohepatitis, with bile ductule proliferation and portal fibrosis. The sections examined were prepared in a way that did not allow visualization of adjacent portal triads. Bridging portal fibrosis was assumed to be present, and the mare's prognosis for full recovery was guarded.

At this point, potential causes included ascending bacterial cholangiohepatitis or hepatotoxin exposure, such as alsike clover or pyrrolizidine alkaloids [2]. The mare had no history of ingestion of these plants, nor did the farm have any previously known hepatotoxin exposure. Thus, idiopathic bacterial cholangiohepatitis with associated cholelithiasis was the final but unconfirmed diagnosis. Biopsy and laboratory findings suggested that acute and chronic processes were occurring. A possible explanation was chronic ascending cholangitis, which led to stone formation and eventual hepatic disease and acute onset of hepatocellular damage. Surgical removal of choleliths is described [10,11,13] but is not considered the treatment of choice [2,5,7]. This option was discussed with, and declined by, the client.

On day 4, because of a better appetite, fluid therapy was stopped. Blood work revealed mild anemia, an even higher GGT concentration, increased ID and AST concentrations, and normal bilirubin concentration. The triglyceride level was normal, indicating adequate lipid metabolism (see Table 2). Per a lameness consultation, shoes and wedge pads were placed on the mare's front feet to provide better sole support and decrease the risk of developing laminitis. Phenylbutazone therapy was started, with a regimen of 1.5 g in the morning and 1 g in the evening for 3 to 5 days.

The mare's improved appetite and attitude became consistent, and sporadic fever was not recorded from days 5 through 9. Thus, the horse was discharged after 9 days in the clinic. Prescribed treatment consisted of trimethoprim-sulfamethoxazole (TMS; 25 mg/kg administered orally twice daily) for at least 30 days, and a diet of free-choice mixed grass hay and 3.5 to 4.5 kg of sweet feed (12% protein) daily. On day 37, a CBC and chemistry panel showed improved but still elevated GGT and ID concentrations (see Table 2). The globulin value climbed in the 5-week interim, and TMS was continued. The mare continued to experience intermittent episodes of anorexia, fever, and depression. Flunixin meglumine (0.5–1.1 mg/kg administered intravenously) was given as needed. The mare was artificially inseminated on two occasions during the first 60 days at home but failed to conceive. Monitoring of blood work values showed a gradual improvement in globulins and liver enzymes (see Table 2). After 18 weeks of therapy, the GGT concentration was only slightly out of the reference range, and TMS therapy was discontinued. During this period, the mare intermittently experienced recurrent episodes of mild depression and lameness.

References

[1] Henneke DR, Potter GD, Kreider JL, et al. Relationship between condition score, physical measurements and body fat percentage in mares. Equine Vet J 1983;15(4):371–2.

[2] Barton MH. Disorders of the liver. In: Reed SM, Bayly WM, Sellon DC, editors. Equine internal medicine. 2nd edition. St. Louis (MO): WB Saunders; 2004. p. 951–94.

[3] Jones SL, Blikslager AT. Disorders of the gastrointestinal system. In: Reed SM, Bayly WM, Sellon DC, editors. Equine internal medicine. 2nd edition. St. Louis (MO): WB Saunders; 2004. p. 769–801, 937–49.

[4] Reef VB, Johnston JK, Divers TJ, et al. Ultrasonographic findings in horses with cholelithiasis: eight cases (1985–1987). J Am Vet Med Assoc 1990;196(11):1836–40.

[5] Peek SF, Divers TJ. Medical treatment of cholangiohepatitis and cholelithiasis in mature horses: 9 cases (1991–1998). Equine Vet J 2000;32(4):301–6.

[6] Traub JL, Rantanen N, Reed S, et al. Cholelithiasis in four horses. J Am Vet Med Assoc 1982;181(1):59–62.

[7] Johnston JK, Divers TJ, Reef VB, et al. Cholelithiasis in horses: ten cases (1982–1986). J Am Vet Med Assoc 1989;194(3):405–9.

[8] Pearson EG. Diseases of the hepatobiliary system. In: Smith BP, editor. Large animal internal medicine. 3rd edition. St. Louis (MO): Mosby; 2002. p. 790–823.

[9] Peek SF. Liver disease. In: Robinson NE, editor. Current therapy in equine medicine 5. St. Louis (MO): WB Saunders; 2003. p. 169–73.

[10] Ryu SH, Bak UB, Lee CW, et al. Cholelithiasis associated with recurrent colic in a Thoroughbred mare. J Vet Sci 2004;5(1):79–82.

[11] Laverty S, Pascoe JR, Williams JW, et al. Cholelith causing duodenal obstruction in a horse. J Am Vet Med Assoc 1992;201(5):751–2.

[12] Gerros TC, McGuirk SM, Biller DS, et al. Choledocholithiasis attributable to a foreign body in a horse. J Am Vet Med Assoc 1993;202(2):301–3.

[13] Traub JL, Grant BD, Rantanen NW, et al. Surgical removal of choleliths in a horse. J Am Vet Med Assoc 1983;182(7):714–6.

ELSEVIER
SAUNDERS

Vet Clin Equine 22 (2006) 117–126

VETERINARY
CLINICS
Equine Practice

Liver Disease in a 9-year-old Arabian Stallion

Janyce Seahorn, DVM, MS

Equine Veterinary Specialists, 629 Craig Lane, Georgetown, KY 40324, USA

History

A 9-year-old Arabian stallion presented with a history of weight loss and anorexia of 30 days' duration (Fig. 1). There was an acute onset of weakness, tachycardia, and dehydration. Injected, icteric mucous membranes were observed by the referring veterinarian. Hematocrit was reported to be 70% (normal, 32%–53%), and serum urea nitrogen (BUN) was lower than 10 mg/dL (normal, 13–29 mg/dL). Twelve liters of lactated Ringer's solution were administered, and the animal was referred to the teaching hospital. Additional information included a negative Coggin's test 30 days earlier, a 30-day alternating deworming program, a current vaccination status (including tetanus, encephalitis, *Streptococcus equi bacterin*), and a diet consisting of Kleingrass hay free choice and 10 pounds of 10% protein sweet feed daily. Two of the 20 other horses on the same premise were showing signs of anorexia and mild weight loss.

Physical examination

The stallion was thin, depressed, and markedly icteric. The temperature was 38.5°C (101.3° F), heart rate was 60 beats/minute, and respiratory rate was 16 breaths/minute. The horse was estimated to be 6% dehydrated based on decreased skin turgor, injected mucous membranes, and a capillary refill time of 2.5 seconds. Dry, mucus-covered feces were passed during the examination, and gastrointestinal sounds were decreased. The stallion had a retained right testicle.

E-mail address: Jcseahorn@aol.com

0749-0739/06/$ - see front matter © 2006 Elsevier Inc. All rights reserved.
doi:10.1016/j.cveq.2005.12.014
vetequine.theclinics.com

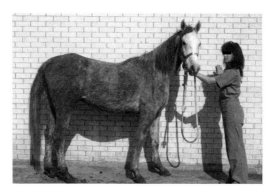

Fig. 1. Horse presented in this case.

Initial assessment

Abnormalities identified included icterus, anorexia, weight loss, tachycardia, dehydration, scant and dry feces, and a retained right testicle. Hepatic disease was suggested by the icterus and reported low BUN. Other possibilities included abdominal abscess or neoplasia, peritonitis, lymphosarcoma, and equine infectious anemia, all of which could influence weight loss and secondary anorexia and icterus. A hemolytic crisis was considered, but the reported hematocrit did not support this possibility. Tachycardia, decreased gastrointestinal sounds, and the acute onset were suggestive of colic.

Diagnostic plan and assessment of results

The diagnostic plan included a complete blood cell count, serum chemistry profile (with direct bilirubin, sorbitol dehydrogenase [SDH], and lactate dehydrogenase [LDH]), blood ammonia, bromosulfophthalein (BSP) clearance time, coagulation profile, routine urinalysis, abdominocentesis, rectal palpation, ultrasonography, and liver biopsy.

Complete blood cell count

A stress leukogram was indicated by the presence of a neutrophilia, lymphopenia, and eosinopenia (Table 1). All subsequent leukograms were within normal limits except for lymphopenia, which persisted through day 3. Polycythemia (packed cell volume 59%; normal, 32%–53%) and increased hemoglobin were assumed to be relative because of hemoconcentration, but the normal plasma protein (Table 2) prompted these considerations: (1) hemoconcentration with an actual low protein; (2) minimal hemoconcentration exacerbated by splenic contraction; (3) polycythemia. Polycythemia persisted despite return to normal hydration status, making relative polycythemia unlikely. There was no evidence of absolute polycythemia. Chronic

Table 1
Complete blood cell count, fibrinogen, and coagulation parameters

Parameters	Day 1	Day 3	Day 8	Day 56	Normal values
Packed cell volume/ hemoglobin	59%/21.7	61%/21.7	54%/19.1	46%/18	32%–53%/ 11–19 g/dL
Red blood cell count $\times$ 10^6	10.7				6.8–12.9
Red blood cell morphology	Normal	Normal	Normal	Normal	
Platelets	Adequate	Adequate	Adequate	Adequate	100–350 $\times$ 10^3/mL
Total white cell count/μL	14,300	10,800	10,100	7100	5400–14,300
Neutrophil count/μL	12,727	8964	7878	2751	2260–8580
Lymphocyte count/μL	1430	1404	1818	1136	1500–7700
Monocyte count/μL	143	108	404	182	0–1000
Eosinophil count/μL	0	0	0	71	0–850
Fibrinogen	300	300	200	200	
Prothrombin time		9.3 s			9–10.5 s
Activated partial prothrombin time		43.2			40–60 s
Fibrin degradation products		<10			<10

hypoxia caused by pulmonary or cardiovascular disease was not evident, ruling out secondary appropriate polycythemia. Secondary inappropriate polycythemia caused by increased erythropoietin production has been reported in association with certain hepatic tumors, some benign and malignant renal disorders, and certain endocrine diseases [1–4]. Erythropoietin assay might have confirmed increased levels in this horse, but the assay was not available when this horse was managed. Erythropoietin is produced in the kidneys, in response to hypoxia and some other stimulants, and possibly in the liver. In this animal, theoretically, hepatic changes may have induced hepatic production of erythropoietin, systemic alterations secondary to hepatic disease may have influenced renal production by some unknown mechanism, or an unidentified erythropoietin-producing tumor could have been present. Polycythemia secondary to a renal disorder was considered, but the absence of azotemia and abnormalities on ultrasound examination made this possibility unlikely.

Serum chemistry

Elevated gamma-glutamyl-transferase (GGT), alkaline phosphatase (ALP), aspartate aminotransferase (AST), total and direct bilirubin, and blood ammonia, with the decreased BUN, supported a diagnosis of primary hepatic disease (Table 2). Increased ammonia and decreased BUN may occur with liver disease because of decreased hepatocyte capacity to convert ammonia to urea and may indicate chronicity [5]. Blood ammonia values may vary greatly because of diet and bacterial population; thus the increased

Table 2
Serum chemistry parameters

Parameter	Day 1	Day 3	Day 8	Day 12	Day 56	Normal values
BUN (mg/dL)	11	8	6	9	13	13–29
Creatinine (mg/dL)	1.3	1.3	1.0	1.0	1.2	1.0–2.2
Serum GGT (U/L)	415	188	138	131	71	6.5–24.5
Serum ALP (U/L)		379	333	291	131	91–289
Serum AST (U/L)	1130	497	337	247	175	80–228
LDH (U/L)		470				139–450
SDH (U/L)		445	305	172		30–300
Creatine phosphokinase (U/L)	320	313	276	116	67	71–307
Total bilirubin (mg/dL)	6.4	4.8	3.9	2.6	2.1	0.5–2.2
Direct bilirubin (mg/dL)	3.3	1.2	1.0	1.0	0.9	0.04–0.44
Total protein (g/dL)	7.3	6.3	6.2	6.4	6.8	5.4–7.6
Albumin (g/dL)		2.9	2.7 g	2.7	3.2	2.4–3.5
Globulin (g/dL)		3.4	3.5	3.7	3.6	3.0–4.0
Glucose (mg/dL)	79	73	83	76	140	60–100
Sodium (mEq/L)	140					132–146
Potassium (mEq/L)	3.1					3.0–4.7
Cloride (mEq/L)	109 mEq/L					99–104
Calcium (mg/dL)		12	11.2	11.2	11.8	9.0–13.0
Phosphorus (mg/dL)		3.4	3.3	3.4	3.3	2.9–6.0
BSP clearance (min)		3.5				2.0–3.7
Ammonia (µg/dL)	184			336		
Ammonia (control) µg/dL	20			3.4		

GGT, ALP, and conjugated (direct) bilirubin (51.5% of total) suggested a cholestatic disorder. GGT and ALP are induced enzymes that increase in response to increased intracanalicular pressure. Hepatocellular leakage enzymes, SDH, LDH, and AST, were only mildly elevated. By day 12, SDH had returned to normal, and AST was only slightly above normal limits, reflecting the longer half-life of this hepatic enzyme [5]. Both GGT and ALP remained elevated but decreased steadily during hospitalization; only GGT remained elevated at the time of reevaluation, 56 days following initial presentation. Increases in GGT have been reported to be more persistent in chronic hepatic disease, especially with cholestasis [6]. These laboratory value trends supported a cholestatic rather than an hepatocellular disorder.

Blood ammonia concentration was quite elevated in this horse and increased from day 1 to day 12 (Table 2). Daily blood ammonia levels vary widely in normal horses [7]. Ammonia values are influenced by the bacterial population in the gastrointestinal tract and the diet. The increase in blood ammonia for this horse noted on day 12 probably reflected the return of appetite and normal food consumption. There is no correlation between blood ammonia concentration and severity of liver disease, although elevated levels have been significantly associated with both hepatoencephalopathy

(HE) and the presence of disease [7]. Blood ammonia is only one of the many factors incriminated in development of HE; thus, the absence of central nervous system signs in this horse was not surprising. The pathogenesis of HE remains unclear but is probably multifactorial and includes the following suggested mechanisms: gastrointestinal-derived neurotoxins; false neurotransmitter accumulation associated with amino acid imbalance; augmented γ-aminobutyric acid activity in the brain; increased permeability of the blood–brain barrier; and impaired energy metabolism in the central nervous system [5].

Urinalysis

Bilirubinuria (Table 3) was attributed to the marked increase in the more soluble conjugated bilirubin [5]. The mild proteinuria may have been influenced by semen constituents present or might have represented mild renal glomerular changes. A false positive caused by alkalinity was ruled out, and the acid urine was assumed to be caused by anorexia. Isosthenuria and glucosuria were caused by sample collection after initiation of dextrose-containing fluid therapy. Subsequent urinalyses indicated normal concentrating ability and absence of glucosuria.

Bromosulfophthalein clearance time

BSP clearance time was 3.5 minutes (normal, 2.0–3.7 minutes). BSP conjugating ability may have remained normal because unconjugated bilirubin, with which it competes for hepatocyte uptake, was only mildly elevated, and data indicated minimal active hepatocellular damage. Thus, the liver may have retained normal BSP conjugating ability. The normal BSP clearance time was surprising, however, because conjugated BSP will reflux back into plasma by the same route as conjugated bilirubin. This case was managed 20 years ago. Since that time, serum bile acid concentration has replaced foreign dye clearance as an assessment of liver function. Normal liver removes more than 90% of bile acids from hepatic circulation; thus, bile acid concentration increases in the presence of liver disease [5]. Fasting and fed bile acids are not typically performed in horses because of intestinal

Table 3
Urinalyses

Parameter	Day 1	Day 8	Day 56	Normal values
Source	Voided	Voided	Voided	–
Specific gravity	1.012	1.028	1.031	1.010–1.050
pH	6.0	8.0	8.0	7.0–8.0
Protein	30	negative	negative	<30 mg/dL
Glucose	100 mg/dL	negative	negative	negative
Bilirubin	2 +	1 +	negative	negative

fill. Therefore, a single sample is submitted for analysis. Normal serum bile acid levels in horses are less than 15 umol/L.

Rectal palpation

Rectal palpation revealed a retained, small, soft right testicle and no other significant findings. This absence of significant findings, along with a normal abdominal fluid analysis, made gastrointestinal crisis, abdominal abscess, or neoplasia less likely.

Ultrasonography

The liver was normal in size, contour, and echogenicity; no masses or choleliths were detected. The kidneys were normal in appearance, size, and echogenicity.

Liver biopsy

On day 5 a liver biopsy was performed. Results included wide bands of immature connective tissue that seemed to span from central vein to central vein (bridging fibrosis) (Figs. 2–4). Finer bands of connective tissue can be seen to dissect through the hepatic cords. Adjacent to the wide bands of connective tissue are aggregates of large cuboidal to polygonal cells that frequently orient in an acinar arrangement, interpreted as foci of hepatocellular regeneration. There are several scattered foci of hepatocellular vacuolar degeneration. Based on these findings, a diagnosis of chronic, diffuse, and dissecting hepatic fibrosis with nodular regeneration was made. The cause could not be determined, but lesions most closely resembled a toxic hepatopathy.

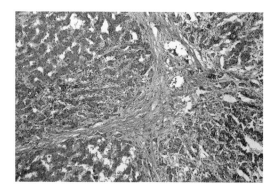

Fig. 2. Hematoxylin and eosin (H&E) stain of liver biopsy. Finer bands of connective tissue can be seen to dissect through the hepatic cords. Adjacent to the wide bands of connective tissue are aggregates of large cuboidal to polygonal cells that frequently orient in an acinar arrangement, interpreted as foci of hepatocellular regeneration. There are several scattered foci of hepatocellular vacuolar degeneration.

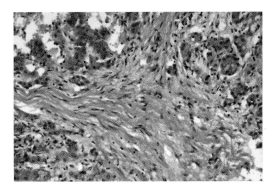

Fig. 3. H&E stain of liver biopsy: Close-up view of Fig. 2.

On day 56 a second biopsy was made. At this time there was moderate fibrosis around the portal areas. Biliary epithelium was moderately hyperplastic, and the hepatocytes were moderately vacuolated. There was no evidence of active inflammation.

Based on these findings, a diagnosis of portal hepatic fibrosis was made. The fibrosis was much less evident in this sample than in the previously submitted biopsy for this animal. If this biopsy is representative of hepatic change, then the fibrosis seemed to be regressing.

Therapeutic management

The fluid deficit was calculated to be 24 L; 12 L of lactated Ringer's solution was administered to provide 50% of the deficit before initiating 5% dextrose therapy. This treatment would rapidly expand the plasma volume without promoting osmotic diuresis and excessive insulin release from rapid

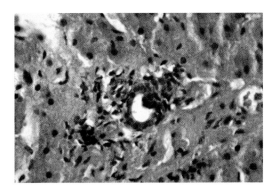

Fig. 4. H&E stain of liver biopsy from a normal, healthy horse.

administration of dextrose. Fifty-two liters of 5% dextrose were administered over 24 hours to alleviate the liver's role in gluconeogenesis. Four liters of mineral oil were administered for its cathartic effects, because gastrointestinal stasis was indicated by the decreased intestinal sounds and dry, mucus-covered feces. Vitamins A, D, and E were administered parenterally because fat emulsification, necessary for absorption of these vitamins, may have been deficient in this horse secondary to cholestasis.

Hydration status normalized, and appetite improved within 24 hours. Dextrose therapy was gradually decreased and was stopped on day 6. Clinically, the horse was bright, and vital signs were normal. The horse was consuming approximately 8 pounds of grass hay and 8 pounds of 10% sweet feed daily.

The horse was discharged on day 14 with instructions to feed free choice grass hay, 8 pounds of 10% sweet feed, and a B-vitamin supplement. Access to pasture was recommended but only at night to avoid photosensitization. Dietary goals were to supply adequate carbohydrates and minimal amounts (8%–10%) of high-quality protein. Dietary supplementation with branched-chain amino acids (BCAAs) has been reported to affect clinical improvement in equine hepatic disease and was discussed but was not incorporated into the diet because this horse improved during hospitalization without major dietary modification. A mixture of beet pulp and cracked corn (2:1 ratio) in molasses provides a rich source of BCAAs. [8] Sorghum, bran, or milo may be substituted for the beet pulp [8]. Formulations of BCAAs are commercially available [5]. B-vitamin supplement was added to assure adequate B-vitamin intake, because hepatic storage may be decreased with hepatic disease. Because Kleingrass has been demonstrated to cause hepatic disease in sheep [9], the owner was instructed to stop feeding the hay and to avoid pastures containing the grass. Therapeutic intervention that has been suggested to slow hepatic fibrosis includes pentoxifylline (8 mg/kg every 12 hours by mouth), colchicine (0.01–0.03 mg/kg every 24 hours by mouth), and cyclosporine [5]. The usefulness of these drugs in the treatment of equine hepatic disease has not been fully evaluated, however. These drugs were not considered at the time when this case was managed, in 1985.

Reassessment on day 56 revealed normal vital signs; mucous membranes were pink. Hematocrit and hemoglobin were normal, as were all hepatic-related enzymes with the exception of serum GGT. Elevated direct bilirubin indicated a persisting degree of cholestasis. Biopsy results indicated resolution of the previously identified pathology. The horse was reported to be in normal body condition 6 months later.

Discussion

Two younger stallions on the same premise and diet were presented for weight loss and anorexia of 3 months' duration when this horse was reassessed. (The feeding of Kleingrass hay had been discontinued for all horses on the farm at the time of presentation). Laboratory results, including biopsies, were strikingly similar to the case discussed. These horses also demonstrated marked clinical improvement after the Kleingrass hay was removed from their diets. Known hepatotoxins, such as mycotoxins, plants, chemicals, and drugs [5], could not be related to this case. There was no evidence of biliary calculi on ultrasonographic evaluation. The histologic lesions did not resemble classically described hepatopathies, such Theiler's disease or megalocytic (pyrrolizidine alkaloid) poisoning but did show a similarity to chronic active hepatitis, a traditionally described category of equine hepatic disease of unknown cause.

This horse had chronic hepatic disease with an acute manifestation of signs at presentation. Successful response to supportive therapy was possible because the inciting cause was identified and removed; adequate normal liver tissue remained to allow regeneration. A subsequent prospective clinical study demonstrated a causal relationship between the feeding of Kleingrass hay and development of hepatic disease with similar hepatic pathology in horses [9]. Kleingrass is found in the southwestern United States [9,10].

Two recent studies have suggested that liver biopsy provides the most reliable information for diagnosis and prognosis of hepatic disease [11,12]. Although the presence of HE, increased GGT, ALP, total bilirubin, and bile acids, hyperglobulinemia, and hypoalbuminemia were identified as useful noninvasive tests for the presence of liver disease, none could fully discriminate between horses with and without biopsy-confirmed liver disease.

References

[1] Sellon DC. Disorders of the hematopoietic system. In: Reed S, Bayly W, Sellon D, editors. Equine internal medicine. 2nd edition. St. Louis (MO): W.B. Saunders; 2004. p. 721–68.

[2] Duncan JR, Prasse KW. Erythrocytes. In: Duncan JR, Prasse KW, editors. Veterinary laboratory medicine clinical pathology. 2nd edition. Ames (IA): Iowa State University Press; 1986. p. 3–30.

[3] Lennox TJ, Wilson JH, Hayden SW, et al. Hepatoblastoma with erythrocytosis in a young female horse. J Am Vet Med Assoc 2000;216:718–20.

[4] Roby KA, Beech J, Bloom JC, et al. Hepatocellular carcinoma associated with erthrocytosis and hypoglycemia in a yearling filly. J Am Vet Med Assoc 1990;196:465–7.

[5] Barton MH. Disorders of the liver. In: Reed S, Bayly W, Sellon D, editors. Equine internal medicine. 2nd edition. St. Louis (MO): W.B. Saunders; 2004. p. 951–94.

[6] Reed S, Andrews FM. The biochemical evaluation of liver function in the horse. Nashville (TN): American Association of Equine Practitioners; 1986. p. 81.

[7] West H. Clinical and pathological studies in horses with hepatic disease. Equine Vet J 1996; 28:146–53.

[8] Divers TJ. Therapy of liver failure. In: Smith BP, editor. Large animal internal medicine. 2nd edition. St. Louis (MO): Mosby-Year Book Inc.; 1996. p. 948–50.

[9] Cornick JL, Carter GK, Bridges CH. Kleingrass-associated hepatotoxicosis in horses. J Am Vet Med Assoc 1988;193:932–5.

[10] Divers TJ. Liver failure and hemolytic anemia. In: Orsini JA, Divers TJ, editors. Manual of equine emergencies treatment and procedures. 2nd edition. Philadelphia: W.B. Saunders; 2003. p. 315–38.

[11] Durham AE, Smith KC, Newton JR, et al. Development and application of a scoring system for prognostic evaluation of equine liver biopsies. Equine Vet J 2003;35:534–40.

[12] Durham AE, Smith KC, Newton JR. An evaluation of diagnostic data in comparison to the results of liver biopsies in mature horses. Equine Vet J 2003;35:554–9.

VETERINARY
CLINICS
Equine Practice

Vet Clin Equine 22 (2006) 127–143

Clostridial Myositis and Collapse in a Standardbred Filly

Allison J. Stewart, BVSc(Hons), MS

Assistant Professor, Department of Clinical Sciences, College of Veterinary Medicine,
1500 Wire Road, Auburn University, AL 36849, USA

Case summary

A 2-year-old, 450-kg Standardbred filly used as a racehorse was presented for evaluation. The filly was the third of five horses vaccinated 5 days previously for influenza and rhinopneumonitis (EHV1 and EHV4) in the left cervical musculature from a five-dose vial. One day after vaccination, the filly was depressed, and a swelling 15 cm in diameter marked the vaccination site. The referring veterinarian administered dexamethasone (0.1 mg/kg intravenously), flunixin meglumine (1.1 mg/kg intravenously), phenylbutazone (4.4 mg/kg by mouth, every 12 hours for 4 days) and procaine penicillin-G (20,000 IU/kg intramuscularly every 12 hours for 4 days). After 48 hours, severe swelling of the head began to cause occlusion of the nasal passages. The referring veterinarian inserted a nasopharyngeal tube in the right nostril and gave tripelennamine (1 mg/kg intramuscularly every 12 hours for 2 days), dimethyl sulfoxide (DMSO) (0.6 g/kg in 5 L lactated Ringer's solution intravenously every 24 hours for 2 days), gentamicin (6.6 mg/kg intravenously every 24 hours for 2 days), and tetanus toxoid and antitoxin (1500 IU intramuscularly). The filly ate and drank until the day of referral. The referring veterinarian considered the edema an allergic reaction and because of its severity advised euthanasia. The insurance company required a necropsy, so the filly was referred to The Ohio State University.

The five horses had been purchased 5 months previously from yearling sales. This was their first known vaccination. The other four horses had remained normal. All horses were stabled in the mid-Atlantic region, fed free choice hay and oats (3 kg every 12 hours), and had been dewormed with ivermectin 20 days prior.

E-mail address: stewaaj@vetmed.auburn.edu

Physical examination

The filly was markedly depressed. The head was twice its normal size. A nasopharyngeal tube was sutured in the right nostril. Tissue swelling occluded the left nasal passage and obscured both orbits, rendering the filly unable to see (Fig. 1). The filly was disoriented, moved reluctantly with low head carriage, and showed weakness (stumbling, knuckling, and toe-dragging). Oral mucous membrane color (mmc) was dark pink with a normal refill time of 2 seconds. The vulvar mmc was a normal pink. Rectal temperature, pulse, and respiratory rate were 100.4°F (38°C), 42 beats/minute, and 12 breaths/minute, respectively. Pulse quality was good and synchronous with a regular heartbeat. No auscultable pulmonary abnormalities were detected. A rebreathing examination was not performed. Borborygmi and rectal palpation were normal. Head elevation and palpation of the nose and lips were resented, precluding any dental examination. The ventral neck was diffusely swollen, but no focal pain or crepitus was palpable. No lymphadenopathy or dermatologic abnormalities were present, and sinus percussion was unremarkable.

Assessment and case management

Euthanasia was not considered immediately necessary because the horse was systemically stable with normal vital parameters. Primary problems identified were marked facial swelling with left nasal passage obstruction, mechanical blindness caused by edema, inability to assess ocular function and integrity because of lid edema, dark-pink oral mmc, weakness, depression, pain, history of neck swelling from intramuscular vaccination and

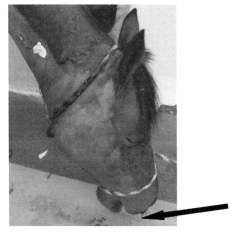

Fig. 1. The filly at presentation, with severe swelling of face and ventral head carriage. A nasopharyngeal tube is in the right nostril (*arrow*).

excessive administration of non-steroidal anti-inflammatory drugs (NSAIDs). Complications of intramuscular injections include type I hypersensitivity, mild local pain and inflammation, iatrogenic contamination with abscess formation, or, rarely, diffuse cellulitis or myositis and fulminant systemic toxemia.

The hyperemic oral mmc was probably caused by venous congestion and lymphatic obstruction from facial swelling and dependent edema. Causes of swelling include diffuse cellulitis or myositis extending from the vaccination site, dependent edema from head positioning, or unrelated angioedema. The basic causes of edema include increased hydrostatic pressure, decreased oncotic pressure, inflammation, and decreased lymphatic drainage. Because the swelling was limited to the head and neck, decreased oncotic pressure was not considered likely. Bilateral jugular vein thrombosis can cause head swelling secondary to increased hydrostatic pressure, but both jugular veins filled normally. The neck was painful to palpation; therefore swelling was probably related to inflammation and possible secondary lymphatic obstruction and venous congestion.

The extreme reluctance to move and the obscured eyeballs limited neurologic evaluation. The depression and inability to raise the head were attributed to neck pain, weakness, and absence of sight. Toxemia, metabolic disease, and electrolyte derangements can result in weakness and depressed mentation. Toxemic weakness can occur with myositis, cellulitis, endotoxemia, and sepsis. Additional differentials for weakness and stumbling include central nervous system disease such as cervical cord compression (trauma, osteomyelitis, abscess, vertebral malformation), or meningoencephalitis (Alphavirus and Flavivirus encephalomyelitides, rabies, EHV1). Rabies was unlikely, but gloves were initially worn.

A low dose of butorphanol (0.015 mg/kg intravenously) was administered for analgesia. The filly stood quietly with the head down and did not seem to be in distress. A cephalic catheter was placed, and a complete blood cell count, serum chemistry profile, fibrinogen concentration, venous blood gas, urinalysis, and ultrasound examination were performed. Urinalysis was important, because NSAIDs and aminoglycosides can be nephrotoxic, and early recognition before azotemia occurs is warranted.

Imaging of the swollen lips, cheeks, eyelid, and forehead was performed using a 5-MHz linear scanner, and findings were consistent with edema. Fluid was observed dissecting between the tissue planes resulting in subcutaneous tissue swelling ranging from 1 to 6 cm in thickness. Loculations of fluid were small, and no focal fluid pockets or compartmentalization was apparent. Imaging of the left cervical musculature from the mandible to the level of C4 was performed using a 3.5-MHz sector scanner. A cavitating area 8 cm long by 5 cm wide by 3 cm deep located in the cervical musculature 2.5 cm from the skin surface dorsal and superimposed over the mid-cervical vertebrae was observed. The borders were indistinct, with no echogenic encapsulation. The fluid seemed to dissect between tissue planes,

being hypoechoic with flocculent echodensities. There were diffuse hyperechoic free gas echoes suggestive of anaerobic infection (Fig. 2). Volatile fatty
acids are produced by anaerobes such as the gram-negative *Fusobacterium*
or *Bacteroides* rods, gram-positive *Peptococcus* and *Peptostreptococcus*
cocci, gram-positive spore-forming *Clostridium* sp rods, or non–spore forming *Propionibacterium* and *Eubacterium* gram-positive rods [1].

   After blocking the skin with lidocaine (5 mL subcutaneously), ultrasound-guided aspiration of the imaged emphysematous fluid dorsal to
C3-C4, (at the vaccination site) using a 14-gauge needle revealed pungent,
serosanguinous exudate. The fluid was submitted for Gram's staining, aerobic and anaerobic culture, and sensitivity. With local anesthesia (lidocaine,
10 mL subcutaneously), the abscess was lanced, a Penrose drain was placed,
and the wound was flushed with dilute betadine (Fig. 3).

   The Gram's staining was performed immediately and showed abundant
chains of large gram-positive bacilli and filamentous organisms as well as
a few spores, consistent with clostridial organisms. The only differential
would be contaminant environmental bacilli, which was not considered
likely by the microbiologist considering the means of sample collection
and presence of gas. The rapid progression of abscess formation and severe
tissue swelling after intramuscular injection with identification of large, gas-
producing, spore-forming, gram-positive rods led to the presumptive diagnosis of clostridial myositis. Direct fluorescent antibody stains were not
available but can be used for definitive diagnosis of some clostridial species
[2,3]. Malignant edema caused by *C septicum, C perfringens, C chauvoei, C
fallax,* and *C novyi* has a poor-to-good prognosis [1,3]. Bacterial culture in
this case was negative, possibly because of the previous antibiotic therapy.
Although the head edema was severe, normal vital signs suggested minimal
toxemia and thus a better prognosis.

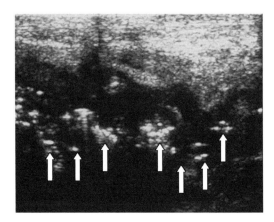

Fig. 2. Two-dimensional sonogram obtained using a 3.5-MHz sector scanner. There are diffuse
hyperechoic free gas echoes (*arrows*) suggestive of anaerobic infection within the echolucent abscess fluid.

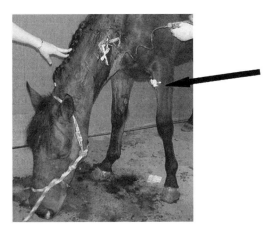

Fig. 3. The abscess has been lanced, Penrose drains placed, and the wound is being flushed with dilute betadine. A cephalic catheter is present in the left leg (*arrow*).

It was planned to replace the nasopharyngeal tube with a temporary tracheostomy tube. The tracheostomy site had been clipped, surgically prepared, and a subcutaneous lidocaine bleb preplaced. Because the filly was breathing without difficulty, a quick examination of the pharynx and larynx was performed after removal of the nasopharyngeal tube and before placement of the tracheostomy tube. To view the pharynx by endoscopy, the head was elevated 50 cm. After a 10-second view of the larynx (which was normal other than diffuse edema), the filly recoiled backward, dog-sat, then collapsed in lateral recumbency. Vital signs remained normal. Although breathing rate and effort and vulval mmc remained normal, the tracheostomy was performed with the filly in recumbency. The filly remained immobile and hyporesponsive to audible and tactile stimuli for the next 2 hours (Fig. 4). Anal and patellar reflexes were normal, but there was minimal response to digital pressure to the ear canal or lips. Palpebral reflex was present but reduced because of the severe eyelid swelling. There was no aversion when hemostats were applied to the plantar pastern region or perineum. The horse appeared as if under general anesthesia.

The obtundation before collapse and semiconscious state suggested possible cerebral deficits. There was also the possibility of cervical spinal cord compression or simply severe neck pain. Neurologic differentials included meningitis (with possible elevation of intracranial pressure), meningoencephalitis, fractured cervical vertebrae, abscess within cervical musculature with or without cervical spinal cord compression, or direct communication with the spinal canal and osteomyelitis. Non-neurologic differentials included acute toxic or bacterial shower from abscess disruption, severe pain (impossible to assess if the horse had a "headache/migraine," if she remained immobile because doing so was less painful than moving, or if there

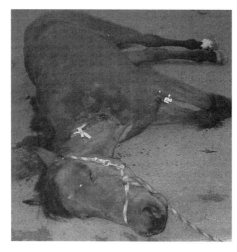

Fig. 4. After collapsing, the filly remained recumbent and unresponsive for 3 hours. Vital parameters remained within normal limits.

had been some reaction to the butorphanol). The source and dosage of butorphanol administered was rechecked and considered appropriate.

Several of the differentials could cause an increase in the intracranial pressure resulting in obtundation and immobility. The filly's collapse was not attributed to the butorphanol, but, because the cause of the obtundation and semicomatose state was uncertain, further sedatives were withheld for the next 2 hours. In hindsight, more aggressive analgesic therapy (additional butorphanol [up to 0.1 mg/kg] or morphine [0.3–0.66 mg/kg intravenously with xylazine to prevent excitement], or even a morphine/lidocaine/ketamine infusion) was warranted. Because the filly had already received 2 g of phenylbutazone every 12 hours for the last 4 days, including a dose that morning before referral, administration of additional NSAIDs was contraindicated until renal function could be assessed (results of urinalysis and serum biochemistry were still pending).

The filly's immobility enabled rapid lumbosacral cerebrospinal fluid collection for cytology and culture. Risk of general anesthesia for atlanto-occipital cerebrospinal fluid collection was unjustified. Equipment was not readily available in this emergency situation to measure intracranial pressure. A right lateral radiograph of the cervical spine was taken. No evidence of cervical vertebral canal stenosis, osteoarthritis, osteomyelitis, or fracture was observed radiographically, but a second irregular marginated region of gas lucency dorsal to C5 was seen (Fig. 5). External evidence of this gas filled abscess was undetectable.

Ultrasonographic imaging of the left cervical musculature caudal to the previously drained abscess was performed. A large 12 cm by 5 cm by 3 cm hyperechoic free-gas cavitating area was observed 20 cm caudal to the

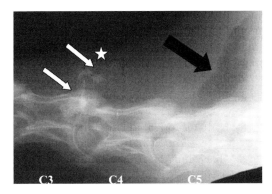

Fig. 5. Right lateral radiograph of the cervical spine after draining the abscess at the level of C3-C4 and placement of two Penrose drains (*white arrows*). The site of the prior vaccination is marked with a star. A large, gas-filled, previously undetected abscess is present dorsal to C5 (*black arrow*).

previously drained abscess. The new caudal abscess was located 5 cm deep to the skin. Before drainage, the skin was blocked with lidocaine (10 mL subcutaneously distributed in four sites). Ultrasound-guided aspiration using an 18-gauge spinal needle, 60-cm^3 syringe, and three-way stopcock obtained 500 mL of pungent gas and 200 mL of serosanguinous fluid with fibrin clots before surgical drainage and placement of two more Penrose drains. No other abscesses were detected by thorough ultrasonographic reexamination of the uppermost right facial, cervical, and thoracic musculature. It was uncertain if the second abscess communicated with the spinal canal, leading to possible meningitis, extradural cord compression, or disruption of cerebrospinal fluid flow leading to increased intracranial pressure. The reason for the filly's recumbency and immobility was still considered uncertain.

The results of the complete blood cell count (Table 1) revealed a very mild leukocytosis with a mature neutrophilia and monocytosis consistent with infection, inflammation, or a stress leukogram. Elevation of the acute phase protein fibrinogen and the presence of reactive lymphocytes were attributed to the myonecrotic abscesses. The results of the serum biochemical profile (Table 2) indicated an elevated alkaline phosphatase of 390 IU/L (reference range: 80–187), which was considered of minor significance, with biliary obstruction unlikely because the gamma-glutamyltransferase was normal. There was no reason for the intestinal isoform of alkaline phosphatase to be elevated, but alkaline phosphatase release from activated neutrophils or osteoblasts in metabolically active bone was possible because of the location of the abscess over the cervical vertebrae. The slightly elevated unconjugated bilirubin (3.0 mg/dL; reference range: 0.6–1.8) was probably caused by inappetence because there was no hemolysis, and with normal sorbitol dehydrogenase and gamma-glutamyltransferase, hepatic and posthepatic causes were unlikely. Absorbed bacteria or toxins from necrotic muscle could cause liver damage, but significant liver disease was not

Table 1
Hematology

Value	Day 1	Day 3	Reference values
Packed cell volume (%)	37	40	37–52
Red blood cell count ($\times 10^{12}$/L)	9.2		5.1–10.0
MCV fl	44		43–55
MCHC (g/dL)	35.8		34.4–36.9
White blood cells ($\times 10^9$/L)	11.4		4.7–10.6
Band neutrophils ($\times 10^9$/L)	0		0- 0.1
Seg. neutrophils ($\times 10^9$/L)	7.1		2.4–6.4
Lymphocytes ($\times 10^9$/L)	3.3		1.0–4.9
Monocytes ($\times 10^9$/L)	1.0		0–0.5
Leukocyte morphology	Reactive lymphocytes		
Platelets ($\times 10^9$/L)	151		125–310
Fibrinogen (mg/dL)	985		193–422

Abbreviations: MCHC, mean corpuscular hemoglobin concentration; MCV, mean corpuscular volume.

considered present. Aspartate aminotransferase (AST) was mildly elevated (487 IU/L; reference range: 170–370) and is a nonspecific indicator of tissue necrosis, but in conjunction with elevated creatine kinase (1190 IU/L; reference range: 150–360), myonecrosis was the likely cause. Elevations in creatine kinase and AST were minimal considering the degree of myonecrosis. Urinalysis was normal (Table 3) other than a trace of protein (30 mg/dL) that was detected by urine dipstick. Urine protein was not directly measured, but trace dipstick protein is normal in concentrated alkaline urine. With normal serum albumin, glomerular loss of albumin was an unlikely explanation. Catecholamine and glucocorticoid release from stress and pain could explain the mild hyperglycemia (glucose = 130 mg/dL; reference range: 83–114). Normal vital signs and minimal laboratory abnormalities were inconsistent with septic shock, toxemia, endotoxemia, or dehydration.

The rapid progression of abscess formation and severe tissue swelling after intramuscular injection with identification of large, gas-producing, spore-forming, gram-positive rods led to the presumptive diagnosis of clostridial myositis. Filamentous gram-positive organisms are not typical of clostridia, but in the opinion of the microbiologist they were probably clostridial organisms lacking septa because of inhibited cell wall synthesis that occurred as a result of penicillin concentrations below mean inhibitory concentration or in the absence of an essential nutrient within the abscess environment.

Treatment

Intravenous penicillin-G (20,000–60,000 IU/kg every 2–4 hours intravenously, then at a reduced dose for several weeks) is the recommended treatment for clostridial infections [1]. Although penicillin treatment, with and

Table 2
Serum biochemistry

Value	Day 1	Day 2	Day 4	Reference values
Serum urea nitrogen (mg/dL)	13	13	25	13–27
Creatinine (mg/dL)	1.7	1.4	1.7	0.8–1.7
Alkaline phosphatase (IU/L)	390			80–187
Aspartate aminotransferase (IU/L)	487			170–370
SDH (IU/L)	7.2			4–13
Creatine phosphokinase (IU/L)	1190			150–360
Total bilirubin (mg/dL)	3.0			0.6–1.8
Direct bilirubin (mg/dL)	0.1			0.1- 0.5
Glucose (mg/dL)	130			83–114
Sodium (mEq/L)	139	142	138	132–142
Potassium (mEq/L)	3.7	4.3	3.9	2.4–4.6
Chloride (mEq/L)	97	104	99	97–105
Calcium (mg/dL)	12.0	11.9	11.5	11.1–13.0
Phosphorus (mg/dL)	3.2	4.8	4.2	1.2–4.8
Bicarbonate (mEq/L)	27	21	22	21–31
Osmolality (mOsmol/kg)	280			266–286
Total protein (g/dL)	6.5	6.5		6.4–7.9
Albumin (g/dL)	2.9	2.8	2.8	2.8–3.6
Globulin (g/dL)	3.6	3.7		3.6–4.3
Cholesterol (mg/dL)	96			51–97
Venous pH	7.422			7.32–7.45
P_vO_2 (mm Hg)	39			24–39
P_vCO_2 (mm Hg)	43.4			34–53
vHCO$_3$ (mEq/L)	27.8			23–31
Total vCO$_2$ mEq/L	29.1			24–32
Venous base excess (mEq/L)	3.3			−1–5.0

Abbreviations: P_vCO_2, partial pressure of carbon dioxide, vein; P_vO_2, partial pressure of oxygen, vein; SDH, sorbitol dehydrogenase; vCO$_2$, venous carbon dioxide; vHCO$_3$, venous bicarbonate.

without surgical fenestration, has resulted in survival, mortality from gas gangrene is high in horses [1]. Experimentally, penicillin is a poor antibiotic choice, being noncurative with frequent relapse and death [4,5]. In a murine *C perfringens* gas gangrene model, clindamycin, metronidazole, rifampin, and tetracycline were all more effective treatments than penicillin, which resulted in survival rates no different than untreated controls [5]. Protein synthesis inhibitor–antimetabolite antibiotics suppressed clostridial toxin production, whereas *C perfringens* alpha toxin production increased in the presence of penicillin [4]. Tetracycline and metronidazole are standard treatment for clostridial myositis at The Ohio State University, being inexpensive, safe, and anecdotally more efficacious. Treatment with oxytetracycline (6.6 mg/kg intravenously every 24 hours in 500 mL 0.9% NaCl) and metronidazole (20 mg/kg per rectum for two doses, then by mouth every 6 hours) was commenced. The daily cost was $16/day, compared with $360/day for 60,000 IU of penicillin-G potassium administered every 4 hours. Finances were limited in this case. Because cardiovascular parameters seemed stable, analgesia was

Table 3
Urinalysis

Value	Day 1	Day 3	Day 4 (on intravenous fluids)	Day 5 (on oral fluids)	Day 7	Reference values
Source (eg, catheter or free catch)	free catch	catheter	catheter	free catch	free catch	
Color	yellow	yellow	light yellow	light yellow	yellow	yellow
Appearance	opaque	opaque	slightly opaque	slightly opaque	opaque	opaque
Specific gravity	1.045	1.050	1.015	1.018	1.030	1.020–1.050
pH	8.0	8.0	8.0	8.5	8.0	7.5–9.0
Protein (mg/dL)	30	30	< 30	< 30	< 30	< 30
Glucose	negative	negative	negative	negative	negative	negative
Acetone	negative	negative	negative	negative	negative	negative
Bilirubin	negative	negative	negative	negative	negative	negative
Blood	negative	1 +	negative	negative	negative	negative
Casts						
Hyaline casts	negative	1–2 /LPF	1 cast/slide	few casts	negative	negative
Granular casts	negative	negative	negative	negative	negative	negative
Other casts	negative	negative	negative	negative	negative	negative
Leucocytes/HPF	6–8	4–5	0–1	0–1	0–1	0–10
Epithelial cells/HPF	2–4	3–5	2–3	0–2	0–1	0–5
Erythrocytes/HPF	4–5	4–5	2–3	0–1	0–1	0–5
Crystals	CaCO$_3$, Ca oxalate	CaCO$_3$, Ca oxalate			CaCO$_3$, Ca oxalate	CaCO$_3$, Ca oxalate Ca phosphate
Bacteria	negative	not seen	not seen	not seen	not seen	negative
Other	lots of mucus	lots of mucus				mucus

provided with butorphanol (0.01 mg/kg intravenously every 4 hours for 72 hours).

The filly was still recumbent and unresponsive. The severe eyelid swelling prevented any assessment of eye expression or ocular reflexes, which made assessment of mentation difficult. The filly certainly had severe clostridial myositis, which is a very painful condition that can result in systemic toxemia. Because vital parameters (heart rate, palpable pulse pressure, respiratory rate, rectal temperature, and vulval mmc) had remained within normal limits, systemic toxemia seemed unlikely. With possible elevated intracranial pressure, DMSO (1 g/kg in 5 L lactated Ringer's solution intravenously) and 3% hypertonic saline (60 mL/kg/day over 12 hours) were given. Ideally, the definitive cause of obtundation should have been determined before empiric therapy, but osmotic effects of DMSO and hypertonic saline may have helped reduce the facial edema. DMSO also has anti-inflammatory, anti-ischemic, antibacterial, and analgesic effects.

Nursing care and case management

Several clinicians believed the filly should be euthanized, but with the owners' permission the filly was transported on a down-horse skid to a heavily bedded stall. The head was elevated 30° and hourly cold-packing was performed to reduce facial edema. The filly was unresponsive for 2 more hours; then she suddenly stood, drank water (osmoreceptor stimulation from hypertonic saline), and looked for food! The collapse and immobility were attributed to severe pain from compression of the second abscess by head elevation during endoscopy. No other explanation could be determined. Overnight, the head was kept elevated by tethering the horse using a padded halter to an overhead wire for periods of 90 minutes followed by 30 minutes untethered.

Day 2

By the following morning, 60% of the edema had resolved. The eyes were visible, cranial nerve examination was normal, and there was no corneal uptake of fluorescein stain. The filly was still depressed and moved stiffly but was markedly improved. Meningitis was considered unlikely because cerebrospinal fluid cytology, cell count, and protein were normal (Table 4), and culture was subsequently negative. The 3% hypertonic saline was replaced by intravenous lactated Ringer's solution (60 mL/kg/day, 1 L/hour).

By afternoon, only 10% of the facial edema remained. The tracheostomy tube was removed. Selected serum chemistry profile (see Table 2) indicated normal renal parameters (serum urea nitrogen and creatinine) and electrolyte concentrations (despite the 3% NaCl). The filly's measured water intake was normal (28 L in 24 hours), and the intravenous fluids were discontinued. The filly's neck was still very painful, so phenylbutazone (2.2 mg/kg by

Table 4
Cerebrospinal fluid cytology (day 1)

Characteristic	Reference	Day 1
Source of specimen		lumbosacral
Color before centrifugation	colorless	colorless
Clarity before centrifugation	clear	clear
Cerebrospinal fluid protein (mg/dL)	20–80	55
White blood cells/μL	0–5	2
Red blood cells/μL	0–5	0
Neutrophils (%)	0	0
Monocytes or macrophages (%)	~30%	24
Small lymphocytes (%)	~70%	76
Eosinophils (%)	0	0
Other (%)	0	No cytologic abnormalities

mouth every 12 hours) was administered. The neck was evaluated by ultrasound daily, the fenestrated area was hot-packed, and wounds were flushed with 1% povidone iodine every 8 hours.

Day 3

The filly was more depressed. Water intake (5 L in 12 hours) and appetite were reduced. Urinalysis (see Table 3) revealed a slight proteinuria (pH = 8), moderate occult blood with few red blood cells, rare hyaline casts, and hypersthenuria (urine specific gravity = 1.050). Renal concentrating function was appropriate for the mild dehydration caused by the reduced water intake. In concentrated alkaline urine, there is often a false-positive protein detected by dipstick analysis. Differentials for pigmenturia include myoglobinuria from myonecrosis (day 1 creatine kinase and AST were only mildly elevated), hemoglobinuria caused by hemolysis from DMSO, or immune-mediated hemolysis as is occasionally reported with clostridial infections. There was no gross pigmenturia or pink plasma, and PCV was 40%, so further investigation was not performed. The few red blood cells, pigmenturia, and cylindruria may indicate early tubular damage. Hyaline casts (Tamm-Horsfall mucoprotein precipitation) occur with hyperosmolarity, decreased tubular flow, pigmenturia, tubular damage, or glomerular disease. Decreased renal blood flow occurs with dehydration, and inhibition of prostaglandin E_2 and prostaglandin I_2 by NSAIDs leads to further reduction in renal perfusion, which can cause ischemic medullary or papillary necrosis. Ischemia and nephrotoxins (aminoglycosides, NSAIDs, myoglobin, hemoglobin, mercury, vitamin D or K_3) can lead to acute tubular necrosis. The cylindruria, maximized urine specific gravity with coincident reduced water intake, and the risk of drug nephrosis were of concern. To allow NSAIDs to be given safely, treatment with intravenous lactated Ringer's solution (90 mL/kg/day, intravenously, 1.5 L/hour) was commenced. Treatment with phenylbutazone was discontinued, and flunixin meglumine (0.5 mg/kg intravenously every 12 hours for 6 days), being a safer NSAID, was commenced.

Day 4

The filly was quiet and alert. Other than a single hyaline cast (which can be normal), the renal serum chemistry and urinalysis were normal (see Tables 2, 3). Isotonic maintenance oral electrolyte solution (21 L of water with 10 g NaCl, 15 g NaHCO$_3$, 75 g KCl, and 60 g KH$_2$PO$_4$ added) at 90 mL/kg/day was administered through an 8-mm diameter nasoesophageal feeding tube. Intravenous fluid therapy was discontinued because finances were now limited.

Day 5

The filly looked brighter. There were a few casts detected on urinalysis (see Table 3). Ultrasonographic imaging of the neck was performed using a 3.5-MHz sector scanner and a 5-MHz linear scanner. A loculated pocket of fluid 2 cm from the skin surface, approximately 6 cm in diameter, was observed 8 cm from the caudal-most Penrose drain. After the skin was blocked with lidocaine (7 mL subcutaneously), ventral drainage was established, and a Penrose drain was placed between the previous site and new incision. There was still potential for osteomyelitis because of the proximity of the abscess cavity to transverse vertebral processes.

Days 6 through 8

The filly was drinking, and there was resolution of renal casts (see Table 3). Supplemental oral fluids were discontinued. The neurologic examination was normal, but neck pain was still present. The cranial incisions had healed. On day 7, urinalysis was normal. On day 8, treatment with oxytetracycline was discontinued, and treatment with doxycycline (10 mg/kg by mouth, every 12 hours for 5 days) was commenced. The metronidazole was continued for a further 5 days. The filly was discharged with orders for wound flushing every 12 hours and for the Penrose drain to be removed by the referring veterinarian after 2 days.

Day 12

The owner reported that the vital signs and attitude were normal, and the wound discharge was minimal.

Day 40

The filly returned to training and was racing 6 months later.

Discussion

Clostridial myositis results from a rapidly progressive necrosis of muscle from infection with clostridial organisms, often with fatal consequences. The majority of equine cases are iatrogenic secondary to intramuscular injections or as a result of direct contamination of deep wounds with bacterial growth in an anaerobic environment. The most common injected substances associated with clostridial myositis in horses include flunixin meglumine, xylazine, antihistamines, vaccines, dipyrone, prostaglandin $F_2\alpha$, ivermectin, and B-complex vitamins [1]. Infection results in local inflammation, often with severe pain and swelling, and can progress to a state of systemic inflammatory response with fever, depression, tachycardia, progressive toxemic shock, disseminated intravascular coagulation, and death. There is often rapid progression, and in severe cases, even with early and aggressive therapy, a guarded-to-poor prognosis should be given.

Malignant edema, clostridial myositis/cellulitis/fasciitis, and gas gangrene are a continuum of conditions caused by infection of the subcutis, fascia, or muscle [2]. There is often fulminant tissue necrosis, with disintegration of tissue and serosanguinous exudate with bubbles of gas or free gas caused by infection with gas-producing anaerobic clostridial organisms.

The pathogens

C perfringens, C septicum, C chauvoei, C fallax, C sordelli, and *C novyi* are the principal pathogens [1,6,7]. They are large gram-positive, obligatory anaerobic rods that are ubiquitous in the soil and environment. They are also commensals of the skin, oral cavity, and intestinal tract. There is also evidence for the presence of dormant clostridial spores in equine skeletal muscle [8]. Clostridial organisms form spores, which allow the organism to survive until germination and growth can occur. Germination of spores and vegetative growth occurs in suitable anaerobic conditions.

Clinical signs

In acute cases, animals may be found recumbent or dead. Painful muscular swellings, often with crepitus, may be felt. The overlying skin may initially be hot and inflamed but becomes cool and insensitive with progressive necrosis. If systemic toxemia occurs, the horse will become profoundly depressed and show signs of systemic inflammatory response (tachycardia, tachypnea, fever, and leukocytosis or leukopenia) [6].

The extent of tissue necrosis and surrounding edema can be observed ultrasonographically. A distinction between edema and cellulitis can sometimes be difficult. Edema is characteristically located in the subcutaneous tissue, dissects along tissue planes, and is anechoic and loculated in appearance. Cellulitis usually appears as an echogenic, homogeneous thickening of the subcutaneous tissues, also dissecting along tissue planes. Sometimes hypoechoic pockets are seen in an area of cellulitis, but loculations are not typically seen. In anaerobic infections, gas shadowing is often observed.

Aspiration of nonclotting, malodorous fluid (with or without gas) is typical. Volatile fatty acids are produced by anaerobes such as the gram-negative *Fusobacterium* or *Bacteroides* rods, gram-positive *Peptococcus* and *Peptostreptococcus* cocci, gram-positive spore-forming *Clostridium* spp. rods or non–spore-forming *Propionibacterium* and *Eubacterium* gram-positive rods. Gram's stain can provide a presumptive diagnosis of clostridial myositis with the detection of large gram-positive rods, with or without spores [9]. Anaerobic (and aerobic) culture is also recommended. Direct fluorescent antibody stains can be used for definitive diagnosis of some clostridial species, but this test is limited in its availability [9].

Clinicopathologic changes are nonspecific. Muscle enzyme activities are usually moderately elevated but often not to the extent expected for the degree of myonecrosis present [10]. Changes typical of septic–toxic conditions include leukocytosis or leukopenia, often with elevation of the band neutrophil count and fibrinogen concentration. There may be hyperproteinemia with a long-standing walled-off abscess, but more typically hypoproteinemia occurs because of exudative losses into the necrotic tissue. With the development of toxic shock, there is hemoconcentration, azotemia, and often coagulopathies with thrombocytopenia and disseminated intravascular coagulation. Rarely, there is anemia from autoimmune-mediated anemia secondary to antibody formation against red blood cells originating from an immune response against the clostridial antigens [11,12].

Treatment and prognosis

Intravenous penicillin-G (20,000 to 60,000 IU/kg every 2–4 hours intravenously, then at a reduced dose for several weeks) is the historically recommended treatment for clostridial infections [1,2]. Although penicillin treatment, with and without surgical fenestration, has resulted in survival, mortality with gas gangrene is unacceptably high. Some authors give only a 25% chance of survival [1]. Of 38 cases of clostridial myositis in horses reported in the literature before 2001, only 12 survived [6]. A recent retrospective study reported a survival rate of 73% for all cases of clostridial myositis, with a slightly higher survival rate of 81% for cases infected with *C perfringens* [3]. Experimentally, in rodent models of gas gangrene, penicillin was found to be a poor antibiotic choice, being noncurative with frequent relapse and death [5]. In a murine *C perfringens* gas gangrene model, clindamycin, metronidazole, rifampin, and tetracycline were all more effective than penicillin, which had survival rates no different from those in untreated controls [5]. Of these antibiotics, tetracycline, rifampin, and metronidazole can be safely administered to horses. Protein synthesis inhibitor–antimetabolite antibiotics suppressed clostridial toxin production, whereas *C perfringens* alpha toxin production continued in the presence of penicillin [4]. Based on treatment of about 20 cases (at The Ohio State University and Auburn University), tetracycline and metronidazole are the standard treatments for clostridial myositis, being inexpensive, safe, and anecdotally more efficacious. The author and colleagues' approximate combined success rate would be higher than 80% using metronidazole and oxytetracycline. Dosages are variable: oxytetracycline (6.6 mg/kg) can be given intravenously every 12–24 hours in 500 mL 0.9% NaCl, and metronidazole (20 mg/kg) can be given by mouth every 6 hours, or 15 mg/kg can be given intravenously every 6 hours). The author tends to use the twice-per-day oxytetracycline dose and initially one dose of intravenous metronidazole. The daily cost is approximately now $30/day, compared with more than $400/day for 60,000 IU penicillin-G potassium given every 4 hours. Although definitive experimental efficacy trials have not been performed in the horse, anecdotal evidence suggests that this alternative therapy is safe, is as efficacious, if not more so, than penicillin, and certainly is more economic. Long-term antibiotic therapy is essential, and horses are discharged on metronidazole and doxycycline (10 mg/kg every 12 hours) for a total of 10 to 25 days of antibiotic therapy.

Wound fenestration to allow oxygenation of the anaerobic necrotic environment and drainage of exudates is generally recommended [2,6,7]. Extensive skin sloughing may occur if skin viability is lost. Often, limb wounds result in massive swelling, with the entire leg expanding to three times its normal diameter. The massive swelling of tissues causes pressure necrosis and loss of vascular supply to overlying skin, resulting in skin sloughing. With neck infections, edema fluid and sometimes dissemination of the infection spreads ventrally, resulting in pectoral, thoracic, and even limb edema. If the head is held low because of neck pain or depression, severe head edema can occur, often resulting in airway obstruction. Tracheostomy may be required [13]. Cold-hosing or cold-packing of the surrounding tissue can help with the resolution of edema. Hyperbaric oxygen therapy involves the exposure of affected tissues to increased concentrations of oxygen under pressure and has been used in dogs and humans to treat clostridial infections. Hyperbaric oxygen chambers for horses now are available at a number of institutions.

Clostridial myositis can be a rapidly progressing and life-threatening condition. The author has seen one horse present in severe distress with purple mucus membranes, heart rate above 120 beats per minute, and with entire body crepitus 12 hours after vaccination. Another case died from disseminated intravascular coagulation 36 hours after a vitamin B_{12} injection. In other cases, the myositis has been controlled, but the animals have died from hemolytic anemia. With rapid treatment, when signs of systemic toxemia are minimal, the prognosis can be good with aggressive medical and surgical therapy.

References

[1] Moore RM. Pathogenesis of obligate anaerobic bacterial infections in horses. Compend Contin Ed Pract Vet 1993;15(2):278–87.

[2] Perdrizet JA, Callihan DR, Rebhun WC, et al. Successful management of malignant edema caused by Clostridium septicum in a horse. Cornell Vet 1987;77:328–38.

[3] Peek SF, Semrad SD, Perkins GA. Clostridial myonecrosis in horses (37 cases 1985–2000). Equine Vet J 2003;35(1):86–92.

[4] Stevens DL, Maier KA, Mitten JE. Effect of antibiotics on toxin production and viability of Clostridium perfringens. Antimicrob Agents Chemother 1987;31(2):213–8.

[5] Stevens DL, Maier KA, Laine BM, et al. Comparison of clindamycin, rifampin, tetracycline, metronidazole and penicillin for efficacy in prevention of experimental gas gangrene due to Clostridum perfringens. J Infect Dis 1987;155(2):220–8.

[6] Jeanes LV, Magdesian KG, Madigan JE, et al. Clostridial myositis in horses. Comp Contin Educ Pract Vet 2001;23(6):577–87.

[7] Peek SF, Semrad SD. Clostridial myonecrosis in horses. Equine Vet Educ 2002;14(3):163–8.

[8] Vengust M, et al. Preliminary evidence for dormant clostridial spores in equine skeletal muscle. Equine Vet J 2003;35(5):514–6.

[9] Topley WWC. Clostridium: the spore-bearing anaerobes. In: Collier L, Balows A, Sussman M, editors. Microbiology and microbial infections. London: Oxford University Press; 1998. p. 731–55.

[10] Rebhun WC, Shin SJ, King JM, et al. Malignant edema in horses. J Am Vet Med Assoc 1985; 187(7):732–6.

[11] Reef VB. Clostridium perfringens cellulitis and immune-mediated hemolytic anemia in a horse. J Am Vet Med Assoc 1983;182(3):251–4.

[12] Weiss DJ, Moritz A. Equine immune-mediated hemolytic anemia associated with Clostridium perfringens infection. Vet Clin Pathol 2003;32(1):22–6.

[13] Brehaus BA, Brown CM, Scott EA, et al. Clostridial muscle infections following intramuscular injections in the horse. Equine Vet Sci 1983;3(2):42–6.

ELSEVIER
SAUNDERS

VETERINARY
CLINICS
Equine Practice

Vet Clin Equine 22 (2006) 145–156

Polysaccharide Storage Myopathy in a 4-Year-Old Holsteiner Gelding

Jennifer M. MacLeay, DVM, PhD

*Department of Clinical Sciences, Colorado State University, 300 West Drake Road,
Fort Collins, CO 80523, USA*

A 4-year-old Holsteiner gelding used for dressage and trained to first level had a history of exercise-associated muscle cramping that occurred 4 to 5 weeks before presentation. The horse was dewormed every 8 weeks, most recently 4 weeks ago with ivermectin, and was vaccinated for eastern and western equine encephalitis, tetanus, influenza, and rhinopneumonitis 12 weeks previously. The horse was exercised for approximately 1 hour 5 days a week and was turned into a small paddock for 4 hours 3 days a week. The gelding is fed a free-choice grass/alfalfa hay mix and a total of 2 kg of sweet feed twice daily. Muscle cramping was also reported to have occurred multiple times in the past. At the time of the most recent episode of muscle cramping, the referring veterinarian confirmed muscle damage (rhabdomyolysis) by documenting elevations in serum levels of creatine kinase (CK) and aspartate aminotransferase (AST), although the exact values were not known by the horse's owner. After the first episode, the horse was stall rested for several days and attempts were made to reintroduce it to work; however, each time, it had another episode of muscle cramping. The horse was presented for evaluation and therapeutic options.

Physical examination

On physical examination, temperature and heart and respiratory rates were within reference limits. Auscultation of the heart, lungs, and intestinal tract failed to detect any abnormalities. Visual inspection of the horse revealed no asymmetry of the major muscle groups, but a slightly smaller profile of the right biceps femoris was noted. Deep palpation of the muscles

Adapted from MacLeay JM. Polysaccharide storage myopathy in a Holsteiner horse. Vet Forum 2005;22:46–51; with permission.

E-mail address: jmacleay@colostate.edu

of the neck, back, and hind limbs was within normal limits. Manipulation of the neck revealed good flexibility, and the horse demonstrated no pain or discomfort in response to palpation. A neurologic examination was performed, and no abnormalities were noted. Observation of the horse at the walk and trot in a straight line and on a 20-m circle on a longe line in both directions on concrete revealed no evidence of lameness or neurologic deficits.

Case assessment

Causes of poor performance include lameness, neurologic disease, upper airway obstruction, lower airway disease, and myopathies. No evidence of lameness was seen on the initial evaluation, and it had not been reported by the owner or referring veterinarian. Neurologic causes of poor performance include cervical vertebral malformation or instability, trauma to the central nervous system or peripheral nerves, vestibular disease, equine herpes myelitis, equine motor neuron disease, and equine protozoal myelitis. Neurologic abnormalities were ruled out on the basis of the neurologic examination.

Common upper airway obstructions include intermittent dorsal displacement of the soft palate, epiglottal entrapment, arytenoid chondritis, dynamic pharyngeal collapse, space-occupying lesions (eg, ethmoid hematoma, cyst), space-occupying lesions of the sinuses with deformation of the nasal passage, tumors of the nasal passage or sinuses, and left laryngeal hemiplegia. No evidence of inspiratory or expiratory stridor was found on the initial evaluation, and there was no history of exercise-associated respiratory noise or cough. Lower airway respiratory diseases, including pneumonia and reactive airway disease, were ruled out on the basis of lack of cough and lack of increased respiratory rate or respiratory distress associated with exercise.

Myopathies associated with decreased performance include infectious (eg, clostridial myositis; sarcocystis infection; other bacterial infections, including but not limited to staphylococcal or streptococcal infections; viral), autoimmune streptococcal-related myositis, acute traumatic injury (eg, muscle strain), fibrosis of muscle caused by chronic traumatic injury (fibrotic myopathy), vitamin E or selenium deficiency (equine motor neuron disease), malnutrition, and exertional rhabdomyolysis ("tying up") (Box 1). Acute muscle strains and fibrosis of muscle secondary to trauma result in consistent alterations of gait and were unlikely in this case based on the lack of lameness (Box 2). The chronicity of the disorder and overall health of the horse argued against a diagnosis of autoimmune and infectious myositis or malnutrition. The most likely diagnosis at this time was chronic exertional rhabdomyolysis based on the clinical history and the absence of another abnormality on examination.

Procedures

Between episodes of exertional rhabdomyolysis, horses appear without obvious abnormalities; therefore, a standardized protocol to document exertional rhabdomyolysis was followed. The initial evaluation included a complete blood cell count (CBC), serum chemistry profile, urinalysis, serum vitamin E concentration, and triiodothyronine (T3) and thyroxine (T4) levels as well as calculation of fractional excretions of sodium, chloride, and potassium. Fractional excretions were calculated as follows based on values obtained from urine chemistry and serum chemistry, where collection of each was taken at the same time:

$$\text{Fractional clearance} = \frac{\text{Urine [X]}}{\text{Serum [X]}} \times \frac{\text{Serum [Cr]}}{\text{Urine [Cr]}} \times 100$$
$$X = \text{Na, Cl or K concentration}$$
$$\text{Cr} = \text{Creatinine Concentration}$$

where X indicates sodium, chloride, or potassium concentration, and Cr indicates creatinine concentration.

In addition, a standardized exercise test and muscle biopsy of the middle gluteal and right biceps femoris muscles were performed.

Laboratory results revealed normal values for the CBC, serum vitamin E concentration, T3 and T4 levels, urinalysis, and fractional excretions of electrolytes (Table 1). Serum chemistry demonstrated elevated CK and AST activity (CK = 3021 U/L, normal: 100–470 U/L; AST = 550 U/L, normal: 185–375 U/L). CK is a muscle-specific enzyme, whereas AST can be released into the circulation in response to liver or muscle damage. The half-life of CK in the horse is brief, approximately 90 minutes, and peaks approximately 4 to 6 hours after muscle insult, provided that the insult is not ongoing. AST has a longer half-life, approximately 24 hours. In the absence of elevations of enzymes specific for liver damage, such as gamma-glutamyltransferase (GGT) and sorbitol dehydrogenase (SDH), muscle damage was the likely cause for the elevation in AST. The horse was stabled overnight to negate any adverse effects of transport to the hospital. Horses recently transported may have mild elevations in CK activity. In this author's experience, the elevation in CK activity is still typically less than 1000 U/L in healthy horses. On the second day of hospitalization, a standardized exercise test was performed. The test consisted of taking a baseline serum CK, followed by 15 minutes of exercise on a longe line at a trot. A second CK level was measured 4 hours after the exercise test. The CK activity before exercise was 1870 U/L, and the CK activity after exercise was 4640 U/L. Similar exercise tests performed by horses without a history of exertional rhabdomyolysis show elevations of CK of less than 200 U/L in the author's experience. After the 4-hour blood draw, a muscle biopsy was taken at a standard site and depth from the middle gluteal

Box 1. Classification of equine myopathies according to etiology

1. Neurogenic: may be hereditary or environmental in origin, acquired or congenital
   a. Disorders of anterior horn cells
   b. Disorders of motor nerve roots
   c. Peripheral neuropathies
   d. Disorders of neuromuscular transmission
      i. Botulism
      ii. Tetanus
2. Myogenic
   a. Traumatic
      i. Fibrotic myopathy
      ii. Gastrocnemius muscle rupture
      iii. Serratus ventralis muscle rupture
   b. Inflammatory
      i. Sore or "pulled" muscles
   c. Infectious
      i. Bacterial
         (1) Clostridial myositis
         (2) Streptococcal species
            (a) Abscessation
            (b) Autoimmune
               (i) Purpura hemorrhagica
               (ii) IgG mediated
               (iii) IgA mediated (Henoch-Schönlein purpura)
         (3) Staphylococcal species
         (4) *Corynebacterium* pseudotuberculosis
      ii. Viral
      iii. Parasitic
         (1) Sarcocystis
         (2) *Trichinella spiralis*
   d. Toxic
      i. *Cassia occidentalis*
      ii. White snake root
      iii. Ionophores
   e. Hormonal
      i. Hypothyroidism (unsubstantiated)
   f. Circulatory
      i. Postanesthetic myositis
      ii. Aortic-iliac thrombosis

g. Genetic
  i. Mitochondrial enzyme deficiencies
  ii. Glycogen branching enzyme deficiency
  iii. Myotonias
    (1) Hyperkalemic periodic paralysis
    (2) Myotonia congenita
    (3) Myotonia dystrophica
  iv. Glycogen storage disorders
    (1) Polysaccharide storage myopathy in Quarter Horses
    (2) Equine polysaccharide storage myopathy in draught horses
  v. Recurrent exertional rhabdomyolysis in Thoroughbred horses
h. Nutritional
  i. Vitamin E
    (1) Equine motor neuron disease
    (2) Equine degenerative myelopathy
  ii. Selenium
  iii. Malnutrition
  iv. Carbohydrate overloading
  v. Thiamine deficiency
  vi. Electrolyte deficiency
i. Exercise-related, overexertion and the exhausted horse syndrome
j. Cachectic atrophy secondary to chronic disease
k. Disuse atrophy
l. Malignancy: muscle tumors
m. Miscellaneous or idiopathic
  i. Atypical myoglobinuria
  ii. Polymyopathy

Modified from MacLeay JM. Disorders of the muscular system. In: Reed S, Bayly W, Sellon D, editors. Equine internal medicine. Philadelphia: WB Saunders; 2003. p. 477.

muscle using a 6-mm modified Bergstrom needle. If this specialized needle is not available, a 2-cm × 1-cm × 1-cm muscle biopsy of the semimembranosus muscle can be taken by open biopsy approximately 4 to 6 inches below the anus.

Evaluation of the muscle biopsy was done by frozen section at a veterinary neuromuscular laboratory specializing in equine muscle biopsies (University of Minnesota Neuromuscular Diagnostic Laboratory) and

Box 2. Problem-based approach to horses with muscle disease

1. Profound muscle cramping with exercise, "tying up" syndrome, elevated plasma/serum CK activity after exercise.
   a. Horses with underlying myopathy
      i. Recurrent exertional rhabdomyolysis in Thoroughbred horses
      ii. Polysaccharide storage myopathy of Quarter Horses
      iii. Equine polysaccharide storage myopathy of draught horses
      iv. Idiopathic chronic exertional rhabdomyolysis
      v. Mitochondrial myopathy
   b. Horses without underlying myopathy
      i. Overexertion
      ii. Vitamin E or selenium deficiency
      iii. Electrolyte depletion
2. Horses with altered gait but without underlying myopathy and without muscle cramping, with or without elevated CK
   a. Acute: muscle strain, sprain, tear
   b. Chronic: fibrotic myopathy
3. Muscle weakness
   a. Hyperkalemic periodic paralysis
   b. Myotonia congenita and dystrophica
   c. Equine motor neuron disease
   d. Equine polysaccharide storage myopathy in draught horses (demonstrate primarily weakness)
4. Muscle wasting
   a. Generalized, may be accompanied by mild elevations in CK activity
      i. Equine motor neuron disease
      ii. Streptococcal immune-mediated myositis, IgG mediated
      iii. Cachectic atrophy
      iv. Disuse atrophy
   b. Segmental
      i. Neurogenic
      ii. Disuse atrophy
      iii. Fibrotic myopathy
5. Acute rhabdomyolysis, swollen painful musculature, with or without recumbency, with or without death
   a. Severe acute exercise-related rhabdomyolysis as from 1a and 1b
   b. Malignant hyperthermia or postanesthetic myopathy
   c. Clostridial myositis

d. Sarcocystitis
e. Streptococcal immune-mediated myositis, Henoch-
Schönlein (IgA) purpura
f. Aortic-iliac thrombosis
g. Toxic plants
i. *Cassia occidentalis*
ii. White snake root
h. Ionophore toxicity
6. Disorders of the neonate
a. White muscle disease or nutritional
myodegeneration
b. Foal rhabdomyolysis
c. Glycogen branching enzyme deficiency
d. Arthrogryposis
7. Other miscellaneous disorders
a. Atypical myoglobinuria
b. Postanesthetic myasthenia
c. Polymyopathy
d. Abscesses
e. Tumors
Disorders are grouped according to similar clinical appearance.
Please note that no category is mutually exclusive. Disorders
are grouped by the most common clinical presentation. The
reader is directed to the text for more extensive discussion for
each disorder or disease.

Modified from MacLeay JM. Disorders of the muscular system. In: Reed S,
Bayly W, Sellon D, editors. Equine internal medicine. Philadelphia: WB Saunders;
2003. p. 478.

included periodic acid–Schiff (PAS) and hematoxylin and eosin stains. Histochemistry revealed damaged cells being removed by infiltrations of macrophages. Smaller cells with more centrally located nuclei were consistent with regenerating cells and previous muscle damage. Some cells had an abnormal amount of PAS-positive staining material in them. The staining pattern was identical to that documented in Quarter Horses with polysaccharide storage myopathy and human beings with glycogen storage disorders. Analysis of the material isolated from Quarter Horses has shown it to be an abnormal form of glycogen. There was no increase in fibrous tissue, and the blood vessels appeared normal. These findings were consistent with a diagnosis of polysaccharide storage myopathy (PSSM). Electromyography was not available for use on this patient but has been performed before and after exercise in individuals with documented PSSM. In these individuals, electromyographic abnormalities were not documented.

Table 1
Laboratory results

	Result	Normal range
Complete blood cell count		
Total white blood cell count	8700	5550–10,500
Neutrophil	5200	3000–7000
Lymphocyte	3100	1500–4000
Eosinophil	100	0–600
Monocyte	300	0–600
Total protein	6.6	5.8–7.8 g/dL
Packed cell volume	42	30–45%
Chemistry Profile		
BUN	22	5–28 mg/dL
Creatinine	1.7	0.7–1.8 mg/dL
Creatine kinase		100–470 IU/L
Presentation	3021	
Before-exercise	1870	
After-exercise	4640	
AST	550	185–375 IU/L
GGT	13	8–22 IU/L
SDH	8	0–12 IU/L
Sodium	137	130–142 mEq/L
Potassium	4.0	2.5–4.6 mEq/L
Chloride	101	95–108 mEq/L
Fibrinogen	300	0–400 g/dL
T3	46	27.9–67 ng/dL
T4	2.25	1.16–3.24 µg/dL
Serum vitamin E	2.1	Greater than 1.5 mg/mL
Urinary fractional excretion		
Sodium	35	0%–46%
Chloride	1.35	0.48%–1.64%
Potassium	54	23.9%–75%

Abbreviations: AST, aspartate aminotransferase; BUN, blood urea nitrogen; GGT, γ-glutamyltransferase; SDH, sorbitol dehydrogenase; T3, triiodothyronine; T4, thyroxine.

Discussion of differential diagnosis

Other causes of myopathy that were considered include bacterial and viral infection, sarcocystosis, trauma and nutritional myodegeneration because of vitamin E or selenium deficiency, sporadic exertional rhabdomyolysis, and the chronic exertional myopathies (including PSSM, recurrent exertional rhabdomyolysis [RER], and idiopathic exertional rhabdomyolysis) (Box 3).

Infectious myopathies are usually acute in onset and cause severe progressive muscle damage as in *Clostridium* spp– or *Streptococcus* spp– associated myositis. Streptococcal infections can be complicated by autoimmune reactions. These can lead to elevated CK concentrations secondary to vasculitis as in purpura hemorrhagica or can occur as the result of primary myositis that is IgG or IgA mediated [1]. These were ruled out based on the chronic history, physical examination findings, normal CBC results, and muscle biopsy findings.

Box 3. Differential diagnosis of chronic muscle cramping (or altered gait) and elevated serum creatine kinase activity in horses

1. PSSM in Quarter Horses, draft horses, and warmblood horses
2. RER in Thoroughbred horses
3. Idiopathic chronic exertional rhabdomyolysis
4. Chronic electrolyte deficiency
5. Repeated episodes of overexertion
6. Vitamin E deficiency/equine motor neuron disease
7. Mitochondrial myopathy (rare)

Mild stiffness has been associated with equine herpesvirus type 1 and equine influenza A2 infections. These were ruled out based on an adequate vaccination history, chronicity of signs, lack of upper respiratory tract signs, and normal CBC results. Animals heavily infested with *Sarcocystis* spp may also show muscle stiffness [2]. Sarcocystosis is an uncommon cause of myopathy. Sarcocystosis is usually seen in horses older than 8 years of age, which must be heavily infected to show clinical signs. This was ruled out based on the lack of organisms seen on muscle biopsy. Traumatic causes of myopathy include fibrotic and ossifying myopathy secondary to trauma or infection and compartment syndrome, which occurs in down animals. These were ruled out on the basis of history and physical examination.

Nutritional myodegeneration (white muscle disease) is associated with vitamin E or selenium deficiency, especially in the dam during gestation, and is typically diagnosed in young animals [3]. Animals with nutritional myodegeneration have signs that are recognized during the first months to year of life and have muscle weakness that progresses to stiffness as fibrosis occurs within the muscles. This was ruled out on the basis of the lack of weakness, lack of fibrosis in the muscle biopsy, and age of the horse.

Mature horses that consume a vitamin E–deficient diet can develop equine motor neuron disease because of chronic oxidative stress, leading to degeneration of peripheral nerves and primary myopathy [4–7]. Clinically, these horses have poor muscle mass, stand with a low head carriage and base narrow, and may have an elevated tail base. They can also have tremors when standing as opposed to when walking. This is because muscles rich in type I fibers are primarily affected and are most active in maintaining posture over the type II–rich muscles of locomotion. Horses may also have mild elevations in serum CK activity. Equine motor neuron disease was ruled out in this case because of the lack of tremors and normal muscle mass, stance, muscle biopsy, and serum vitamin E concentration.

Exercise-related myopathies occur in most breeds and may be sporadic or chronic, and muscle cramping is a common clinical presentation for horses with sporadic or chronic exertional rhabdomyolysis [8]. Sporadic myopathies are associated with a high plane of nutrition combined with increased exercise after several days of rest or may occur after exercise beyond the horse's level of fitness, leading to electrolyte depletion from excessive sweating and exhaustion. The horse presented here had a chronic history of muscle cramping after less than half an hour of exercise at a mild to moderate pace and thus was unlikely to have had repeated episodes of sporadic exertional rhabdomyolysis.

Chronic exertional rhabdomyolysis is characterized by muscle cramping in response to brief periods of exercise and is not associated with fitness level; therefore, it implies an underlying myopathy. Three forms have been described as causes for exercise-associated muscle cramping and elevated CK activity: PSSM, RER, and idiopathic chronic exertional rhabdomyolysis. RER has been described in Thoroughbreds and is characterized by muscle cramping during aerobic exercise. Affected horses are often described as having a nervous temperament, and episodes are associated with race or speed training, high grain intake, and exercise after a period of stall rest [9,10]. Muscle contractility testing supports that RER is likely caused by a defect in calcium regulation within the cell, resulting in increased sensitivity to caffeine and halothane-induced contraction and faster times to peak contraction and 50% relaxation [11,12]. Histopathologic examination reveals evidence of current or past rhabdomyolysis with macrophages removing damaged myofibers and centrally located nuclei in regenerated myofibers. PAS staining for glycogen is normal [13]. RER was ruled out in this case based on the breed and the results of the muscle biopsy.

Idiopathic exertional rhabdomyolysis is an open diagnosis in which the horse experiences multiple bouts of exercise-associated muscle cramping but the signalment and muscle biopsy do not support a diagnosis of RER or PSSM. Because of the limited knowledge about exertional myopathies in horses, a subset of horses cannot be firmly diagnosed. Typically, recommendations include management of these horses similar to cases with RER and PSSM to determine if the horse responds favorably. This open diagnosis was not necessary in this case, because the biopsy supported a diagnosis of PSSM.

PSSM has been described in Quarter Horses, draft horses, and warmblood breeds. It has been proposed that although storage of abnormal glycogen in myofibers is seen in each of these breeds on muscle biopsy, it is unknown whether an identical genetic defect is responsible [8,14–16]. The etiology of PSSM is unknown, but a defect in glucose metabolism resulting in increased uptake of glucose by muscle cells has been proposed in a study examining Quarter Horses [17]. This increased glucose uptake results in increased storage of glycogen, and the abnormal form of glycogen stains positively on the PAS stain. The diagnosis of PSSM as the cause of chronic exertional rhabdomyolysis in this individual was based on the clinical history of muscle cramping associated with exercise, increased CK and AST at baseline and after exercise, and the pathologic findings seen on muscle biopsy.

Treatment of acute episodes of muscle cramping attributable to exercise depends on the circumstances and underlying cause in individual horses. Horses with mild to moderate signs that do not have concurrent electrolyte and fluid deficiencies can be managed conservatively by allowing them to stand quietly for 15 to 30 minutes until the cramping begins to abate and then walking if the horse is willing. More severe episodes may be additionally treated with nonsteroidal anti-inflammatory drugs (NSAIDs), such as phenylbutazone (2 mg/kg), flunixin meglumine (1 mg/kg), or ketoprofen (2 mg/kg), or with acepromazine (0.04 mg/kg) to provide pain relief and muscle relaxation, respectively. These medications should not be given to electrolyte-depleted dehydrated horses because NSAIDs may cause renal papillary necrosis and acepromazine may exacerbate hypotension and poor renal perfusion.

Treatment and outcome

Management of horses with PSSM involves changes in the diet and exercise regimen of the affected horse. Dietary changes include feeding good-quality grass or oat hay [17]. In addition, a balanced electrolyte, vitamin, and mineral supplement (including vitamin E and selenium) should be provided. For many horses exercising at minimal levels, this diet is adequate to maintain health. If additional calories are needed, they should not be provided as a high-carbohydrate feed, such as sweet feed. Corn oil, diets rich in rice bran (20% fat), or other commercially available high-fat feeds are excellent sources of calories provided as fat. Rice bran products are high in phosphorus and may be calcium balanced during processing or may necessitate a supplemental calcium source supplied by the manufacturer. Rice bran supplements can be fed at 1 to 4 lb/d for adult horses. Corn oil is a less expensive alternative and can be fed at 1 to 4 cups per day for adult horses. Some horses find large amounts of corn oil unpalatable, however. Several commercial feed companies now have rice bran–based feeds on the market, and these may also be used.

Changes to the exercise regimen should include daily exercise. Living at pasture is ideal; however, if unavailable, regular turnout, riding, longing, or walking on a hot walker daily is beneficial. When the exercise regimen is being increased to increase the horse's fitness, changes in intensity should be made gradually. A change in diet combined with daily exercise is much more effective at decreasing the incidence of muscle cramping than either change alone (S. Valberg, DVM, PhD, personal communication, 2005). The owner was counseled that the goal of intervention was to decrease the incidence of episodes of muscle cramping, because no treatment can eliminate the disorder.

Dietary changes were implemented over 3 weeks; during this time, the horse was turned out in a paddock. At the end of the 3-week period, serum CK levels were verified to be within normal range by the referring veterinarian. Reintroduction to light exercise then began. Exercise consisted of hand walking and then riding as the horse was reintroduced to work. Horses with PSSM do best when they are exercised daily and are turned out as much as possible. Regular exercise in horses with PSSM improves glucose metabolism [17]. The owners implemented this protocol, and ride 60 to 90 minutes or turn the gelding out daily. The horse is fed grass hay and 4 lb of rice bran with 3 oz of a vitamin and mineral supplement added daily. Twelve months after presentation, the owners reported good progress in the horse's training program.

References

[1] Valberg S, Bullock P, Hogetvedt W, et al. Myopathies associated with Streptococcus equi infections in horses. Proc Am Assoc Equine Pract 1996;42:292–3.
[2] Traub-Dargatz J, Schlipf JJ, Granstrom D, et al. Multifocal myositis associated with Sarcocystis sp in a horse. J Am Vet Med Assoc 1994;205:1574–6.
[3] Higuchi T, Ichijo S, Osame S. Studies on serum and tocopherol in white muscle disease of foals. Jpn J Vet Sci 1989;51:52–9.
[4] Jackson C, De La Hunta A, Cummings J, et al. Spinal accessory nerve biopsy as an ante mortem diagnostic test for equine motor neuron disease. Equine Vet J 1996;28:215–9.
[5] Jackson C, Riis R, Rebhun W, et al. Ocular manifestations of equine motor neuron disease. Proc Am Assoc Equine Pract 1995;41:225–6.
[6] Jackson M. Intracellular calcium, cell injury and relationships to free radicals and fatty acid metabolism. Proc Nutr Soc 1990;49:77–81.
[7] Jackson M, Jones D, Edwards R. Techniques for studying free radical damage in muscular dystrophy. Med Biol 1984;62:135–8.
[8] MacLeay J. Diseases of the musculoskeletal system. In: Reed S, Bayly W, Sellon D, editors. Equine internal medicine. 2nd edition. St. Louis (MO): WB Saunders; 2004. p. 461–522.
[9] MacLeay J, Sorum S, Valberg S, et al. Epidemiological factors influencing recurrent exertional rhabdomyolysis in Thoroughbred racehorses. Am J Vet Res 1999;60:1560–3.
[10] MacLeay J, Valberg S, Pagan J, et al. Effect of ration on plasma creatine kinase activity and lactate concentration in Thoroughbred horses with recurrent exertional rhabdomyolysis. Am J Vet Res 2000;61:1390–5.
[11] Lentz L, Valberg S, Herold L, et al. Myoplasmic calcium regulation in myotubes from horses with recurrent exertional rhabdomyolysis. Am J Vet Res 2002;63:1724–31.
[12] Mlekoday J, Mickelson J, Valberg S, et al. Calcium sensitivity of force production and myofibrillar ATPase activity in muscles from Thoroughbreds with recurrent exertional rhabdomyolysis. Am J Vet Res 2001;62:1647–52.
[13] Valberg S, Mickelson J, Gallant E, et al. Exertional rhabdomyolysis in Quarter horses and Thoroughbreds: one syndrome, multiple etiologies. Equine Vet J Suppl 1999;30:533–8.
[14] Valentine B. Polysaccharide storage myopathy in draft and draft related horses and ponies. Equine Pract 1999;21:16–9.
[15] Valentine B, Hintz H, Freels K. Dietary control of exertional rhabdomyolysis in horses. J Am Vet Med Assoc 1998;212:1588–93.
[16] De La Corte F, Valberg S, MacLeay J, et al. Developmental onset of polysaccharide storage myopathy in 4 Quarter Horse foals. J Vet Intern Med 2002;16:581–7.
[17] De La Corte F, Valberg S, Mickelson J, et al. Blood glucose clearance after feeding and exercise in polysaccharide storage myopathy. Equine Vet J Suppl 1999;30:324–8.

VETERINARY
CLINICS
Equine Practice

Vet Clin Equine 22 (2006) 157–162

Excessive Drowsiness Secondary to Recumbent Sleep Deprivation in Two Horses

Joseph J. Bertone, DVM, MS

Equine Medicine College of Veterinary Medicine, Western University of Health Sciences,
309 East Second Street, Pomona, CA 91766, USA

Case I

Signalment and history

A 12-year-old Quarter Horse gelding was presented with a complaint of weight loss. The horse had been used as a successful Western pleasure horse for the last 8 years. Within the last 6 months, the horse had gradually lost a massive quantity of weight, but an accurate scale or tape weight was not collected. The horse had shown no other clinical signs. There was some suspicion that the horse did not aggressively forage and was slow in consuming hay and feed.

Case assessment

The diagnostic strategy was aimed at the chief complaint of weight loss. The horse was emaciated. All thoracic ribs were evident, and the tuber coxae and thoracic and lumbar spinous processes were prominent. He was quiet but did not seem depressed. The horse was 16.1 hands and weighed 940 pounds (427 kg). An estimated normal weight for a horse of his stature was 1250 pounds (568 kg). There was a 2- to 3-cm alopecic callus over both front fetlocks. All other physical examination parameters were within expected limits.

A screening serum chemistry profile, plasma fibrinogen concentration, and complete blood cell count were submitted. No parameters were outside the reference ranges. The complete blood cell count, however, tended to a stress leukogram with a neutrophil count near the upper end of normal

E-mail address: jbertone@westernu.edu

doi:10.1016/j.cveq.2005.12.020
vetequine.theclinics.com

and a lymphocyte count near the lower end of the range. An analysis of abdominal fluid collected on abdominocentesis was within normal limits. Rectal examination was within normal limits.

Thoracic and abdominal radiography and ultrasonography were considered. On the walk from the horse's stall to radiography and ultrasound, a noise was noted coming from the horse's abdomen. The noise occurred only as the horse walked. It sounded like rocks in a stream colliding under water. A thoracic radiograph was performed, and the thoracic cavity was considered normal, but a curious density was noted caudal to the diaphragm in the cranial abdominal cavity. The radiographic view was repositioned, and the unit was reset. The density on the thoracic radiograph was identified as the cranial partner of a pair of enteroliths (Fig. 1). In addition, several small metal linear densities were evident cranial to the

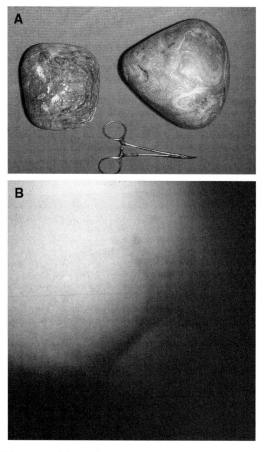

Fig. 1. (*A*) Enteroliths removed from a horse with enterolithiasis and primary hypersomnia. (*B*) Radiograph of horse with enterolithiasis and primary hypersomnia.

masses. They were embedded in soft tissue. It was believed that collisions of the two stones caused the noise heard while the horse was walked. Based on these findings an abdominal exploratory was planned for the following day.

The diagnostic procedures occurred over the course of 3 days. An interesting phenomenon was noted after a few minutes whenever the horse was placed in his quiet stall. The horse's eyelids would begin to close, and the lower lip would begin to droop. After a few more seconds, the horse's head would slowly drop to the ground. As the horse's head came within inches of the ground, the horse would begin to collapse. It was noted that on several occasions, as the horse neared collapse, his fetlocks lost extensor rigidity and flexed under the horse's weight at the small ground-to-limb angle (Fig. 2). It was believed that the dorsal fetlock calluses were secondary to this maneuver. Multiple episodes of this activity were observed.

Treatment and outcome

At surgery it was noted that the large colon could not be easily exteriorized because of adhesions of the sternal and diaphragmatic flexure to the diaphragm. It was elected to break down these tight adhesions bluntly. Additionally, the enteroliths (see Fig. 1A) were too large to remove through the pelvic flexure and were taken through a ventral colon enterotomy. The horse recovered uneventfully.

One hour after being placed back into his stall, the horse was seen lying down for the first time since the horse's arrival in the clinic. The horse remained quietly recumbent for nearly 12 hours. Because the horse evidenced no distress, he was observed but not disturbed. Thereafter the horse was seen resting recumbent at least two to three times per day. He was discharged 10 days postoperatively.

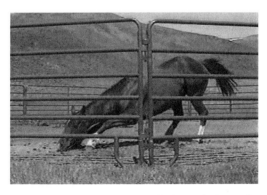

Fig. 2. A horse evidencing primary hypersomnia. (This is not the horse discussed in the text of this article.)

Six months later the horse was scale weighed at 1290 pounds (586.4 kg). The dorsal fetlock calluses had resolved. The owners indicated that they often found the horse recumbent in his stall and noted that before surgery and after the weight loss issue began, they had not seen him lie down. It was theorized that the adhesions of the large colon to the diaphragm made it difficult and painful for the horse to lie down, and the horse was deficient in paradoxical recumbent sleep. The cause of the weight loss was not specifically identified, but a combination of lack of recumbent sleep, the adhesions, the chronic peritonitis, and the enteroliths may have been additive.

Case II

Signalment and history

An 8-year-old Quarter Horse gelding recently purchased as a pleasure horse was referred for narcolepsy-cataplexy secondary to equine protozoal myeloencephalitis. The collapsing episodes were on going for nearly 8 months. The horse was kept out in pasture but could be seen by the owner from the kitchen window of their home. The horse was seen nearly collapsing, as in Fig. 2, multiple times during each day. A cerebral spinal fluid analysis was collected for submission for Western immunoblot assay for equine protozoal myeloencephalitis. A cytologic examination of the sample was not performed. The test indicated that the spinal fluid was positive for *Sarcocystis neurona*. The horse was treated with a multiple regimen of antiprotozoal medication with no improvement.

Case assessment

The horse was in good body condition. He was quiet but not overtly depressed. The horse was 15.3 hands and weighed 1040 pounds (472.7 kg). There was a 2- to 3-cm partially alopecic, excoriated area over both front fetlocks. All other physical examination parameters were within expected limits. The horse was not lame. In addition, a neurologic examination revealed no abnormalities.

A screening chemistry panel, fibrinogen, and complete blood cell count were completed. No parameters were outside the reference ranges. An analysis of abdominal fluid collected on abdominocentesis and a rectal examination were both within normal limits. Thoracic and abdominal radiography and ultrasonography were within normal limits.

It was decided to probe the client further. It was already known that the horse had been purchased about 30 days before the initial episode of near collapse. Further interrogation indicated that the horse was purchased from a farm with nearly 100 horses located in one pasture. The horse was moved to the client's new home and pasture, where he was the sole occupant of a 10-acre field located near an interstate highway.

Treatment and outcome

The author's 23-year-old Miniature Horse was borrowed and used as a pasture partner for the gelding. In the first few days of the pairing, the gelding was seen lying down approximately 50% of the time. The gelding's episodes of collapse resolved, and he seemed to function normally subsequent to the excessive days of sleep. Two more horses were purchased as companions for the gelding. The old Miniature Horse sleep aide was returned to its caretaker.

Discussion of excessive drowsiness secondary to recumbent sleep deprivation

Horses need a period of recumbent sleep that can be avoided for several days but eventually must be taken [1]. Hypersomnia, or sleeping for frequent excessive periods of time, was seen in both cases after resolution of the assumed underlying cause of recumbent sleep deprivation. The author places cases of excessive drowsiness into three categories [2].

1. Pain-associated excessive drowsiness is defined as those cases in which horses do not lie down because it is painful to do so. Most often these horses have musculoskeletal issues that create pain or mechanical difficulties on attempts at recumbency or rising to stand. In addition, horses have episodes of excessive sleepiness in association with thoracic or abdominal pain (as assumed in case I) that is elicited with recumbency or on attempting to stand.

2. Environmental insecurity–associated excessive drowsiness is the condition in which horses do not lie down because they are psychologically uncomfortable doing so; horses will lie down only when they are environmentally comfortable [1]. One can assume that this behavior stems from horses being prey and from herd behavior. The author has treated several horses with this condition by adding a friend to the pasture or stall, by moving the horse to an area where there are more horses, or by removing an aggressive horse from a group in which several horses may have the problem. This condition would also include horses in an insecure environment that may simply require a larger stall or paddock and horses near loud, harassing noise, such as fireworks or speedways.

3. Monotony-induced excessive drowsiness is best exemplified by the horse in crossties being braided that begins to lower its head to the point of near collapse. This behavior is assumed to be caused by the horse moving from slow-wave to paradoxical sleep [1,2]. This behavior may be seen more commonly at the odd hours that owners tend to braid horses. The horse is often very comfortable in its environment, and near-sleep is simply induced.

Excessive drowsiness secondary to recumbent sleep deprivation in horses with partial collapse upon motor function loss is often labeled as narcolepsy in horses. In the presented cases, both horses were labeled as narcoleptics, but neither horse collapsed completely to the ground. Narcolepsy is associated with episodes of full sleep and cataplexy (reversible loss of motor function). In horses, this would mean complete recumbency, not partial collapse. In human patients and horses, narcolepsy-cataplexy most often occurs when patients are fully engaged in a task or behavior. Narcolepsy and cataplexy are exceedingly rare in humans and in horses as well. In human patients, episodes are frequently elicited by emotions such as laughter, excitement, anger, or surprise [3]. In horses, narcolepsy-cataplexy is rare and breed associated, and episodes are elicited by feed presentation, excitement, and exercise [4]. Horses should not be diagnosed as having narcolepsy-cataplexy unless they meet the criteria of the clinical syndrome as listed in this paragraph. Labeling horses as narcoleptics leads one to look at pathophysiologic mechanisms and therapies that have little to do with the more prevalent condition of excessive drowsiness secondary to a recumbent sleep deprivation. This situation is similar to that of human patients who experience disturbed sleep secondary to sleep apnea, multiple movement disturbances, pain, or sleeping with pets. Some may liken the sleep deprivation syndrome in horses to hypersomnia. Hypersomnia, however, requires excessive or inappropriate sleep episodes, whereas these horses lack the ability to sleep in the required recumbent fashion. Idiopathic hypersomnia in human patients is also associated with some unknown central nervous system disorder [5]. These horses have no central nervous system disturbance other than recumbent sleep deprivation. In case I chronic pain and in case II social isolation prevented the horses from having normal recumbent sleep. Once the underlying cause was removed, the horses had a period of excessive sleep (hypersomnia) that resolved the primary recumbent sleep deficiency. It is important to consider causes of sleep deprivation before making a diagnosis of narcolepsy-cataplexy or diagnosing equine protozoal myeloencephalitis in horses.

References

[1] Dallaire A. Rest behavior. Vet Clin North Am Equine Pract 1986;2(3):591–607.
[2] Bertone JJ. Neurological disease in geriatric horses. In: Bertone JJ, editor. Equine geriatric medicine and surgery. St. Louis (MO): WB Saunders; 2006. p. 227–9.
[3] Guilleminault CG, Anagnos A. Narcolepsy. In: Kryger MH, Roth T, Dement WC, editors. Principles and practice of sleep medicine. 3rd edition. St. Louis (MO): W.B. Saunders; 2000. p. 676–86.
[4] Andrews FM, Mathews HK. Seizures, narcolepsy and cataplexy. In: Reed SM, Bayly WM, Sellon DC, editors. Equine internal medicine. St. Louis (MO): W.B. Saunders; 2004. p. 560–6.
[5] Guilleminault CG, Pelayo R. Idiopathic central nervous system hypersomnia. In: Kryger MH, Roth T, Dement WC, editors. Principles and practice of sleep medicine. 3rd edition. St. Louis (MO): W.B. Saunders; 2000. p. 687–92.

VETERINARY
CLINICS
Equine Practice

Vet Clin Equine 22 (2006) 163–175

Left Otitis Media/Interna and Right Maxillary Sinusitis in a Percheron Mare

Lisa Katz, DVM, MS, PhD, MRCVS

University Veterinary Hospital, School of Agriculture, Food Science and Veterinary Medicine,
University College Dublin, Belfield, Dublin 4, Ireland

Temporohyoid osteoarthropathy is a disorder that results in bony proliferation of the tympanic bulla, proximal stylohyoid, and petrous temporal bones, eventually leading to fusion of the temporohyoid joint [1–7]. It has been proposed that the underlying cause of this disease leading to eventual fusion of the temporohyoid joint involves otitis media interna causing osteitis of the bones of the temporohyoid joint [3,4,6] or a primary nonseptic degenerative joint disease [4,5]. Initial clinical signs are often vague and involve nonneurologic abnormalities, such as head shaking, head tossing, and resentment of ear handling [2,4,5,7,8]. Often, these initial clinical signs may be missed or dismissed, such that the earliest clinical abnormalities noted involve the acute onset of neurologic deficits to the facial or vestibulocochlear nerves. Although the onset of these clinical signs is acute, they are indicative of a more advanced stage of the disease, with the development of fractures through bony proliferation thought to be responsible [2–6].

Case history

A 6-year-old 650-kg Percheron mare was referred for evaluation of a 6-day history of a left ear droop, right mucopurulent nasal discharge, and 12-hour duration of ataxia. The mare was on a grass pasture with four horses; was dewormed every 6 weeks with ivermectin; was annually tested for equine infectious anemia; and was vaccinated against tetanus, eastern and western equine encephalitis, and influenza. No new animals had been introduced in 2 years, there was no history of travel or dietary change, and no other animal was ill. There was no history of *Streptococcus equi* infection on the farm. Initially, the mare was noted to have a right

E-mail address: lisa.katz@ucd.ie

doi:10.1016/j.cveq.2005.12.032

mucopurulent nasal discharge and a swollen and drooping left ear with superficial abrasions around the ear base. The referring veterinarian diagnosed right guttural pouch empyema and a left ear infection. The mare was treated with trimethoprim-sulfadiazine (20 mg/kg [9.1 mg/lb] administered orally every 12 hours) and had the right guttural pouch infused with an unknown amount and concentration of gentamicin in sterile water and the left ear flushed with sterile water. No improvement was noted after 4 days; phenylbutazone (3 mg/kg [1.4 mg/lb] administered orally every 12 hours) was added to the treatment regimen, and the right guttural pouch and left ear were treated as before. The mare was then referred for further evaluation.

Clinical examination

On physical examination, the mare was alert and responsive, with a base-wide stance. The rectal temperature, heart rate, and respiratory rate were all within reference ranges. The mucous membranes were pink and moist with a normal capillary refill time, the cardiac rhythm was normal with no murmurs, and all lymph nodes palpated within normal limits (WNL). There was a right, odorless, mucopurulent nasal discharge. Airflow from both nostrils was adequate, and percussion of the paranasal sinuses revealed right-sided dullness; no bony deformities of the head were noted. Auscultation and percussion of the lung fields were normal. The left ear had superficial abrasions around the base, and when it was manipulated, the mare became resentful. Palpation inside the ear revealed no foreign objects. A neurologic examination revealed a left head tilt (poll ventrally deviated toward the left), drooping of the left ear and lower muzzle, ptosis of the left eyelid, and deviation of the muzzle to the right (Figs. 1 and 2). There was ventrolateral deviation of the left eyeball and spontaneous horizontal nystagmus of both eyes, with the fast phase to the right. The results of an ophthalmic examination and pupillary light reflex (PLR) testing of both eyes were WNL. Because of the nystagmus, a fundic examination was not performed. Vision and sensation were intact for the left eye and eyelid, respectively, but there was neither a menace response nor a palpebral reflex. The mare was observed to drink and eat a handful of grass with no obvious dysphagia, although examination of the oral cavity revealed some mild packing of food along the rostral left buccal surface. The horse was reluctant to move, and when asked to walk forward, it was asymmetrically ataxic and preferred to circle and lean to the left, with its body flexed laterally with left concavity. No weakness was noted, and the ataxia was graded 3/5 to 4/5 in all limbs. Proprioception was not evaluated because of the degree of ataxia.

The left ear and muzzle droop, ptosis, buccal food impaction, and deviation of the muzzle to the right were all signs consistent with left-sided facial nerve (cranial nerve [CN] VII) paralysis, with the loss of the menace response and palpebral reflex on the left side likely a result of loss of eyelid movement caused by facial nerve paralysis. The head tilt, strabismus,

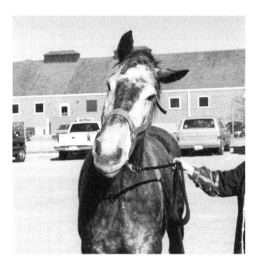

Fig. 1. Six-year-old Percheron mare with a right mucopurulent nasal discharge, left facial nerve paralysis, and a left-sided head tilt. There was ventrolateral deviation of the left eyeball and spontaneous horizontal nystagmus of both eyes, with the fast phase to the right.

nystagmus, and asymmetric ataxia were all characteristic of left-sided peripheral (CN VIII) or central vestibular disease. Based on the neurologic examination, the lesion was localized to the left petrous temporal bone involving CN VII and CN VIII (peripheral) or to the medulla affecting the vestibular and facial nuclei (central). Central vestibular disease was unlikely because of the alert demeanor, strength preservation, and lack of other CN involvement. The main differentials for left-sided peripheral

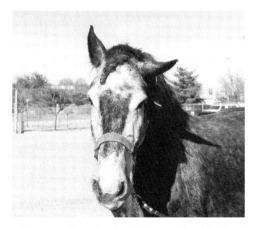

Fig. 2. A closer view of the mare shown in Fig. 1. A superficial skin abrasion involving the base of the left ear can be clearly seen, along with the left facial nerve paralysis and the right mucopurulent nasal discharge.

vestibular disease and facial nerve paralysis include left-sided temporohyoid osteoarthropathy with or without otitis media interna, left petrous temporal bone trauma, left guttural pouch mycosis, equine protozoal myeloencephalitis (EPM), equine herpesvirus I myeloencephalopathy (EHV-1), polyneuritis equi (PNE), and verminous myeloencephalitis. Given the history and physical and neurologic examination findings, PNE and verminous myeloencephalitis were unlikely.

Mucopurulent nasal discharge indicated severe inflammation or infection of the lower respiratory tract or upper respiratory tract (URT) mucosa. Because lung auscultation was WNL and the right paranasal sinuses were dull with the nasal discharge unilateral to the right, the lesion likely involved the URT, with right primary or secondary sinusitis as the most likely cause. Primary sinusitis is usually a sequela to bacterial URT infections (eg, *Streptococcus, Staphylococcus*). Secondary sinusitis can result from dental disease (eg, abscessed tooth root, fractured tooth), a cyst, neoplasia (squamous cell carcinoma), fungal granuloma (eg, *Cryptococcus, Coccidioides*), or trauma. Guttural pouch disease (eg, empyema, mycosis), a laryngeal or pharyngeal abscess, or a foreign body could not be excluded but would not cause dullness of the sinuses.

Causes of a painful ear include temporohyoid osteoarthropathy, inflammation of the middle or inner ear attributable to infection (eg, bacterial, mycotic), trauma, insect hypersensitivity, foreign objects, ectoparasites (ticks), or neoplasia. Based on the results of the physical examination, foreign objects, ectoparasites, and neoplasia were unlikely. The abrasions around the ear base were likely self-inflicted.

Case management

On day 1, a complete blood cell count (CBC), serum chemistry panel, and urinalysis were performed to evaluate the hydration and immune status, electrolyte and protein concentrations, and various organ systems. The CBC revealed normocytic normochromic anemia. The profile revealed elevated lactate dehydrogenase (LDH; 1887 IU/L, reference range: 527–1612 IU/L), hyperglobulinemia (4.6 g/dL, reference range: 2.2–3.7 g/dL), and low normal albumin (2.5 g/dL, reference range: 2.5–3.8 g/dL). The results of the urinalysis were WNL. Reticulocytes are rarely released into equine peripheral blood; thus, classification of anemia as regenerative or nonregenerative is difficult to do without a bone marrow examination. Based on the history and physical examination (mucopurulent nasal discharge) and laboratory findings (hyperglobulinemia), nonregenerative anemia of chronic disease resulting from inhibition of erythropoiesis by cytokines released in response to infection was most likely.

LDH has isoenzymes in various tissues, but large amounts are in skeletal muscle. Thus, the lack of evidence for other diseased organs suggested skeletal muscle damage as the cause of the high LDH level. Because LDH is slower to return to normal than creatine kinase (CK) or aspartate amino-transferase (AST), and the CK and AST levels were WNL, the muscle damage likely had been mild and short and was resolving. Reasons for this included trauma or recumbency associated with the neurologic disorder or a subclinical myopathy (eg, polysaccharide storage disease, equine rhabdomyolysis syndrome). Serial measurement of the serum enzymes was planned, and if the LDH remained elevated, an isoenzyme profile was to be run to determine the specific tissue source. Because this was horse was a draft breed, subclinical polysaccharide storage disease was considered; however, a muscle biopsy was not performed, because if polysaccharide storage disease was present, it was not likely contributing to the clinical problem. The hyperglobulinemia was likely from ongoing and chronic inflammation. Albumin is a negative acute-phase reactant and decreases slightly when globulins are elevated.

Upper airway endoscopy was performed to look for the source of the nasal discharge, to assess the pharyngeal and laryngeal function (evaluating CNs IX, X, and XI), and to examine the guttural pouches and stylohyoid bones. No sedation was used. The appearance and function of the pharynx and larynx were WNL, whereas mucopurulent material was found in the right rostral nasal passage. Both guttural pouches were clean, but there was enlargement of the proximal third part of the left stylohyoid bone and some osseous proliferation noted at the articulation of the temporohyoid joint; the right stylohyoid bone and temporohyoid joint appeared normal. Lateral and dorsoventral standing survey skull and sinus radiographs were taken to evaluate the upper airway (sinuses), the bones associated with the temporohyoid joints, and the skull further. To obtain a dorsoventral view, the mare was sedated with xylazine (75 mg administered intravenously); this resulted in worsening of the ataxia (grade 4+/5), so further sedation was not used. Thickening of the left stylohyoid bone and periosteal proliferation and sclerosis of the left petrous temporal bone were found; no fracture lines were apparent. There were fluid lines in the right rostral and caudal maxillary sinus. No masses or dental involvement was found. While sedated, the mare tolerated a brief otoscopic and endoscopic examination of the left ear canal. Visualization of the tympanic membrane was impeded by debris. No foreign objects or ectoparasites were found.

The left eye was evaluated for corneal ulceration and tear production. The inability to blink can lead to exposure keratitis and corneal ulceration, although some animals learn to retract the globe, allowing the upper and third eyelid to move across the cornea. There was no fluorescein uptake of the left eye, indicating intact corneal epithelium. The lacrimal gland is innervated by parasympathetic nerve fibers that run with CN VII and VIII within the petrous temporal bone [9]. These fibers can be damaged with CN VII and VIII, resulting in decreased tear production, keratoconjunctivitis sicca, and corneal ulceration [10]. The results of Schirmer tear tests were WNL for both eyes.

A tentative diagnosis of left temporohyoid osteoarthropathy with possible otitis media interna and right maxillary sinusitis was made. Based on the radiographs, primary sinusitis was likely, although dental disease could not be completely discounted, because survey radiographs may miss dental problems. The left ear trauma was likely self-inflicted, possibly attributable to an inner ear infection. Transtympanic lavage of the ear for culture of a possible causative organism and collection of cerebrospinal fluid (CSF) from the atlanto-occipital space were not performed. Tympanocentesis is a difficult and low-yield procedure, and the results of analysis of CSF from most horses with otitis media interna are WNL. Both procedures would require general anesthesia, and the risk of brain herniation or a bad recovery because of the ataxia and size of the mare was considered too great in light of the minimal information gained from these procedures. Although unlikely, it was possible that more than one cause existed for the neurologic signs. A lumbosacral tap was considered but not done because of the ataxia, which became more pronounced with sedation. A serum sample was submitted for immunoblot analysis for EPM. Although a positive result only indicates exposure, a negative result would make the likelihood of EPM extremely low. Diagnostics for EHV-1 were not pursued because it was considered unlikely and treatment would not change. Centesis of the right rostral maxillary sinus to obtain a sample for cytology and culture and sensitivity testing and to lavage the sinuses was attempted but aborted because the mare became excited and sedation resulted in the ataxia worsening.

To treat the possible otitis media interna and sinusitis, trimethoprim-sulfadiazine (20 mg/kg, administered orally every 12 hours) was chosen because it provides a broad spectrum of coverage. Phenylbutazone (4.4 mg/kg administered intravenously once and then 4.4 mg/kg administered orally every 24 hours) was used to alleviate inflammation and provide analgesia. Oral medication was used because the mare was not dysphagic and the goal was to send the horse home on long-term medication that the owner could easily give. Dimethyl sulfoxide (90%, 1 g/kg administered intravenously every 24 hours for 3 days) diluted to 10% in intravenous fluids was used for its anti-inflammatory effects as well for its diuretic effects to reduce edema and the scavenging of free radicals associated with ischemia of neuronal tissue. Food and water were offered, and the mouth was rinsed periodically. The neurologic status, food and water intake, fecal and urine output, and fecal consistency were monitored.

On day 2, the mare's neurologic status was basically unchanged, although the horse exhibited a slight improvement in vestibular abnormalities. The head tilt and base-wide stance had decreased slightly in severity, and when asked to walk, the mare was less hesitant and would move in all directions, including a straight line. The mucopurulent nasal discharge had decreased, food and water intake was adequate, the packed cell volume was stable, and the total protein measurement was WNL. By day 3, the mare's neurologic status had improved further, although the horse had started to rub its left ear, traumatizing the abrasions around the ear base even more. Although the facial nerve paralysis remained unchanged, the nystagmus had slowed and the left head tilt was less noticeable. The ataxia was now a grade 3/5, and proprioception was WNL, substantiating the diagnosis of peripheral disease. The improved vestibular signs were likely attributable to visual and limb proprioceptive orientation. A CBC and chemistry profile on day 3 revealed the LDH to be WNL and the anemia and hyperglobulinemia unchanged. By day 4, the nasal discharge had decreased significantly. Repeat skull and sinus radiographs were unchanged, and re-evaluation of the eyes showed normal tear production and no fluorescein stain uptake. On day 5, the nystagmus had resolved and the ataxia improved to a grade 2+/5. On day 7, a Western blot test was reported negative for EPM.

The mare was discharged on day 5 with instructions to continue the trimethoprim-sulfadiazine and phenylbutazone for 8 weeks; to keep the mare in a small area; and to monitor its attitude, fecal consistency, and nasal discharge. Vestibular signs may resolve by 2 to 4 weeks, but facial nerve paralysis is slower to improve. The referring veterinarian saw the mare 5 weeks after discharge. He reported no improvement in CN VII, a mild left head tilt, a grade 1/5 ataxia, and no nasal discharge. Two months after discharge, the owner reported that the horse was healthy, with no nasal discharge and an improvement in CN VII. The mare was scheduled to come back 4 months after discharge for examination, radiographs, a CBC, a chemistry profile, and sinus centesis if indicated.

Discussion

Temporohyoid osteoarthropathy is a disease that primarily causes facial and vestibulocochlear nerve dysfunction [3–5,7,10,11]. The underlying cause of this disease has been proposed to be otitis media interna, resulting in osteitis of the bones of the temporohyoid joint [3,4,6] or a primary nonseptic degenerative joint disease [4,5]. Otitis media interna involves inflammation of the tympanic bulla and neural end organs of the vestibulocochlear nerve and, most commonly, is the result of a microbial infection [4]. It may develop secondary to hematogenous spread of bacteria, ascending infection from the respiratory tract, extension of guttural pouch infection, or extension of otitis media externa [4,5]. Regardless of the initiating cause, early clinical signs of temporohyoid osteoarthropathy are associated with middle ear infection, bony proliferation, and subsequent arthritic changes of the temporohyoid joint and include head shaking, ear rubbing, and resentment of ear manipulation [4,5]. In this case, it was not entirely clear if otitis media interna was present, but there was a strong clinical suspicion of an active inner ear infection because the mare intermittently rubbed the left ear while hospitalized and, on initial presentation, had some superficial skin abrasions around the left ear base indicating past ear rubbing. Diagnostically, looking for the presence of excessive inflammatory fluid accumulation within the tympanic cavity by the use of CT or MRI could have helped to confirm an inner ear infection; however, these modalities were not available. If present, the otitis media interna was likely bacterial in origin, with the most likely source being hematogenous spread, possibly also causing the right sinusitis or originating from the sinus itself. Because the sinusitis was right-sided, an extension of the sinus infection to the left inner ear was unlikely, although there could have been hematogenous spread to the right sinus from the left inner ear, originating as otitis externa. Considering the apparent lack of involvement of dental disease or an obvious mass within the sinus cavity, the sinusitis was likely primary and bacterial in origin, which supports the hypothesis that hematogenous spread of bacteria was involved. It seems that inner ear infections in the horse typically do not result in rupture of the tympanic membrane but, instead, extend ventrally, resulting in chronic inflammation of the tympanic bulla and proximal stylohyoid bone, with eventual resolution of any active inflammation but fusion of the temporohyoid joint [5]. This type of chronic inflammation could explain the mare's painful ear and hyperglobulinemia.

After resolution of the inflammation and fusion of the joint, early clinical signs, such as ear pain and head shaking, are often eliminated. As with the present case, the subsequent presentation is then the acute onset of neurologic signs most commonly affecting the facial and vestibulocochlear CNs. Although neurologic signs of temporohyoid osteoarthropathy appear acutely in horses, they are more indicative of a chronic problem, because the onset of neurologic signs is likely attributable to fracture of the petrous temporal or stylohyoid bone caused by movement of the tongue or larynx. Normal tongue and laryngeal movements, such as swallowing, rely on movement of the hyoid apparatus [5], which supports the tongue, pharynx, and larynx and consists of a basihyoid bone; lingual process; and paired stylohyoid, ceratohyoid, and thyrohyoid bones [5,7,11]. With the temporohyoid joint fused, movement of the tongue or larynx places abnormal forces on the stylohyoid and petrous temporal bones and predisposes horses to fracture of the petrous temporal bone and through any bony proliferation within the temporohyoid joint [2,3,5]. The fracture line is commonly found to extend through the petrous temporal bone, tympanic bulla, and internal acoustic meatus [13] but can involve other bones, such as the basisphenoid and occipital bones [5]. Thickening of the stylohyoid bone is frequently observed with guttural pouch endoscopy and is likely the result of primary infection or remodeling secondary to increased forces on the bone with fusion of the temporohyoid joint. Therefore, the weakened osteomyelitic petrous temporal bone is more frequently fractured.

Fractures are thought to be responsible for the acute onset of neurologic deficits as a result of tearing or stretching of the CNs or because bony proliferation directly impinges on the nerves [5]. The facial and vestibulocochlear nerves are most commonly affected because both nerves are in close approximation to the petrous temporal bone and pass through the internal acoustic meatus [9], whereas the glossopharyngeal and vagus nerves are located much more caudally and are only affected with severe bony proliferation and inflammation [5,11]. Often, vestibular signs may be present several days before facial nerve deficits [4], although in the present case, an ear droop, indicating facial nerve dysfunction, was noted before the onset of vestibular signs. In addition to the involvement of CNs VII and VIII, corneal ulceration may develop because of decreased ability to blink secondary to the facial paralysis or decreased tear production [3,5,12,13]. As stated previously, the lacrimal gland is innervated by parasympathetic nerve fibers that run with CNs VII and VIII within the petrous temporal bone [9]. These fibers can be damaged with CNs VII and VIII, resulting in decreased tear production, keratoconjunctivitis sicca, and corneal ulceration. Thus, corneal staining and a Schirmer tear test should always be part of the evaluation of a horse suspected of having temporohyoid osteoarthropathy, and the eye should be monitored for ulcer development or decreased lacrimation during the treatment period. In some cases, performing a temporary partial tarsorrhaphy may help to protect the eye until some nerve function returns or the horse learns to retract the eye, allowing the third eyelid to lubricate the cornea. If ulceration and dry eye are severe, enucleation may need to be performed.

Guttural pouch endoscopy is currently the best test to confirm a tentative diagnosis of temporohyoid osteoarthropathy [3–5]. It is relatively simple and can be used to detect early changes (Figs. 3 and 4). In addition to assessing both stylohyoid bones for symmetry and enlargement, especially at the temporohyoid joint, the guttural pouches themselves can be evaluated to rule out other diseases, such as guttural pouch mycosis, and the function of the larynx can be more objectively reviewed. In the present case, endoscopy was also warranted to try to determine the source of the right nasal discharge. Sinus endoscopy was also considered so as to explore the sinuses more thoroughly, looking for and taking a biopsy of any masses present. Because the mare would not tolerate sinus centesis and became markedly ataxic with sedation, this procedure was not performed. We also used a pediatric endoscope to visualize the mare's left ear canal. The size of the mare allowed the passage of the pediatric scope, which was easier to manipulate than an otoscope because the horse was only lightly sedated and standing.

Survey radiographs are often performed to confirm the clinical diagnosis of temporohyoid osteoarthropathy and should always include lateral and dorsoventral views so as to allow comparison between the right and left tympanic bulla and temporohyoid joints. Fractures and other subtle changes, such as fluid accumulation within the tympanic cavity, are often missed with this modality, however. It has been reported that horses diagnosed with temporohyoid osteoarthropathy often had fractures missed with survey radiographs that were later identified after death [5]. In the present case, survey radiographs were also indicated for evaluation of the sinuses

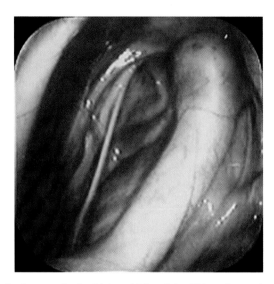

Fig. 3. Endoscopic photograph of a thickened left stylohyoid bone from a horse with left facial nerve paralysis and a left-sided head tilt.

for fluid or masses. Diseased teeth may be missed with survey radiographs, however, especially if the changes are subtle [14]. If available, CT would have been a good alternative in the present case because it provides excellent clarity of bony involvement, and thus would likely have provided the most information concerning the teeth, sinuses, and skull, in addition to detecting

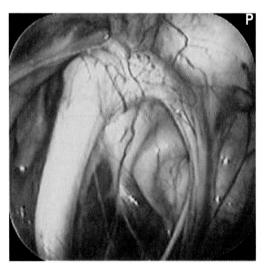

Fig. 4. Endoscopic photograph of a normal right proximal stylohyoid bone and temporohyoid joint from the same horse shown in Fig. 3.

fluid in the middle and external ear canal. It has been previously reported that CT detected petrous temporal bone fractures in two horses that were not found using standard survey radiographs [7], although CT did miss early changes associated with temporohyoid osteoarthropathy in a second report [5]. It has been hypothesized that MRI, the most precise modality available for imaging soft tissue changes and inflammatory fluid accumulation, may have been more appropriate to highlight these early changes [5]. CT and MRI do require general anesthesia, however, which has increased risks, including recovery of an already ataxic animal, especially a draft breed. In the present case, nuclear scintigraphy would have been a good option for further exploration for dental disease [15]. This modality can be performed in standing horses, the equipment is more frequently available than CT or MRI equipment, and, in combination with radiography, the sensitivity and specificity for diagnosing dental disease are high [16]. Interestingly, nuclear scintigraphy was found to be a better screening tool than radiography for cases in which the presence of dental disease was uncertain [16], such as in the current case.

Long-term (30 days or more) broad-spectrum antibiotics and anti-inflammatory drugs are the main treatments for temporohyoid osteopathy and primary sinusitis. Tympanocentesis has been advocated as a way to try to identify the presence of active infection within the inner ear and to isolate the organism causing the infection, but it is technically difficult and requires general anesthesia; thus, it was not performed in the present case. Because it is often difficult to determine if there is active infection, it is recommended to treat horses with broad-spectrum antimicrobials after the onset of clinical abnormalities associated with temporohyoid osteopathy, especially horses with neurologic deficits [5]. Although the CBC parameters and temperature were WNL for the horse in the present case, there was some evidence of chronic active ear pain that may have been attributable to otitis media interna. In addition, appropriate antibiotics and anti-inflammatory drugs were warranted for the treatment of the sinus infection. Performing sinus centesis to obtain a sample for culture and sensitivity testing, in addition to draining and flushing the right sinus, would have been ideal, so that the choice of antibiotics could have been based on the results of culture and sensitivity testing. Because trephination of the sinus could not be performed safely in the current case, no sample could be submitted for analysis and culture, and drainage and lavage of the sinus could not be done. Thus, broad-spectrum antibiotics with good activity against streptococcal species and anti-inflammatory therapy were the main treatments for the sinusitis in the present case.

A partial stylohyoidostectomy has been recommended as a prophylactic treatment in early cases of temporohyoid osteopathy in an effort to prevent fracture of the petrous temporal bone in cases in which the temporohyoid joint has fused [2,7]. This operation is supposed to relieve forces produced by the tongue and laryngeal movement on the ankylosed temporohyoid joint so as to prevent the development of fractures and worsening of clinical signs [2]. A segment of bone is removed from the midshaft of the stylohyoid bone, and a pseudoarthrosis is formed during healing [2]. Whether this operation has any benefit over medical therapy and, if so, exactly when it is most beneficial to perform this operation remain to be determined. Complications of this operation include transection of the lingual artery, injury to the hypoglossal nerve [2], and regrowth of the stylohyoid bone with recurrence of clinical signs [7]. A ceratohyoidectomy has been advocated as an alternative surgical procedure if regrowth of the stylohyoid bone occurs after a partial stylohyoidectomy, and possibly as an alternative prophylactic procedure to a partial stylohyoidectomy in an effort to minimize regrowth of the stylohyoid bone [7]. This type of operation also may have less risk for injury of the hypoglossal nerve [7].

The prognosis for resolution of CN deficits is guarded, with most horses retaining some degree of neurologic dysfunction [4,5]. As in this case, the facial nerve abnormalities are the most common residual deficits, although blindfolding may reveal compensated vestibular deficits [4]. Owners should be made aware that it may take several months to years for the neurologic deficits to improve, although it has been reported recently that 14 of 20 horses returned to their prior athletic use [5]. Owners should be made aware that although the neurologic deficits may improve, these horses still pose a significant risk of harm to handlers and themselves and that manipulation of the head, especially the tongue, may cause the acute onset of neurologic signs with little to no warning [4,5].

References

[1] Geiser DR, Henton JR, Held JP. Tympanic bulla, petrous temporal bone, and hyoid apparatus disease in horses. Compend Contin Educ Pract Vet 1988;10:740–54.

[2] Blythe LL, Watrous BJ, Shires MH. Prophylactic partial stylohyoidostectomy for horses with osteoarthropathy of the temporohyoid joint. J Equine Vet Sci 1994;14:32–7.

[3] Hassel DM, Schott HC, Tucker RL, et al. Endoscopy of the auditory tube diverticula in four horses with otitis media/interna. J Am Vet Med Assoc 1995;207:1081–4.

[4] Blythe LL. Otitis media and interna and temporohyoid osteoarthropathy. Vet Clin North Am Equine Pract 1997;13:21–42.

[5] Walker AM, Sellon DC, Cornelisse CJ, et al. Temporohyoid osteoarthropathy in 33 horses (1993–2000). J Vet Intern Med 2002;16:697–703.

[6] Yadernuk LM. Temporohyoid osteoarthropathy and unilateral facial nerve paralysis in a horse. Can Vet J 2003;44:990–1.

[7] Pease AP, Van Biervliet J, Dykes NL, et al. Complication of partial stylohyoidectomy for treatment of temporohyoid osteoarthropathy and an alternative surgical technique in three cases. Equine Vet J 2004;36:546–50.

[8] Lane JG, Mair TS. Observations on headshaking in the horse. Equine Vet J 1987;19:331–6.

[9] deLahunta A. Veterinary neuroanatomy and clinical neurology. 2nd edition. Philadelphia: WB Saunders; 1983.

[10] Spurlock SL, Spurlock GH, Wise M. Keratoconjunctivitis sicca associated with fracture of the stylohyoid bone in a horse. J Am Vet Med Assoc 1989;194:258–9.

[11] Power HT, Watrous BJ, deLahunta A. Facial and vestibulocochlear nerve disease in six horses. J Am Vet Med Assoc 1983;183:1076–80.

[12] Blythe LL, Watrous BJ. Temporohyoid osteoarthropathy (middle ear disease). In: Robinson NE, editor. Current therapy in equine medicine IV. Philadelphia: WB Saunders; 1997. p. 323–5.

[13] Hardy J, Leveille R. Diseases of the guttural pouches. Vet Clin North Am Equine Pract 2003; 19:123–58.

[14] Henninger W, Frame EM, Willmann M, et al. CT features of alveolitis and sinusitis in horses. Vet Radiol Ultrasound 2003;44:269–76.

[15] Freeman DE. Sinus disease. Vet Clin North Am Equine Pract 2003;19:209–43.

[16] Weller R, Livesy L, Maierl J, et al. Comparison of radiography and scintigraphy in the diagnosis of dental disorders in the horse. Equine Vet J 2001;33:49–58.

ELSEVIER
SAUNDERS

VETERINARY
CLINICS
Equine Practice

Vet Clin Equine 22 (2006) 177–191

Equine Herpes Myeloencephalopathy in a 12-Year-Old American Quarter Horse

David Wong, DVM, MS[a],*, W. Kent Scarratt, DVM[b]

[a]Veterinary Clinical Sciences, College of Veterinary Medicine, Iowa State University,
Ames, IA 50011, USA
[b]Department of Large Animal Clinical Sciences, Virginia-Maryland Regional College of
Veterinary Medicine, Blacksburg, VA 24061, USA

Equine herpesvirus type 1 (EHV-1) is highly contagious in horses and has been responsible for causing respiratory tract infections, abortions, neonatal infection and death, and neurologic dysfunction. Although EHV-1 is ubiquitous in the equine population, with many young horses being infected in the first year of life, the incidence of equine herpes myeloencephalopathy (EHM) is relatively infrequent considering the widespread presence of this virus [1]. Several recent outbreaks of EHM have exemplified the prevalence of EHV-1, its ability to act as an infectious disease, and its potential negative impact on neurologic function in horses, however. This case report describes a case of EHM and highlights various diagnostic and therapeutic options available for EHM; minimal emphasis is placed on specific viral characterization of EHV-1 and its pathophysiologic role in horses.

Case details

History

A 12-year-old American Quarter Horse mare weighing 410 kg was referred for a 1-week history of fever (40.5°C [105°F]), depression, and abnormal right hind limb carriage. Before referral, the mare was treated with penicillin and gentamicin for 7 days. Three days before referral, the rectal temperature had returned to normal reference intervals (38.2°C [100.7°F]) but the right hind limb abnormality was still present. The owner also noted decreased appetite and water consumption for the past 4 days. The mare was vaccinated against tetanus, influenza, eastern and western equine

---

* Corresponding author.
E-mail address: dwong@iastate.edu (D. Wong).

0749-0739/06/$ - see front matter © 2006 Elsevier Inc. All rights reserved.
doi:10.1016/j.cveq.2005.12.003

encephalomyelitis, rabies, and Potomac horse fever 6 months before presentation, and ivermectin was administered every 2 months. The mare's diet consisted of two flakes of grass hay and 1 kg of sweet feed (12% protein) offered twice daily along with free-choice water. None of the other eight horses on the premises demonstrated signs of illness.

Physical examination

On presentation, the mare was depressed but responsive. The horse was in good body condition, with no muscle atrophy noted. Rectal temperature (37.8°C [100.0°F]), heart rate (44 beats per minute), and respiratory rate (20 breaths per minute) were within normal limits, as was auscultation of the heart and respiratory and gastrointestinal tracts. No musculoskeletal abnormalities were noted, including examination of the right hind limb, and no other problems were detected on physical examination. When observed walking, the horse was moderately ataxic in the hind limbs, and during physical examination, the mare postured to urinate twice but voided only small amounts ($\sim$ 300 mL total) of urine. Rectal palpation revealed normal feces and abdominal viscera and a severely distended urinary bladder. Urine could not be expressed, despite moderate pressure placed on the urinary bladder during rectal palpation. Rectal palpation of the pelvis revealed no skeletal abnormalities. On complete neurologic examination, significant findings included asymmetric ataxia (grade 3/4 in right hind limb, grade 2/4 in left hind limb) and asymmetric paresis of the hind limbs along with hypotonia of the tail.

Case assessment, differential diagnosis, and diagnostic procedures

The initial problem list included a history of inappetence, depression, and fever as well as physical examination findings of asymmetric paraparesis and ataxia of the hind limbs, weak tail tone, and bladder dysfunction characterized by dysuria and urine retention. In this case, bladder dysfunction was typical of upper motor neuron (UMN) dysfunction based on the intermittent dribbling of urine and the inability to express the bladder with pressure during rectal examination. Collectively, these deficits suggested a focal or multifocal lesion in the thoracolumbar spinal cord. The differential diagnosis at this time included EHM, equine protozoal myeloencephalitis (EPM), spinal cord trauma, and polyneuritis equi. Nonneurogenic causes of bladder dysfunction were also considered, such as cystic, urethral, or sabulous urolithiasis; bacterial cystitis; and neoplasia.

A complete blood cell count and biochemistry profile revealed no significant abnormalities. Ultrasonographic examination of the urinary tract was performed, along with a urinalysis via bladder catheterization. Ultrasonographic examination revealed an extremely distended urinary bladder with a mild amount of sediment on the ventral aspect of the bladder. On passage of a urinary catheter, 7.5 L of urine was collected. Results of the urinalysis

were within normal limits. The horse was subsequently administered deto-
midine (0.01 mg/kg) and butorphanol (0.01 mg/kg) intravenously, and cerebrospinal fluid (CSF) was collected via a lumbosacral spinal tap.
Xanthochromic CSF was collected and submitted for cytologic analysis, detection of antibodies against *Sarcocystis neurona*, albumin quotient, and
IgG index. In addition, blood samples were submitted for detection of
EHV-1 serum-neutralizing (SN) antibody, antibodies against *S neurona*,
and EHV-1 polymerase chain reaction (PCR) of the buffy coat. CSF abnormalities noted on cytologic analysis included xanthochromia, elevated protein (241.4 mg/dL, reference interval: 50–80 mg/dL), mild elevation in red
blood cells (54 cells/µL, reference interval: 0–10 cells/µL), and a normal total
nucleated cell count (0 cells/µL, reference interval: 0–6 cells/µL).

Treatment and case outcome

Based on the history (fever, inappetence, and depression), clinical signs
(hind limb paresis, ataxia, and bladder dysfunction), and clinicopathologic
findings (CSF abnormalities, including xanthochromia; elevated protein;
and normal white blood cell count), EHM was highly suspected. The horse
was housed in an isolation stall, and continuous intravenous fluid therapy
(lactated Ringer's solution at a rate of 50 mL/kg/d), flunixin meglumine
(1.1 mg/kg administered intravenously every 12 hours), dimethyl sulfoxide
(DMSO; 500 mg/kg administered intravenously every 24 hours diluted in
sterile fluids), and acyclovir (15 mg/kg administered orally every 8 hours)
were initiated on the first day. Rectal temperature, fecal output, heart
rate, and respiration rate were monitored every 6 hours and were normal
throughout hospitalization. A complete ophthalmic examination on day 2
of hospitalization did not reveal uveitis, hypopyon, or retinal hemorrhage,
which can be consistent with EHM. Rectal palpation was performed twice
daily to monitor urinary bladder size. Although the mare urinated small
amounts two to three times a day, catheterization of the bladder was performed twice daily for the first 3 days based on rectal palpation. Urine
was submitted for urinalysis daily to monitor for bacterial cystitis and
evaluate renal function, and the results remained within normal limits.
The mare's appetite was decreased initially but improved to normal by
day 6. The flunixin meglumine and DMSO were discontinued after 3 days
based on the clinical improvement in attitude and appetite and stable
neurologic status.

An EHV-1 SN antibody titer of 1:256 was received on day 4. This titer
was moderately elevated and considered diagnostic for EHM in light of
the history, clinical signs, and CSF color and cytology. The result of PCR
of the buffy coat (EHV-1) was negative. The mare's neurologic status was
stable, with mild improvement noted over the 6-day hospitalization period.
No medications were dispensed, but the owner was instructed to monitor
urine output. The mare was examined 7 days after discharge and was noted

to be bright and alert with a normal attitude and appetite. The bladder was a normal size, and hind limb paresis was improved. Serum was submitted at this time and revealed an EHV-1 SN antibody titer of 1:512. Although not a classic fourfold increase, the rise in serum titer was highly suggestive of EHM. The EPM results, albumin quotient, and IgG index were received after discharge. Within the CSF, an elevated albumin concentration and elevated albumin quotient were noted. These findings suggested increased blood-CSF permeability, which may occur in EHM secondary to vasculitis. The IgG concentration and IgG index of the CSF were also elevated, which suggested increased intrathecal production of IgG. Increased intrathecal production can occur in inflammatory diseases of the spinal cord, such as EPM and bacterial meningitis. No evidence of bacterial meningitis was noted on the neurologic examination or CSF cytology, but the EPM results were positive in serum and CSF. These results could have been caused by iatrogenic contamination of CSF by blood or secondary to central nervous system (CNS) vasculitis. EPM could not be definitively ruled out, but the horse showed clinical improvement over time without the use of antiprotozoal medications. The owner was contacted 4 months after discharge and reported that the mare had no neurologic deficits and was being ridden regularly.

Discussion

Signalment

Single cases and multiple horse outbreaks of EHM have been reported in various breeds and ages. Although some outbreaks have noted increased prevalence in pregnant or lactating mares, EHM has been reported in stallions, geldings, and foals, and neurologic deficits have not been related to gender in other outbreaks [2–4]. No breed predilection has been reported, but some retrospective studies have suggested increased susceptibility in younger (≤ 4 years old) horses [5]. In addition, cases of EHM may be more common in the winter and spring months (January through May) [5,6].

History and clinical signs

Nonspecific signs, such as depression, inappetence, nasal discharge, colic, and distal limb edema, may be noted on physical examination in cases of EHM. There is frequently a history of respiratory disease, abortion, neonatal death, or neurologic disease on the premises, with other horses demonstrating the aforementioned nonspecific clinical signs. The rectal temperature is commonly normal at the time neurologic deficits are noted but may be preceded by a history of fever [5,7]. Experimental studies of EHV-1 have demonstrated febrile episodes 1 to 7 days after experimental inoculation in the absence of neurologic deficits, followed by neurologic deficits 6 to 10 days after infection [8,9]. Because of the multifocal distribution of CNS lesions, clinical signs are variable. Commonly, horses with EHM demonstrate an acute onset of symmetric or asymmetric ataxia and paresis that stabilizes over 24 to 48 hours. Typically, gait deficits in the hind limbs are more pronounced than in the forelimbs, and ataxia and paresis may progress to recumbency in severe cases and serves as a negative prognostic indicator. Conscious proprioceptive deficits, such as toe dragging, stumbling, pivoting, and circumduction of the limb(s) when circling, may be observed. Additional reported neurologic deficits include bladder paresis or atony, weak tail and anal tone, and fecal retention [2,7]. Urine dribbling, which may cause urine scalding of the perineum and hind limbs, may be observed secondary to overflow from a distended atonic bladder [2,4,7,10]. Cranial nerve deficits, such as facial nerve paralysis, head tilt, nystagmus, poor or weak tongue tone, ptosis, blindness, and strabismus, have less commonly been reported [2,4,6,7]. Ophthalmic examination may reveal serous ocular discharge, mydriasis, hypopyon, uveitis, chorioretinitis, retinal hemorrhage or detachment, optic neuritis, or blindness [3,5,11]. Epistaxis has also been reported occasionally, and stallions may demonstrate scrotal and testicular edema and loss of libido [3,10,11].

Diagnostic findings

Typically, horses with EHM have normal hematology and serum biochemical evaluations, but lymphopenia may be noted early in the course of the disease [4,6,11]. Alternatively, derangements in CSF analysis are common and include elevations in protein concentration in the absence of pleocytosis (albumino-cytologic dissociation) [2,5,6,12,13]. Xanthochromia of the CSF is also commonly noted [5,6,12,13]. EHM is characterized by vasculitis of the CNS endothelium, which can potentially result in a compromised blood-CSF barrier [2]. This, in turn, may result in movement of protein across the blood-CSF barrier, leading to elevations of CSF protein [5]. Increased CSF protein concentrations are commonly associated with inflammatory processes of the CNS. Other causes include subarachnoid hemorrhage, viral encephalitis, and neoplasms or abscesses of the CNS [14]. Elevations in CSF red blood cell (RBC) counts can be iatrogenic during sample collection or result from extravasation through a compromised blood-CSF barrier secondary to vasculitis or trauma. Degradation of RBCs and hemoglobin catabolism in the CSF results in the release of two pigments, oxyhemoglobin and bilirubin, eventually causing the xanthochromic discoloration [15]. Other causes of CSF xanthochromia to be considered include jaundice, increased protein concentrations (>150 mg/dL) leading to increased albumin-bound bilirubin in the CSF, bilirubin leakage secondary to high serum bilirubin concentrations (total bilirubin concentration >10–15 mg/dL), or leakage of indirect bilirubin through a compromised blood-brain barrier [15].

In a retrospective study of 10 horses with EHM, 8 horses demonstrated elevations in CSF protein concentrations, with a median protein concentration of 155 mg/dL (range: 78–612 mg/dL, reference range: 5–100 mg/dL), whereas 8 of 10 horses demonstrated normal nucleated cell counts (median nucleated cell count = 3.5 cells/μL, range: 0–63 cells/μL, reference range: <6 cells/μL) [5]. Cytologically, most nucleated cells were mononuclear. In addition, the RBC count was high in all horses (median = 426 cells/μL, range: 6–9240 cells/μL), and xanthochromia was noted in 6 horses. The authors did not detect any significant differences between horses that survived and horses that were euthanized with respect to CSF protein concentrations, nucleated cell counts, or RBC counts. Furthermore, cisternal and lumbar CSF samples were collected concurrently from 2 horses, which demonstrated similar protein concentrations between the two locations, but higher numbers of RBCs were noted from the cisternal CSF when compared with the lumbar CSF. Sequential samples from 2 horses were also collected (days 1 and 8 in the first horse and days 1 and 2 in the other horse), which demonstrated increasing protein concentrations and nucleated cell counts between the collection periods [5]. In some cases, samples collected early in the course of disease lack CSF abnormalities [6,7]. If EHM is highly suspected but the initial CSF analysis is normal, subsequent CSF collection and analysis may demonstrate albumino-cytologic dissociation [5,7].

CSF albumin and IgG reflect and are in proportion to serum values [16]. Elevations in CSF albumin concentration may be associated with hemorrhage into the CSF, persistently elevated serum albumin concentrations, or compromise of the blood-CSF barrier [16,17]. Likewise, elevations in CSF IgG can result from compromise of the blood-CSF barrier or from increased intrathecal production of IgG in individuals with inflammatory neurologic disease [16,17]. To evaluate the integrity of the CNS in health and disease, the CSF albumin quotient (CSF albumin/serum albumin × 100) and IgG index ([CSF IgG/serum IgG] × [serum albumin/CSF albumin]) have been used to evaluate blood-CSF barrier permeability and intrathecal IgG production, respectively [16,17]. These methods have also been evaluated in adult and neonatal foals, and increased albumin quotients with normal IgG indices have been noted in EHM and reflect the underlying vasculitis and protein leakage into the CSF [13,17,18].

Western blot analysis for antibodies to *S neurona* in CSF has been used as a method of antemortem diagnosis of EPM. Although the sensitivity of Western blot analysis for horses with EPM has provided adequate results, the specificity of the Western blot test may yield high numbers of false-positive results [19]. A false-positive result may be caused by iatrogenic introduction of antibodies during sample collection or result from a compromised blood-CSF barrier [17]. Loss of the normal integrity of the blood-CSF barrier can potentially allow serum antibodies to enter the CSF. Therefore, interpretation of Western blot test results for EPM in clinical cases that involve a compromised blood-CSF barrier (ie, EHM) should be interpreted with caution. Although increased virus-specific IgG has been noted intrathecally 6 to 10 days after clinical herpes simplex virus encephalitis in people, the discovery of EHV-1 antibodies within the CSF is likely a result of leakage across the compromised blood-CSF barrier rather than intrathecal production [13,16,20,21]. As noted in the case presented here, the result of the Western blot test for antibodies against *S neurona* was positive in light of a high IgG index and albumin quotient. The EPM finding in this case was likely a false-positive result attributable to leakage of circulating antibodies through a compromised blood-CSF barrier, and the increased IgG within the CSF was likely a result of IgG crossing the compromised blood-CSF barrier secondary to vasculitis rather than primary production of IgG.

A diagnosis of EHM can be supported by history, physical and neurologic examination findings, and CSF derangements. Demonstration of a three- to fourfold increase between acute and convalescent SN or complement-fixing antibodies collected 10 to 14 days apart may be the most readily available antemortem diagnostic test to confirm EHM [7,21]. Additional diagnostics include virus isolation, direct and indirect fluorescent antibody, and PCR for EHV-1 (Table 1); special viral transport media and expeditious transport and processing are necessary for these methods. Gross postmortem findings are inconsistent but may include random multifocal distribution of small areas of hemorrhage throughout the meninges, spinal cord, and brain [2,8,22]. Histologic lesions reflect underlying vasculitis, hemorrhage, thrombosis, and secondary ischemic degeneration of nervous tissue [2,8,22]. Other postmortem methods used to detect EHV-1 include immunoperoxidase, immunofluorescent antibody, and PCR techniques [22,23].

Pathophysiology

Inhalation of EHV-1 is the most likely mode of transmission in horses, although direct contact with aborted fetuses or placental membranes may serve as a possible source of infection. After introduction to the nasal mucosa, viral replication occurs in the nasopharyngeal epithelium and lymphoid tissue. The virus then migrates systemically via mononuclear leukocytes, primarily T lymphocytes, and is considered to be immune privileged despite high circulating antibody titers. The virus can then disseminate to other tissues (ie, respiratory, placental) and, in certain instances, attacks the vascular endothelium of the CNS. Vasculitis subsequently develops, leading to necrosis of the vascular endothelium, hemorrhage, and thrombosis with secondary edema formation, hypoxia, and neuronal cell death. EHV-1, like other herpesviruses, is able to spread directly from one cell to another without an extracellular phase [13]. Unlike herpesvirus infection in people, however, there is no clear evidence that EHV-1 replicates in neurons [6,22]. Clinical signs are associated with vasculitis of CNS endothelium, resulting in thrombosis, hemorrhage, and hypoxic damage to neural tissue.

Table 1
Available diagnostic tests and diagnostic laboratories for equine herpesvirus type 1

Laboratory	Diagnostic test	Specimen	Cost	Address
Cornell University (607) 253-3900 www.diaglab.vet.cornell.edu	Serum neutralization Fluorescent antibody* Virus isolation*	Serum Tissue (sent chilled) Tissue or EDTA whole blood (sent chilled)	$13 $15 $50	Serum sent via mail: Diagnostic Laboratory College of Veterinary Medicine Cornell University PO Box 5786 Ithaca, NY 14852 Federal Express or UPS: Diagnostic Laboratory College of Veterinary Medicine Cornell University Upper Tower Road Ithaca, NY 14853
Colorado State University (970) 491-1281 www.dlab.colostate.edu	Serum neutralization Fluorescent antibody* Virus isolation* PCR*	Serum Tissue (lung or liver sent chilled) Swab or EDTA blood (sent chilled) Nasopharyngeal swab, tissue (lung or liver), or EDTA whole blood (sent chilled)	$8 $5 $40 $30	Mail or UPS: Veterinary Diagnostic Lab Colorado State University 300 West Drake Road Fort Collins, CO 80523 Federal Express: Veterinary Diagnostic Lab Colorado State University 300 West Drake Road Room E-100 Fort Collins, CO 80523

Laboratory	Test	Sample	Price	Shipping
University of Tennessee (865) 974-5643 www.vet.utk.edu/diagnostic/virology	Indirect fluorescent antibody Direct fluorescent antibody* Virus isolation*	Serum or cerebrospinal fluid Tissue or impression smear Tissue (sent chilled)	$15 $15 $55	Serum sent via mail, other tissues sent overnight via Federal Express or UPS: UT-CVM Clinical Virology 2407 River Drive A-239 Knoxville, TN 37996
National Veterinary Service Lab (515) 663-7212 www.aphis.usda.gov/vs/nvsl	Serum neutralization Virus isolation*	Serum Tissue, swab, or whole blood (EDTA or heparin)	$12 $45	Virus isolation samples sent on dry ice: National Veterinary Services Laboratory 1800 Dayton Avenue Ames, IA 50010
Texas A&M University (979) 845-3414 http://tvmdlweb.tamu.edu	Serum neutralization Virus isolation*	Serum Tissue, swab, or whole blood (heparin)	$9 $17	Serum sent via mail: Texas Veterinary Medical Laboratory PO Drawer 3040 College Station, TX 77841 Federal Express or UPS: Texas Veterinary Medical Laboratory #1 Sipple Road College Station, TX 77843

Abbreviations: EDTA, ethylenediaminetetraacetic acid; PCR, polymerase chain reaction; UPS, United Parcel Service.
* Overnight–next day delivery necessary.

Treatment

Numerous EHM outbreaks have been reported previously, and recent hospital outbreaks have demonstrated that horses with EHM can remain contagious to naive horses, thus making isolation of affected horses a prudent measure [4,6,10–13,21,24]. Treatment of horses with EHM entails amelioration of vasculitis and inflammation within the CNS as well as careful supportive care and monitoring. Specific drugs that have been used to decrease inflammation and vasculitis include corticosteroids, nonsteroidal anti-inflammatory drugs (NSAIDs), and DMSO. The use of corticosteroids in light of infectious disease is a controversial issue; however, based on their potent anti-inflammatory effects and ability to stabilize cell membranes, dexamethasone (0.05–0.25 mg/kg given parenterally every 24 hours) or prednisolone acetate (1–2 mg/kg given orally every 24 hours) administered for 2 to 3 days, followed by decreasing doses for 3 to 4 additional days, have been used [3,6,7,13,21]. In the case presented here, we elected not to administer corticosteroids based on the stable neurologic deficits and the potential for immunosuppression and iatrogenic bacterial cystitis associated with repeated catheterization of the urinary bladder. Alternatively, NSAIDs, such as flunixin meglumine (1.1 mg/kg administered intravenously every 12 hours) or phenylbutazone (2.2–4.4 mg/kg administered intravenously every 12 hours), have been administered to decrease CNS inflammation [4,21]. Although the systemic toxicity of DMSO is considered low, the true clinical efficacy of DMSO is debatable [25]. Nonetheless, DMSO has been engrained in equine practice and has been administered intravenously at doses of 0.25 to 1 g/kg, diluted in sterile fluids to a 10% to 20% solution, once to twice daily to reduce inflammation in various conditions of the horse [26,27]. Potential beneficial effects of DMSO include scavenging of free radicals, protection of tissues from ischemic damage, reduction of platelet aggregation, and anti-inflammatory and analgesic actions [25]. Broad-spectrum antimicrobials may be warranted because of the increased risk of bacterial cystitis or other secondary infections. Antimicrobials could have been administered in the case presented here to decrease the risk of bacterial cystitis. The bladder was catheterized aseptically, however, and the urine was monitored frequently for evidence of bacterial cystitis; no untoward complications involving the urinary tract were noted in the case presented here. Intermittent sterile catheterization and decompression of the urinary bladder may be necessary in horses demonstrating incontinence. A closed indwelling urinary catheter system (ie, Foley catheter) may also be used in horses with prolonged urinary dysfunction. Urinalysis should be performed routinely in a horse that has had the bladder decompressed by urinary catheterization to detect evidence of bacterial cystitis or evidence of renal insult secondary to nephrotoxic drugs (eg, NSAIDs, acyclovir). Evacuation of feces from the rectum may be required in horses that are not able to defecate normally. Laxatives, such as mineral oil or psyllium, may also be administered orally to facilitate defecation. Hydration status should be monitored regularly, and intravenous fluids (50–75 mL/kg/d) should be administered if the horse is not drinking voluntarily or dehydration is evident. Provision of good footing can help to avoid self-induced trauma, and a palatable diet should be offered. If the horse is reluctant to eat, feeding a slurry of pelleted feed through a nasogastric tube or parenteral nutrition may be necessary to provide adequate nutrition to the anorectic horse.

Acyclovir is a synthetic purine nucleoside analogue that has antiviral activity against several human herpesviruses and varicella zoster virus. Acyclovir is converted to the active form of the drug by virus-specific thymidine kinase to acyclovir triphosphate, which subsequently interferes with viral DNA polymerase and viral replication [28]. Oral bioavailability of acyclovir is relatively poor in people (15%–30%), and concentrations in CSF are approximately one third to one half of serum concentrations; therefore, intravenous administration of higher doses is recommended in people with herpes simplex virus encephalitis [7,28]. Although injectable forms of acyclovir may be cost-prohibitive in adult horses, one may consider their use in exceptionally valuable horses (approximately $100 per dose of generic acyclovir in a 500-kg horse at a rate of 10 mg/kg administered intravenously; Bedford Laboratories, Bedford, Ohio). Current therapeutic management of herpes simplex encephalitis in people suggests a dosage range of 10 to 20 mg/kg administered intravenously every 8 hours for 14 to 21 days and has demonstrated declining viral loads (assessed by PCR and chemiluminescence assay) after initiation of acyclovir [29–33]. Side effects in people are uncommon, but renal injury (ie, crystalline nephropathy), renal failure, and dose-dependent neurotoxicity have been reported [34–36].

Little information is available with regard to the use of acyclovir in herpesvirus infections in horses, but no adverse affects were noted in one report after oral administration of 10 mg/kg five times a day for 10 days [7]. Acyclovir's in vitro median effective concentration against EHV-1 has been shown to range from 0.3 to 7 µg/mL [37–39], and in one study, it was shown that penciclovir (a nucleoside analogue) had excellent in vitro activity against EHV-1 in tissue culture and in a murine model [40]. In one outbreak of EHM in a herd of 46 riding horses, acyclovir was instituted 3 to 4 days after the onset of neurologic disease in 6 of 19 of the most severely affected horses at a dosage of 20 mg/kg administered orally every 8 hours for 5 days, but clinical efficacy could not be assessed [4]. Another study involving neonatal EHV-1 infection on a Thoroughbred farm used acyclovir at a dosage of 8 to 16 mg/kg administered orally every 8 hours for 7 to 12 days in three foals [24]. Two of the three foals administered acyclovir survived, but it is not possible to know the impact that acyclovir had on survival. In another outbreak in Ohio, plasma concentrations of acyclovir were evaluated in 5 horses with EHM receiving oral acyclovir at a rate of 10 mg/kg five times per day [39]. Three to 4 days after initiation of acyclovir, plasma concentrations of acyclovir were evaluated at 30, 60, and 300 minutes after administration and resulted in serum concentrations ranging from 0.29 µg/mL (range: 0.23–0.87 µg/mL) at 30 minutes, 0.3 µg/mL (range: 0.20–0.38 µg/mL) at 60 minutes, and 0.23 µg/mL (range: 0.17–0.39 µg/mL) at 300 minutes [39]. Interestingly, all 5 horses survived. These results suggest that repeated oral administration of acyclovir may variably reach minimal therapeutic serum concentrations and emphasize the need for frequent (every 5 hours) oral administration; moreover, higher oral doses may be necessary to reach adequate concentrations within the CNS. No adverse affects have been reported with regard to oral administration of acyclovir in horses; however, transient elevation of serum creatinine has been reported in 1 horse administered acyclovir (20 mg/kg given orally every 8 hours), and renal function should be monitored to evaluate for potential renal injury [4].

Recently, pharmacokinetic data with oral and intravenous acyclovir have been gathered in six adult horses [41]. Intravenous administration of 10 mg/kg (diluted in sterile saline, 1 L) over 1 hour resulted in a mean peak serum concentration of 13.74 µg/mL ($\pm$5.88 SD) immediately after infusion was complete and maintained a mean plasma concentration greater than 0.3 µg/mL for 8 hours. Therefore, the authors suggested that twice-daily intravenous administration of acyclovir (10 mg/kg) would provide adequate plasma concentrations ($>$0.3 µg/mL) for the entire treatment interval [41]. In contrast to the previously noted report, plasma concentrations of acyclovir were below limits of detection after single oral administration (20 mg/kg) in all six horses. This may have been attributable to the cumulative affects of repeated (five times daily) oral administration compared with single-dose administration. Further controlled studies evaluating peak CSF concentrations, therapeutic benefits, and side affects are required to determine the effectiveness of acyclovir for the treatment of EHM.

Prognosis

The prognosis for EHM is generally fair to good, with many horses demonstrating stabilization of neurologic deficits after 24 to 48 hours. In a retrospective study of 11 cases of EHM, 5 of 11 horses survived, whereas in another report, 17 of 19 horses with neurologic deficits made a complete recovery [4,5]. Periods of weeks to months may be required before complete recovery from severe neurologic deficits is noted, and some horses may maintain residual neurologic deficits [3,6,10,11,13]. Most mildly to moderately affected mares regain breeding soundness, but the reproductive capabilities of severely affected mares may be limited because of bladder dysfunction [3,13]. Of interest, in the retrospective study of 11 horses with EHM, 5 of the 6 horses that did not survive were recumbent at hospital admission or became recumbent during hospitalization [5]. This reflects the anecdotal findings that affected horses with EHM that remain standing (or can stand with assistance) have a good prognosis for survival, whereas prolonged ($>$24 hours) recumbency suggests a more guarded prognosis [3,6,13]. A few reports of EHM have documented complete recovery after prolonged recumbency (days to weeks) [11,42]. Therefore, euthanasia should not be performed prematurely if the horse's disposition allows prolonged treatment.

Prevention

Vaccines for EHV-1 are commercially available, but current information suggests that vaccination is not protective against the neurologic form of EHV-1. Cases of EHM have been reported in horses vaccinated with killed and modified-live EHV-1 vaccines [6]. Routine vaccination is still recommended to provide circulating antibodies against EHV-1 and theoretically decrease the incidence of respiratory infection and abortion in exposed horses as well as the duration and amount of viral shedding [43]. Control of dissemination of disease in confirmed or suspected cases of EHM may be attempted by routine quarantine, isolation, and disinfection procedures. New horses should be routinely quarantined for at least 3 to 4 weeks before introduction to the remainder of the herd, and horses affected with EHM should be strictly isolated. Subclinical cases of EHV-1 may be detected via serologic evaluation of all horses on the premises, and traffic of horses should be minimized in farms with confirmed cases of EHM for at least 3 weeks after the most recent case [7]. Aborted fetuses and fetal fluids serve as sources of infection and should be properly submitted to a diagnostic laboratory or disposed of immediately (eg, heavy-gauge plastic bag, burning) [13]. Virus transmission can also occur via organic material on clothes, shoes, tack, or other related items; therefore, these items should be thoroughly disinfected.

References

[1] Ostlund EN. The equine herpesviruses. Vet Clin North Am Equine Pract 1993;9:283–94.
[2] Jackson TA, Osburn BI, Cordy DR, et al. Equine herpesvirus 1 infection of horses: studies on the experimentally induced neurologic disease. Am J Vet Res 1977;38:709–19.
[3] McCartan CG, Russell MM, Wood JL, et al. Clinical, serological and virological characteristics of an outbreak of paresis and neonatal foal disease due to equine herpesvirus-1 on a stud farm. Vet Rec 1995;136:7–12.
[4] Friday PA, Scarratt WK, Elvinger F, et al. Ataxia and paresis with equine herpesvirus type 1 infection in a herd of riding school horses. J Vet Intern Med 2000;14:197–201.
[5] Donaldson MT, Sweeney CR. Herpesvirus myeloencephalopathy in horses: 11 cases (1982–1996). J Am Vet Med Assoc 1998;213:671–5.
[6] Kohn CW, Fenner WR. Equine herpes myeloencephalopathy. Vet Clin North Am Equine Pract 1987;3:405–19.
[7] Donaldson M, Sweeney C. Equine herpes myeloencephalopathy. Compend Contin Educ Pract Vet 1997;19:864–71.
[8] Mumford JA, Edington N. EHV1 and equine paresis. Vet Rec 1980;106:277.
[9] Jackson T, Kendrick JW. Paralysis of horses associated with equine herpesvirus 1 infection. J Am Vet Med Assoc 1971;158:1351–7.
[10] Crowhurst FA, Dickinson G, Burrows R. An outbreak of paresis in mares and geldings associated with equid herpesvirus 1. Vet Rec 1981;109:527–8.

[11] Greenwood RE, Simson AR. Clinical report of a paralytic syndrome affecting stallions, mares and foals on a thoroughbred studfarm. Equine Vet J 1980;12:113–7.

[12] Platt H, Singh H, Whitwell KE. Pathological observations on an outbreak of paralysis in broodmares. Equine Vet J 1980;12:118–26.

[13] Wilson WD. Equine herpesvirus 1 myeloencephalopathy. Vet Clin North Am Equine Pract 1997;13:53–72.

[14] Jerrard DA, Hanna JR, Schindelheim GL. Cerebrospinal fluid. J Emerg Med 2001;21:171–8.

[15] Shah KH, Edlow JA. Distinguishing traumatic lumbar puncture from true subarachnoid hemorrhage. J Emerg Med 2002;23:67–74.

[16] Reiber H, Peter JB. Cerebrospinal fluid analysis: disease-related data patterns and evaluation programs. J Neurol Sci 2001;184:101–22.

[17] Miller MM, Sweeney CR, Russell GE, et al. Effects of blood contamination of cerebrospinal fluid on Western blot analysis for detection of antibodies against Sarcocystis neurona and on albumin quotient and immunoglobulin G index in horses. J Am Vet Med Assoc 1999;215: 67–71.

[18] Andrews FM, Geiser DR, Sommardahl CS, et al. Albumin quotient, IgG concentration, and IgG index determinations in cerebrospinal fluid of neonatal foals. Am J Vet Res 1994;55: 741–5.

[19] Daft BM, Barr BC, Gardner IA, et al. Sensitivity and specificity of Western blot testing of cerebrospinal fluid and serum for diagnosis of equine protozoal myeloencephalitis in horses with and without neurologic abnormalities. J Am Vet Med Assoc 2002;221: 1007–13.

[20] Schultze D, Weder B, Cassinotti P, et al. Diagnostic significance of intrathecally produced herpes simplex and varicella-zoster virus-specific antibodies in central nervous system infections. Swiss Med Wkly 2004;134:700–4.

[21] Reed SM, Toribio RE. Equine herpesvirus 1 and 4. Vet Clin North Am Equine Pract 2004; 20:631–42.

[22] del Piero F, Wilkins P, Delahunta A, et al. Fifteen cases of equine herpesvirus-1 (EHV-1) encephalomyelopathy in horses: pathologic and immunoperoxidase histochemical findings. Vet Pathol 1998;35:441.

[23] Schultheiss PC, Collins JK, Hotaling SF. Immunohistochemical demonstration of equine herpesvirus-1 antigen in neurons and astrocytes of horses with acute paralysis. Vet Pathol 1997;34:52–4.

[24] Murray MJ, del Piero F, Jeffrey SC, et al. Neonatal equine herpesvirus type 1 infection on a thoroughbred breeding farm. J Vet Intern Med 1998;12:36–41.

[25] Brayton CF. Dimethyl sulfoxide (DMSO): a review. Cornell Vet 1986;76:61–90.

[26] Stewart RH, Griffiths JP. Medical management of spinal cord disease. Vet Clin North Am Equine Pract 1987;3:429–36.

[27] Sullins KE, White NA, Lundin CS, et al. Prevention of ischaemia-induced small intestinal adhesions in foals. Equine Vet J 2004;36:370–5.

[28] Wagstaff AJ, Faulds D, Goa KL. Acyclovir. A reappraisal of its antiviral activity, pharmacokinetic properties and therapeutic efficacy. Drugs 1994;47:153–205.

[29] Kamei S, Takasu T, Morishima T, et al. Serial changes of intrathecal viral loads evaluated by chemiluminescence assay and nested PCR with acyclovir treatment in herpes simplex virus encephalitis. Intern Med 2004;43:796–801.

[30] Fonseca-Aten M, Messina AF, Jafri HS, et al. Herpes simplex virus encephalitis during suppressive therapy with acyclovir in a premature infant. Pediatrics 2005;115:804–9.

[31] Whitley RJ, Kimberlin DW. Herpes simplex: encephalitis children and adolescents. Semin Pediatr Infect Dis 2005;16:17–23.

[32] Tyler KL. Herpes simplex virus infections of the central nervous system: encephalitis and meningitis, including Mollaret's. Herpes 2004;11(Suppl 2):57A–64A.

[33] Kimberlin D. Herpes simplex virus, meningitis and encephalitis in neonates. Herpes 2004; 11(Suppl 2):65A–76A.

[34] Sodhi PK, Ratan SK. A case of chronic renal dysfunction following treatment with oral acyclovir. Scand J Infect Dis 2003;35:770–2.

[35] Perazella MA. Drug-induced renal failure: update on new medications and unique mechanisms of nephrotoxicity. Am J Med Sci 2003;325:349–62.

[36] Becker BN, Fall P, Hall C, et al. Rapidly progressive acute renal failure due to acyclovir: case report and review of the literature. Am J Kidney Dis 1993;22:611–5.

[37] De Clercq E, Holy A, Rosenberg I, et al. A novel selective broad-spectrum anti-DNA virus agent. Nature 1986;323:464–7.

[38] Rollinson EA, White G. Relative activities of acyclovir and BW759 against Aujeszky's disease and equine rhinopneumonitis viruses. Antimicrob Agents Chemother 1983;24:221–6.

[39] Wilkins P. Acyclovir in the treatment of EHV-1 myeloencephalopathy. Presented at the 22nd American College of Veterinary Internal Medicine Forum, Minneapolis, MN, 2004. p. 170–2.

[40] de la Fuente R, Awan AR, Field HJ. The acyclic nucleoside analogue penciclovir is a potent inhibitor of equine herpesvirus type 1 (EHV-1) in tissue culture and in a murine model. Antiviral Res 1992;18:77–89.

[41] Wilkins P, Papich M, Sweeney R. Pharmacokinetics of acyclovir in adult horses. J Vet Emerg Crit Care 2005;15:174–8.

[42] Charlton KM, Mitchell D, Girard A, et al. Meningoencephalomyelitis in horses associated with equine herpesvirus 1 infection. Vet Pathol 1976;13:59–68.

[43] Burrows R, Goodridge D, Denyer MS. Trials of an inactivated equid herpesvirus 1 vaccine: challenge with a subtype 1 virus. Vet Rec 1984;114:369–74.

ELSEVIER
SAUNDERS

Vet Clin Equine 22 (2006) 193–208

VETERINARY
CLINICS
Equine Practice

Perinatal Asphyxia Syndrome in a Quarter Horse Foal

Lisa Katz, DVM, MS, PhD, MRCVS

University Veterinary Hospital, School of Agriculture, Food Science and Veterinary Medicine, University College Dublin, Belfield, Dublin 4, Ireland

Case history

A 2-day-old Quarter Horse filly weighing 61 kg was presented for generalized seizures of 12 hours' duration. The mare delivered standing and had to have the filly pulled at the end of parturition. The filly was large and stood within 2 hours of delivery, nursing normally. Examination by the referring veterinarian (rDVM) revealed contracted forelimbs, which were treated with an unknown amount of intravenous oxytetracycline and bandages. At approximately 17 hours of age, the suckle reflex and affinity for the dam were lost, with the filly becoming weak and disorientated. The following day, the filly developed generalized seizures that could not be controlled with diazepam (10 mg administered intravenously twice) and was then treated with phenobarbital (1 g administered intravenously), which successfully controlled the seizures for approximately 1 hour. A cerebrospinal fluid (CSF) tap performed by the rDVM was reported to appear normal; the sample in ethylenediaminetetraacetic acid (EDTA) was sent with the filly. Before referral, the filly had been treated intravenously with ketoprofen (100 mg) and gentamicin sulfate (330 mg) and given 90% dimethyl sulfoxide (DMSO; 50 g) and mare's milk (16 oz) per nasogastric intubation. The mare had been housed in a field alone and fed grass hay and a 14% Purina sweet feed mix (Purina Mills, LLC, USA). The mare had been dewormed with ivermectin and vaccinated for rhinopneumonitis at 6, 9, and 11 months of gestation and given tetanus toxoid, eastern and western equine encephalitis, and influenza boosters during the last month of pregnancy. There had been no dietary or management changes, and the dam had a healthy gestation of 340 days. The filly's umbilicus had been dipped with 2% iodine, and the filly had passed meconium. Immunoglobulin levels measured using the CITE

E-mail address: lisakatz@ucd.ie

doi:10.1016/j.cveq.2005.12.007

(IDEXX Inc, Portland, Maine) foal assay revealed concentrations greater than 800 mg/dL, indicating adequate passive transfer of antibodies. The filly was the mare's second foal.

Clinical examination

On presentation, the filly was in right lateral recumbency, exhibiting generalized tonic-clonic convulsions. It was unconscious, thrashing, and paddling all four limbs violently, with repetitive eye blinking and rapid eye movements. The filly was treated with diazepam (5 mg administered intravenously once), which quickly controlled the seizures for approximately 1 hour, after which it had another generalized seizure and was again treated with diazepam (5 mg administered intravenously once). The filly's temperature was 34.8°C (94.6°F) (reference range: 37.2°C–38.9°C [99.0°F–102°F]), and the heart and respiratory rate, taken after treatment with diazepam, were 64 beats per minute (bpm; reference range: 80–120 bpm) and 40 breaths per minute (brpm; reference range: 20–40 brpm), respectively. The mucous membranes were pink and moist, with a capillary refill time of approximately 2 seconds. There was mild bilateral forelimb flexor tendon contracture, the joints all palpated within normal limits, and the umbilicus was dry. The gastrointestinal sounds were normal in all four quadrants, and auscultation of the lungs revealed crackles and inspiratory wheezes bilaterally. A neurologic examination revealed a depressed nonresponsive filly with no suckle response.

The primary problems identified were generalized seizures, depression, hypothermia, decreased heart rate, bilaterally contracted forelimb flexor tendons, and generalized lower respiratory crackles and wheezes. Causes of generalized seizures in a neonate were broken down into extracranial and intracranial diseases. The differential diagnosis for extracranial causes included metabolic derangements (hyponatremia, hypernatremia, hypoxia, and hypoglycemia) as well as toxins and infectious causes (septicemia, endotoxemia, fever, and tetanus), whereas the differential diagnosis for intracranial diseases included congenital abnormalities (hydrocephalus and benign epilepsy), infection (bacterial meningitis, abscess, and encephalitis), trauma, perinatal complications (hypoxic-ischemic encephalitis [HIE]), and toxicity (moldy corn). Based on the signalment and history, metabolic disease, infection, and HIE seemed to be the most likely causes. The differential diagnosis for depression of a large animal neonate is extensive and was narrowed down into disorders that could be related to generalized seizures. These included bacterial infection (septicemia), metabolic derangements (hypoglycemia, hyponatremia, hypokalemia, acidosis, and hypocalcemia), central neurologic lesions (HIE, meningitis, and trauma), hepatitis, and renal failure. The crackles and wheezes indicated lower airway disease, such as pneumonia (viral, bacterial, or fungal), lung abscess, pulmonary edema, and small airway inflammation. Based on the signalment and history, bacterial pneumonia was considered likely as well as pulmonary involvement, such as atelectasis, hyaline membrane formation, and pulmonary hypertension secondary to perinatal asphyxia syndrome (PAS). Differentials for the low body temperature and heart rate included environmental influences, hypoglycemia, septicemic shock, and drug-induced (diazepam) and central neurologic diseases resulting in damage to the regulatory centers in the hypothalamus. Specific causes of flexural contractures are unknown but may possibly be attributable to malpositioning of the fetus in utero.

Case management

On day 1, blood was submitted for a complete blood cell count (CBC), serum chemistry panel, arterial blood gas (ABG), and blood culture. The bladder was catheterized, and an extremely small amount of urine was obtained for urinalysis. The CSF tap collected by the rDVM was submitted for cytology. The CBC showed neutropenia with a degenerative left shift (Table 1), whereas the chemistry profile revealed hyponatremia, hyperkalemia, hypochloremia, elevated blood urea nitrogen (BUN) and creatinine (azotemia), and mildly elevated lactate dehydrogenase (LDH) (Table 2). The urinalysis revealed a dilute urine specific gravity, proteinuria, and a large amount of blood. Acute neutropenia usually occurs because of a shift of neutrophils from the circulating to the marginating pools as a result of endotoxin, whereas chronic neutropenia can be caused by reduced survival or increased use of circulating neutrophils (endotoxemia or sepsis), reduced production of neutrophils, increased ineffective granulopoiesis, and idiopathic factors (secondary to infection). Based on the presence of the degenerative left shift and in light of the history and clinical examination results, margination and consumption or decreased survival as a result of sepsis seemed to be the most likely explanation for the neutropenia. The mildly elevated LDH was likely secondary to muscle damage secondary to the seizure activity and poor circulation from endotoxemic shock. Because the urine specific gravity was low before the administration of fluids, the azotemia was classified as renal, although prerenal and postrenal azotemia could not be completely discounted. Although neonates can adequately concentrate their urine, they normally have dilute urine (range: 1.001–1.006) because of their almost completely liquid (milk) diet. This can make the use of urine specific gravity as a way to differentiate among different causes of azotemia difficult. This filly had signs of maldistributive shock secondary to sepsis, which likely contributed to some prerenal azotemia. Because the filly likely had not been taking in a normal amount of fluid for the 12 hours before presentation, however, the urine specific gravity should have been elevated if prerenal abnormalities were the sole cause of the azotemia. Considering the filly's age, renal azotemia

Table 1
Complete blood cell count results

	Normal values	Day 1	Day 2	Day 3	Day 4	Day 5	Day 6	Day 7	Day 9	Day 11
PCV (%)	28–46	31	30	28	27	30	30	30	29	30
White blood cell count	5100–10,100	3400	1200	4100	4100	5800	4300	5370	5600	6600
Bands	0–150	408	24	164	164	174	43	0	0	0
Segmented neutrophils	3210–8580	2380	1200	1435	1435	3364	3010	3550	3668	4488
Lymphocytes	730–2170	476	1176	2296	2296	2204	1161	1700	1656	1716
Monocytes	80–580	136	0	205	205	58	86	7	184	264
Leukocyte morphology		2+ toxic	3+ toxic	2+ toxic	2+ toxic	2+ toxic				
Platelets	105,000–353,000	176,000	165,000	143,000	143,000	114,000	101,000	118,000	264,000	384,000
Fibrinogen (mg/dL)	200–400	300	300	300	300	400	300	300	300	400

Abbreviation: PCV, packed cell volume.

Table 2
Serum biochemistry results

	Normal values	Day 12:00 am	Day 6:00 pm	Day 2	Day 3	Day 4	Day 5	Day 6	Day 7	Day 8	Day 9	Day 11
BUN (mg/dL)	2–29	50	53	57	60	60	62	50	26	14	7	4
Creatinine (mg/dL)	0.4–3.6	7.1	8.4	9.8	9.4	9.4	7.0	4.7	3.8	2.6	2.4	2.1
Glucose (mg/dL)	101–226	132	100	121	116	116	165	145	144	106	128	120
Sodium (mmol/L)	132–144	112	113	115	130	130	142	144	151	135	137	135
Potassium (mmol/L)	2.7–4.8	6.4	7.2	6.4	4.1	4.1	2.9	3.1	3.9	3.3	3.1	3.3
Chloride (mmol/L)	94–103	79	79	84	90	94	105	103	123	107	109	107
Total protein (g/dL)	4.4–7.6	4.8	4.9	4.5	5.6	5.1	5.1	5.7	5.3	5.1	4.8	5.1
Albumin (g/dL)	2.0–3.7	1.9	1.9	1.9		2.0	2.0	2.2	2.0	2.3	1.8	1.9
Globulin (g/dL)	2.1–3.9	2.9	3.0	2.6		3.1	3.1	3.5	3.3	2.8	3.1	3.2

Abbreviation: BUN, blood urea nitrogen.

likely indicated acute renal failure (ARF), although postrenal azotemia secondary to a rupture in the urinary tract was also a strong consideration. The proteinuria was considered secondary to glomerular damage or as a result of colostral absorption and subsequent protein excretion. The hematuria was considered most likely secondary to ARF as a result of acute tubular necrosis (ATN), or traumatic hemorrhage into the urine secondary to a rupture in the urinary tract. To evaluate the renal system further, calculation of the fractional excretion of electrolytes (sodium, potassium, and chloride) and the gamma-glutamyltransferase (GGT)/creatinine ratio was planned but not performed. The GGT/creatinine ratio (>25 is abnormal) is calculated based on the measurement of urine GGT and creatinine using the following equation:

$$\frac{\text{Urinary GGT}}{\text{Urinary Cr} \times 0.01}$$

GGT is found in the epithelial cells lining the renal tubules, with its activity increasing with tubular damage. An abnormal GGT/creatinine ratio is considered to be an early indicator of renal tubular damage, although it may not have been useful in the current case, because even one dose of a nephrotoxic drug may elevate the ratio and the filly had already received gentamicin, ketoprofen, and oxytetracycline.

The fractional excretion, E, of electrolytes, such as chloride, sodium, or potassium is based on the simultaneous measurement of urine and plasma electrolytes using the following equations:

$$\frac{[\text{Urine E}] \times [\text{Plasma Cr}]}{[\text{Plasma E}] \times [\text{Urine Cr}]} \times 100$$

These clearances are used to evaluate the kidney's ability to secrete or re-absorb electrolytes, with abnormalities pointing toward early tubular dys-function. Unfortunately, the amount of the initial urine sample collected was insufficient to measure these substances, and attempts at subsequent urine collection were unsuccessful, such that the calculations could not be completed before the initiation of fluid therapy. In light of the azotemia, the hypocalcemia, hyponatremia, and hypochloremia were likely the result of renal tubular damage or sequestration of sodium-containing fluid within the abdomen secondary to rupture of the urinary tract. Because this was a large filly and there was a history of dystocia, the latter could not be dis-counted, although based on the history and physical examination results, oliguric ATN secondary to asphyxia and hypoxic-ischemic damage, exacer-bated by the use of oxytetracycline, a nephrotoxic drug, was a strong possi-bility. Although the pathogenesis is unclear, in utero hypoxia can result in renal impairment and generalized edema with oliguria as a result of redistri-bution of fetal cardiac output and decreased renal perfusion [1]. Renal blood flow is extremely sensitive to asphyxia, with fetal adaptations to an in utero hypoxic environment including stimulation of fetal compensatory mecha-nisms and redistribution of blood flow, resulting in preferential perfusion of organs like the heart and brain at the expense of blood flow to organs like the kidneys, gut, and lungs [2]. Increased serum creatinine concentration or profound azotemia detected at birth is suggested to be related to placental insufficiency and neonatal asphyxia [2,3]. It seemed likely that both contrib-uted to the current filly's renal disease given the history and associated clin-ical signs, with the use of oxytetracycline possibly contributing to the problem. The amount of oxytetracycline used to treat flexural contractions is approximately four times the amount needed for its use as an antibiotic, with subsequent increased toxicity to the kidneys. Therefore, it was likely that renal compromise was more likely attributable to the administration of oxytetracycline than that of gentamicin or ketoprofen; however, all three of these drugs are potentially nephrotoxic.

The ABG (see Table 2) indicated profound hypoxemia and primary met-abolic acidosis with respiratory compensation. The hypoxemia was second-ary to diffusion limitations or ventilation/perfusion mismatch, whereas the compensated metabolic acidosis was likely from a combination of poor pe-ripheral perfusion resulting in lactic acid accumulation and ARF. The acidosis was likely worsening the hyperkalemia, because intracellular potas-sium is exchanged for extracellular hydrogen ions as the body attempts to buffer the acidosis. Thoracic radiographs taken to evaluate the pulmonary system further revealed diffuse patchy alveolar and heavy unstructured interstitial opacities throughout the lung fields with an underlying bronchial pattern, indicating diffuse bronchopneumonia, whereas skull radiographs revealed no bony evidence of trauma or congenital defects. A transtracheal wash (TTW) was planned to characterize the cause of the pneumonia further but was not performed, because it was believed that the filly was too unstable to handle the procedure. It was planned to place the filly on broad-spectrum antibiotic therapy and monitor response to treatment and to perform a TTW if no improvement was noted. The cytologic findings of the CSF tap were within normal limits; thus, it was decided not to perform a second CSF tap to obtain a sample for culture and sensitivity testing. Abdominal and renal ultrasonography was performed to evaluate the urinary tract further. The urinary tract appeared intact with no appreciable free fluid found within the abdominal cavity, whereas the kidneys appeared mildly edematous bilaterally with some loss of the corticomedullary junction definition. Abdominocentesis was performed with fluid submitted for cytology and measurement of peritoneal creatinine levels. Based on the peritoneal creatinine/serum creatinine ratio being close to 1:1 (>2:1 indicates urinary tract rupture) and the normal findings on abdominal ultrasonography, a rupture of the urinary tract was considered unlikely. Based on the history as well as the clinical examination and laboratory findings, a presumptive diagnosis of HIE and ARF was made.

Treatment on day 1 included intravenous fluid therapy (lactated Ringer's solution with 50% dextrose [100 mL] added to make a 5% solution administered at a rate of 300 mL/h) so as to address hydration, electrolyte balances, ongoing losses, and tissue and organ perfusion. A dextrose-containing solution was chosen in an attempt to drive potassium into the cells so as to bring down serum potassium concentrations. The filly's exact sodium deficit was not calculated but could have been using the following formula: mEq Na^+ Needed $= (125 - \text{Measured } [Na^+]) \times \text{Body Weight (kg)} \times 0.6$.

Because it was unknown as to how long the filly's sodium concentrations had been less than 120 mEq/L, it was believed that caution was required so as not to return the serum sodium concentrations to normal concentrations too quickly for fear of worsening cerebral abnormalities via inducing cerebral edema. This is why we used the value of 125 mEq in the previous equation in place of the normal serum value of 140 mEq/L. It was possible that the hyponatremia alone was the cause of the seizures, especially if the drop in sodium was acute, such as might occur secondary to ARF, and associated with extracellular fluid (ECF) volume depletion with subsequent hypotonic volume expansion. Because mare's milk is so low in sodium, it is possible that ingesting this may have contributed to a hypotonic volume expansion in the current case, even though the filly was not drinking a normal volume of milk. To evaluate serum osmolality, it could have been calculated using the following formula: Osmolality $= 2[Na^+] + ([\text{Glucose}]/18) + (BUN/2.8)$.

Although acute hyponatremia (<120 mEq/L after 48 hours) associated with ECF volume depletion can cause neurologic problems, such as seizures, because of movement of water into brain cells, there was some concern that the hyponatremia was a more chronic problem, with intracellular conditions having adjusted to extracellular conditions with the formation of osmolytes. If this were the case, this would mean that rapid resolution of the sodium could contribute to further neurologic damage in the present case. Because HIE was still highly considered to be involved, the presence of cerebral edema as a result of HIE was a concern. Therefore, it was decided initially to try to correct the sodium deficit cautiously and then to become more aggressive if the clinical and laboratory results indicated the need. Thus, lactated Ringer's solution, a relatively balanced solution containing little potassium (4 mEq/L) but having a high sodium concentration (130 mEq/L), was chosen to try to bring the sodium concentrations up slowly. Although a fluid solution containing no potassium at all, such as sodium chloride, given at a lower fluid rate may have been a better choice, it was decided to use lactated Ringer's solution initially because it had slightly less sodium and to switch to a potassium-free solution later, because a higher than maintenance fluid rate was chosen to try to increase renal perfusion. In addition, the filly likely had a total body deficit of potassium despite the elevated serum concentration because of decreased dietary intake. Therefore, with increased circulating volume and resolution of acidosis, it was anticipated that hypokalemia might occur. To avoid fluid overload, which could potentially worsen any cerebral edema or result in pulmonary edema, the amount of intravenous fluids given was only one and a half times the calculated maintenance dose of 80 mL/kg/d. Calculations of maintenance fluid requirements for neonates have since been modified, with the recommendation now [4] as follows:

First 10 kg: 100 mL/kg/d
Second 10 kg: 50 mL/kg/d
Rest of body weight (kg): 25 mL/kg/d

For this filly, which weighed 61 kg, maintenance fluid requirements would thus have been calculated to be 105 mL/h, half of the original maintenance calculations.

To support the filly nutritionally, a small nasogastric tube (Mila International, Inc, Florence, Kentucky) was placed in the distal esophagus and sewn into place at the nares after confirmation that it was in the proper place by visualizing the tube entering the esophagus with use of a pediatric endoscope. Tube placement was also confirmed later when thoracic radiographs were taken. The filly was fed milk (200 mL) every hour, which was just less than 10% of the filly's body weight in kilograms, resulting in a total fluid rate of two and a half maintenance (500 mL/h). Even though the nutritional requirement for a normal foal is approximately 25% of the body weight in kilograms, less was chosen for this filly because it was thought that the filly would be unable to tolerate the increased fluid volume and the enteral feeding. It is common that 10% to 15% of the foal's body weight be fed in the first 24 hours and then increased as the foal's tolerance permits. Sick neonates, including foals with PAS, often have problems associated with the gastrointestinal tract (GIT) [5], which may be exacerbated by constant feeding in the face of dysfunction and hypoxia [4]. Damage to the GIT is often subtle and may lag behind other clinical abnormalities for days to weeks [4]. The most common signs of GIT abnormalities include colic, decreased motility and fecal output, decreased weight gain, and ulceration, and some foals may develop necrotizing enterocolitis (NEC) or intussusception [4]. It has been recommended to hold off allowing enteral feeds until vital signs are stable in foals with PAS so as to minimize the risk of NEC [2]. Enteral feeding can be done in a constant or pulsed fashion [6–8], with the most current recommendation being pulsed feeding through a small indwelling tube [4]. These small tubes are ideal, because foals that are able to nurse can do so around them [4]. Because equine neonates should gain 1 to 2 lb/d, the filly was weighed before and every day after the initiation of drug and fluid therapy so as to adjust doses accordingly and to monitor hydration and adequate caloric intake. Because of the possibility of HIE, 90% DMSO (1 g/kg administered intravenously every 24 hours for 3 days) diluted to a 10% solution was used to decrease any cerebral edema and inflammation. DMSO and vitamin E–selenium (E-Se; 1 mL/45 kg administered intramuscularly once) were also given for their antioxidant and free radical scavenging effects. Commercial fresh-frozen plasma (J5; 2 L administered intravenously once) was given to provide additional immunoglobulins, clotting factors, enzymes, and transport proteins as well as to help prevent any systemic effects of endotoxin released. Because of the strong possibility of a bacterial bronchopneumonia and septicemia, the filly was placed on broad-spectrum antibiotics (potassium penicillin G, 22,000 U/kg, administered intravenously every 6 hours; ceftiofur sodium, 4.4 mg/kg, administered intravenously every 12 hours). Retrospectively, sodium penicillin, which contains sodium (2 mEq) per penicillin (1 million U), may have been a better choice than potassium penicillin, which contains potassium (1.7 mEq) per penicillin (1 million U) in an effort to reduce the potassium further and increase the sodium intake in the filly. In reality, however, this amount of potassium is small and likely not of clinical relevance. Ceftiofur was chosen over an aminoglycoside because it is less nephrotoxic but still had some gram-negative coverage, because gram-negative organisms, such as *Klebsiella* spp, *Actinobacillus* spp, and *Escherichia coli*, are commonly implicated as causative agents in equine neonatal infectious diseases. Antiulcer medication (omeprazole, 4 mg/kg, per nasogastric tube administered every 24 hours) was begun, and because of the hypoxemia, the filly was started on oxygen therapy consisting of nasal insufflation at 5 L/min. Because the filly could not stand on its own, it was flipped to the opposite side every 2 hours so as to minimize pulmonary consolidation and pressure sores.

A chemistry profile repeated 12 hours after the initiation of treatment revealed that the BUN, creatinine, and sodium concentrations were unchanged (see Table 2); thus, the intravenous fluids were changed to 0.9% sodium chloride. The packed cell volume (PCV), total protein (TP), and ABG were monitored through the night.

No seizures were observed through the night, and on day 2, the filly seemed to be more responsive and could rise and stand on its own for a short period. When recumbent, the filly was still difficult to arouse and still had no suckle response. An ABG revealed resolving hypoxia; thus, the nasal insufflation was discontinued. Despite fluid therapy, the filly had only urinated once during the night, and a repeat CBC and chemistry profile revealed that the white blood cell count had dropped; the BUN, serum creatinine, and LDH had increased; and the sodium, potassium and chloride concentrations remained unchanged (see Tables 1 and 2). In an attempt to increase the serum sodium level further and bring the potassium level down, the intravenous fluids were changed to a solution containing sodium (total of 234 mEq/L) with bicarbonate and dextrose to drive potassium intracellularly ($NaHCO_3$; 90 mEq added to 10% dextrose in isotonic [0.9%] saline, 1 L). The fluids were maintained at the same rate as previously determined. Additionally, to try to promote urine output and increase renal blood flow, the filly was treated with a diuretic (furosemide, 1 mg/kg, administered intravenously once) and placed on a continuous dopamine drip (1 μg/kg/min administered intravenously). Low-dose dopamine stimulates dopaminergic receptors, resulting in an improvement in renal perfusion, and may augment blood flow in other vascular beds [9], whereas furosemide, a loop-diuretic, supposedly works synergistically with dopamine to produce renal vasodilation and diuresis [10,11]. Blood pressure and urine output need to be carefully monitored so as to avoid stimulating α_1-adrenergic receptors, which would cause peripheral vasoconstriction, increased arterial blood pressure, and reduce renal blood flow [2]. Monitoring indirect blood pressure was attempted but was unsuccessful in the present case because of lack of proper equipment; thus, the filly's PCV, TP, heart rate, and pulmonary system were all monitored closely. Within 1 hour of treatment with dopamine and furosemide, the filly urinated. A repeat urinalysis revealed no changes except glucosuria, which was likely from damaged renal tubules, because there was no evidence of hyperglycemia. Because the filly seemed to be able to tolerate an increase in fluids and showed no clinical signs of GIT abnormalities, the amount of milk fed was increased (300 mL/h), although the intravenous fluid rate remained unchanged. The filly continued to improve neurologically; by day 3, the filly seemed to be alert and aware of its surroundings, and by day 6, it was nursing from the mare. An ABG taken on day 3 was within normal limits, and a CBC and chemistry profile taken on days 3 through 9 showed a daily improvement in the white blood cell count, BUN, creatinine and electrolyte concentrations; by day 11, all values were within normal limits (see Tables 1 and 2). The amount and rate of a variety of different sodium-containing intravenous fluids decreased daily as the amount of milk fed increased, and by day 6, all intravenous fluids were discontinued. A renal ultrasound scan was repeated on day 7 and revealed bilaterally normal kidneys. Thoracic radiographs were repeated on day 7 and exhibited evidence of resolving pneumonia. By day 10, the filly was bright and alert and had gained 12 lb since admission. It was taken off of all antibiotics on day 10 and discharged on day 12 with instructions to maintain the mare and filly within a small area and to monitor the filly's urine output closely. It was recommended to minimize the use of any nephrotoxic drugs in the future because of the possibility of residual defects.

Discussion

HIE, known in the past as neonatal maladjustment syndrome or dummy foal syndrome, is part of a syndrome now commonly referred to as PAS or peripartum asphyxia syndrome [2,12]. HIE is the most common manifestation of PAS, but the kidneys and GIT are also often affected. Foals with HIE show clinical signs ranging from loss of suckle, depression, wandering, and abnormal vocalization ("barking") to grand mal seizures. Most commonly, foals with from HIE seem normal immediately after parturition, with the onset of central nervous abnormalities beginning within a few hours to a few days later. Foals with HIE may present with historical events consistent with periods of hypoxia, such as dystocia, as described in the current case, premature placental separation, or maternal illness, such as placentitis. Many have not had an obvious event causing hypoxia, however (Box 1).

The exact pathophysiology of HIE in the equine neonate is unknown, with most of the hypothesized pathophysiologic events extrapolated from studies examining this syndrome in human neonates. It is believed that central nervous system (CNS) damage occurs from uterine asphyxia as a result of a decrease in uterine blood flow or oxygen leading to activation of the sympathetic nervous system and redistribution of cardiac output to the central organs, such as the brain and heart [12,13,14]). If the reduction in oxygen supply to the fetus continues, the fetal cardiac output eventually falls, resulting in a decrease in cerebral circulation [12,13]. Decreased blood flow (ischemia) results in a decrease in available oxygen, leading to a decrease in oxidative phosphorylation in the brain and a subsequent decrease in energy production [12]. The Na^+/K^+-ATPase pump at the cell membrane thus cannot maintain the ionic gradients, leading to a loss of the membrane potential and the flow of calcium down concentration gradients into the cells through voltage-dependent ion channels [4]. The calcium overload of the neuron then causes cell damage as a result of activation of calcium-dependent proteases, lipases, and endonucleases [4]. Calcium can also enter the neuron through glutamate-regulated ion channels, whereas glutamate, an excitatory neurotransmitter, is released from presynaptic vesicles after anoxic cellular depolarization [4]. During reperfusion, there is believed to be

---

Box 1. Factors leading to hypoxia in the fetus

Maternal causes
  Reduced maternal oxygen delivery
    Maternal anemia
    Maternal pulmonary disease resulting in hypoxemia
    Maternal cardiovascular disease
  Reduced uterine and umbilical blood flow
    Maternal hypotension
    Maternal hypertension
Placental causes
  Premature placental separation
  Placental insufficiency
  Placental dysfunction
Intrapartum causes
  Dystocia
  Premature placental separation
  Uterine inertia
  Oxytocin induction of labor
  Cesarean section
    General anesthesia, decreased maternal cardiac output, poor
      uterine or umbilical blood flow, effects of anesthetic drugs
      on fetus
  Anything that prolongs stage 2 labor

Adapted from Palmer JE. Perinatal hypoxic-ischemic disease. In: Proceedings of the Sixth International Veterinary Emergency Critical Care Symposium. San Antonio (TX): Veterinary Emergency and Critical Care Society; 2000. p. 717–8.

---

a second wave of cell death thought to be attributable to the production and release of oxygen radicals, nitric oxide, and inflammatory mediators [4,12,15]. There is strong evidence supporting the possibility that toxic events within the brain during HIE may extend and change over several days from the time of injury [12,16,17]. An imbalance between excitatory and inhibitory neurotransmitters may also contribute to HIE [4,12,18] as well as to the neurotoxicity of glutamine, an excitatory neurotransmitter [12,16,17]. As calcium enters the cell, glutamine is released and the activation of N-methyl-D-aspartate (NMDA) glutamate receptors is enhanced [4,12,16,17,19]. Injured neurons also have reduced voltage-dependent Mg^{2+} blockade of NMDA currents, which can be partially restored by increasing extracellular Mg^{2+} concentrations [12,20].

Therapy of HIE is primarily symptomatic, involving correction of any fluid, metabolic, and respiratory abnormalities; control of seizures; and maintenance of peripheral, cerebral, and renal perfusion. It is important to maintain nutrition; to monitor and manage any secondary sepsis; to prevent decubital ulcers from forming; and to keep the foal warm, clean, and dry. Because PAS foals are susceptible to secondary infections, repeat determinations of IgG are recommended as well as prophylactic treatment with broad-spectrum antibiotics.

Minimizing seizures is important, because cerebral oxygen consumption increases by at least fivefold during an episode [12]. During seizure activity, it is vital to protect the foal from injury and to ensure a patent airway. As in the current case, seizures can often be controlled with intravenous diazepam at a dose of approximately 5 mg administered intravenously to a 45-kg foal. Diazepam is fast acting but has a short half-life, so it may need to be administered frequently. If diazepam is not effective at controlling the seizures, phenobarbital given to effect can be used, starting with a loading dose of 10 mg/kg administered intravenously, diluted in saline, and given over a 20-minute period; if needed, this is then followed with oral doses of 12 mg/kg every 12 hours. When monitoring a foal's neurologic function after treatment with phenobarbital, it is important to remember that the half-life of phenobarbital is long in the foal [4,21]. It is recommended that the use of ketamine and xylazine be avoided in foals with HIE because of the possibility of these drugs contributing to increased intracranial pressure. Foals with excessive seizure activity or status epilepticus may benefit from a 12- to 24-hour constant-rate infusion of pentobarbital or midazolam.

It is now believed that in most cases of HIE, the cerebral edema is intracellular rather than interstitial [12,22,23]; thus, drugs that are commonly used to treat interstitial edema, such as DMSO and mannitol, are likely to be minimally effective for the treatment of HIE. Despite this, many clinicians still routinely use DMSO and mannitol in the treatment of HIE. It has been recommended that DMSO be given within the first hour after an acute asphyxial insult to be effective, primarily because of its hydroxyl radical scavenging effects and probable protective effects against ischemic-reperfusion injuries [4,24]. Currently, most equine perinatologists use magnesium sulfate when treating suspected cases of HIE. Although most studies have shown magnesium sulfate to be beneficial in the treatment of cerebral asphyxia, no studies have found it to be detrimental [12]. Some clinicians now give it as a constant-rate infusion over 24 hours after a loading dose given over the first hour [12]. An alternative type of infusion includes the combination of magnesium sulfate, ascorbic acid, and thiamine all mixed in a crystalloid fluid (1 L); these substances are believed to be neuroprotective, by blocking NMDA receptors (magnesium and ascorbic acid) or acting as antioxidants (ascorbic acid, thiamine) [25]. Thiamine supports various metabolic processes, such as mitochondrial metabolism and Na^+/K^+-ATPase involved in maintaining cellular fluid balance, and preserves aerobic brain metabolism [4,26,27]. Vitamin E and C are antioxidants and are also commonly used to treat HIE.

Foals with HIE are often difficult to rouse, with abnormal sleep and respiratory patterns. Naloxone, an opioid antagonist, has been advocated for use in human babies and foals for the treatment of HIE, with some clinicians believing that it reduces CNS depression. Naloxone has been suggested to prevent disruption to the blood-brain barrier in a lamb model of HIE [12,28,29], although it has also been demonstrated that naloxone worsened hypoxic-ischemic brain injury in rats [4,12,30]. Caffeine is a central respiratory stimulant with minimal side effects and is commonly used at a loading dose of 10 mg/kg given per rectum, followed by 2.5 mg/kg as needed [4,31]. After treatment, foals are more easily aroused with increased awareness of their surroundings; adverse effects mainly include restlessness, hyperactivity, and tachycardia [4].

Ultimately, the aim of fluid therapy in foals with HIE is to maintain cerebral perfusion without fluid overload. This was difficult to do in the present case because of the oliguric ARF. Currently, inotropic and pressor support is often used in addition to fluid support to maintain perfusion. It is important to monitor urine output, mentation, limb perfusion, and GIT function, for example, as well as blood pressure to help determine whether perfusion is acceptable. The use of glucose in HIE foals has also been modified. Because foals have normal periods of postpartum hypoglycemia, it is currently not recommended to use dextrose aggressively in the initial treatment period because of fear of worsening any present neurologic injury [12].

As mentioned previously, the kidneys are commonly injured as a result of asphyxia, with the clinical signs usually a result of the disruption of renal blood flow leading to tubular edema and necrosis [4]. ARF has also been reported after the administration of oxytetracycline for the treatment of contracted tendons [32]. Foals treated with oxytetracycline likely have also experienced some degree of hypoxia because of prolonged parturition precipitated by the flexural deformity. Therefore, it is prudent to evaluate renal function in these foals before treating with oxytetracycline. Neonates with oliguric ARF may develop signs of fluid overload and generalized edema; thus, it is important to balance urine output with intravenous fluids so as to prevent further organ dysfunction associated with edema. There has been some recent evidence suggesting that neither dopamine nor furosemide reverses ARF, although these drugs may be useful in managing volume overload [4,33–35]. The goal with fluid therapy and any adjuvant therapy is not to drive oliguric ARF into a high-output condition but to enhance urine output [4]. If diuretics and pressors are used overabundantly, it may lead to excessive diuresis; this may be counterproductive because it would further increase fluid requirements [4]. Low-dose dopamine at constant-rate infusion (2–5 µg/kg/min) is considered to be effective at inducing diuresis by natriuresis; large doses of dopamine (>20 µg/kg/min) need to be avoided, because this can produce systemic and pulmonary vasoconstriction [4,36]. Furosemide can be given as a bolus (0.25–1.0 mg/kg) or as a constant-rate infusion (0.25–2.0 mg/kg/h), but the electrolyte concentrations and blood gas values need to be monitored closely, because large amounts of calcium and potassium may be lost, resulting in metabolic alkalosis from the loss of strong ion imbalances [4]. In addition, therapeutic drug monitoring should be performed, especially in those foals with renal dysfunction.

Foals with HIE have a fair to good prognosis for short-term survival if there are no complications, with a good to excellent prognosis for full-term PAS foals if the condition is recognized early and treated aggressively [12,37,38]). Up to 80% of these foals survive and lead athletic lives, with similar performance outcomes when compared with normal horses of the same age [37–40]).

References

[1] Cohn HE, Sacks EJ, Heymann MA, et al. Cardiovascular responses to hypoxemia and academia in fetal lambs. Am J Obstet Gynecol 1974;120:817–24.
[2] Vaala WE. Peripartum asphyxia. Vet Clin North Am Equine Pract 1994;10:187–218.
[3] Bernard WV. Jump-starting the dummy foal (neonatal maladjustment syndrome/hypoxic ischemic encephalopathy). In: Proceedings of the 49th Annual Convention of the American Association of Equine Practitioners 2003;49:8–12.
[4] Wilkins PA. Disorders of foals. In: Reed SM, Bayly WM, Sellon DC, editors. Equine internal medicine. 2nd edition. St. Louis (MO): WB Saunders; 2004. p. 1391–431.
[5] Martin-Ancel A, Garcia-Alix A, Gaya F, et al. Multiple organ involvement in perinatal asphyxia. J Pediatr 1995;127:786–93.
[6] Jawaheer G, Shaw NJ, Pierro A. Continuous enteral feeding impairs gallbladder emptying in infants. J Pediatr 2001;138:822–5.
[7] McClure RJ. Trophic feeding of the preterm infant. Acta Paediatr Suppl 2001;90:19–21.
[8] Premji S, Chessell L. Continuous nasogastric milk feeding versus intermittent bolus milk feeding for premature infants less than 1500 grams. Cochrane Database Syst Rev 2001;1: CD001819.
[9] Hosgood G. Pharmacologic features and physiologic effects of dopamine. J Am Vet Med Assoc 1990;197:1209–11.
[10] Lindner A, Cutler RE, Goodman W. Synergism of dopamine plus furosemide in preventing acute renal failure in the dog. Kidney Int 1979;16:158–66.
[11] Lindner A. Synergism of dopamine and furosemide in diuretic-resistant, oliguric acute renal failure. Nephron 1983;33:121–6.
[12] Wilkins PA. Hypoxic ischemic encephalopathy: neonatal encephalopathy. In: Wilkins PA, Palmer JE, editors. Recent advances in equine neonatal care. Ithaca (NY): International Veterinary Information Service; 2003. p. 1–9.
[13] Goetzman BW, Itskovitz J, Rudolph AM. Fetal adaptations to spontaneous hypoxemia and responses to maternal oxygen breathing. Biol Neonat 1984;46:276–84.
[14] Rudolph AM. The fetal circulation and its responses to stress. J Dev Physiol 1984;6:11–9.
[15] Andine P, Jacobson I, Hagberg H. Enhanced calcium uptake by CA1 pyramidal cell dendrites in the postischemic phase despite subnormal evoked field potentials: excitatory amino acid receptor dependency and relationship to neuronal damage. J Cereb Blood Flow Metab 1992;12:773–83.
[16] Sebastiao AM, de Mendonca A, Moreira T, et al. Activation of synaptic NMDA receptors by action potential-dependent release of transmitter during hypoxia impairs recovery of synaptic transmission on reoxygenation. J Neurosc 2001;21:8564–71.
[17] Vexler ZS, Ferriero DM. Molecular and biochemical mechanisms of perinatal brain injury. Semin Neonatol 2001;6:8564–71.
[18] Evrard P. Pathophysiology of perinatal brain damage. Dev Neurosci 2001;23:171–4.
[19] D'Souza SW, McConnell SE, Slater P, et al. Glycine site of the excitatory amino acid N-methyl-D-aspartate receptor in neonatal and adult brain. Arch Dis Child 1993;69:212–5.

[20] Zhang L, Rzigalinski BA, Ellis EF, et al. Reduction of voltage-dependent Mg2 + blockade of NMDA current in mechanically injured neurons. Science 1996;274:1921–3.

[21] Spehar AM, Hill MR, Mayhew IG, et al. Preliminary study on the pharmacokinetics of phenobarbital in the neonatal foal. Equine Vet J 1984;16:368–71.

[22] Kortz GD, Madigan JE, Lakritz J, et al. Cerebral oedema and cerebellar herniation in four equine neonates. Equine Vet J 1992;24:63–6.

[23] Kempski O. Cerebral edema. Semin Nephrol 2001;21:303–7.

[24] Brayton CF. Dimethyl sulfoxide (DMSO): a review. Cornell Vet 1986;76:61–90.

[25] Bain FT. Management of the foal from the mare with placentitis: a clinician's approach. In: Proceedings of the 50th Annual Convention of the American Association of Equine Practitioners 2004;50:162–4.

[26] Watanabe I, Tomita T, Hung KS, et al. Edematous necrosis in thiamine-deficient encephalopathy of the mouse. J Neuropathol Exp Neurol 1981;40:454–71.

[27] Wilkins PA, Vaala WE, Zivotofsky D, et al. A herd outbreak of equine leukoencephalomalacia. Cornell Vet 1994;84:53–9.

[28] Chernick V, Craig RJ. Naloxone reverses neonatal depression caused by fetal asphyxia. Science 1982;216:1252–3.

[29] Ting P, Pan Y. The effects of naloxone on the post-asphyxic cerebral pathophysiology of newborn lambs. Neurol Res 1994;16:359–64.

[30] Young RS, Hessert TR, Pritchard GA, et al. Naloxone exacerbates hypoxic-ischemic brain injury in the neonatal rat. Am J Obstet Gynecol 1984;150:52–6.

[31] Bhatia J. Current options in the management of apnea of prematurity. Clin Pediatr (Phila) 2000;39:327–6.

[32] Vivrette S, Cowgill LD, Pascoe J, et al. Hemodialysis for treatment of oxytetracycline-induced acute renal failure in a neonatal foal. J Am Vet Med Assoc 1993;203:105–7.

[33] Filler G. Acute renal failure in children: aetiology and management. Paediatr Drugs 2001;3: 783–92.

[34] Rudis MI. Low-dose dopamine in the intensive care unit: DNR or DNRx? Crit Care Med 2001;29.1638–9.

[35] Kellum JA, Decker J. Use of dopamine in acute renal failure: a meta-analysis. Crit Care Med 2001;29:1526–31.

[36] Cheung PY, Barrington KJ. The effects of dopamine and epinephrine on hemodynamics and oxygen metabolism in hypoxic anesthetized piglets. Crit Care 2001;5:158–66.

[37] Baker SM, Drummond WH, Lane TJ, et al. Follow-up evaluation of horses after neonatal intensive care. J Am Vet Med Assoc 1986;189:1454–7.

[38] Bryant JE, Bernard W, Wilson WD, et al. Race earnings as an indicator of future performance in neonatal foals treated for neurologic disorders. In: Proceedings of the 40th Annual Convention of the American Association of Equine Practitioners 1994;40:197–8.

[39] Freeman L, Paradis MR. Evaluating the effectiveness of equine neonatal intensive care. Vet Med 1992;87:921–6.

[40] Axon J, Palmer J, Wilkins PA. Short-term and long-term athletic outcome of neonatal intensive care unit survivors. Proc Am Assoc Equine Pract 1999;45:224–5.

ELSEVIER
SAUNDERS

VETERINARY
CLINICS
Equine Practice

Vet Clin Equine 22 (2006) 209–217

Unilateral Pyelonephritis in a Miniature Horse Colt

Emily A. Graves, VMD, MS

Equine Consulting of the Rockies, PO Box 27–1760, Fort Collins, CO 80527–1760, USA

History

A 2-year-old Miniature Horse colt weighing 68 kg was examined initially 5 weeks before presentation because of depression, gradual weight loss, and poor appetite. On examination by the referring veterinarian, the patient was underweight, depressed, and febrile, with a rectal temperature of 38.3°C (101°F). The initial blood work showed mild mature neutrophilia. The colt was given a single dose of flunixin meglumine (1.1 mg/kg administered intravenously) and received a 7-day course of ceftiofur sodium (4 mg/kg administered intramuscularly every 12 hours). Over the next 24 days, the colt's attitude improved slightly but fever persisted, ranging from 38.9°C to 40.0°C (102°F–104°F).

Eleven days before referral, the depression worsened and the colt was admitted to the referring clinic. Respiratory disease was suspected, and trimethoprim-sulfamethoxazole treatment was started empirically (25 mg/kg administered orally every 12 hours). A complete blood cell count (CBC) showed anemia and neutrophilia with a mild regenerative left shift. Serum chemistry profile results showed hypoalbuminemia and hyperglobulinemia as well as decreased sodium, chloride, and phosphorous concentrations. Fever persisted, and antimicrobial treatment was changed to penicillin G benzathine (20,000 IU/kg administered intramuscularly every 24 hours) and gentamicin (6.6 mg/kg administered intramuscularly every 24 hours). Because of further deterioration, the patient was referred for evaluation on day 1.

The colt had been owned by the current owner for 1 year and was dewormed at 4-month intervals with ivermectin or pyrantel. Its diet consisted of free-choice grass hay and Strategy concentrate (a 14% crude protein, high-energy pelleted feed, Purina Mills, LLC, St. Louis, Missouri) (0.5 kg every 24 hours). Testing for equine infectious anemia 7 months before referral had negative

---

E-mail address: dr.egraves@gmail.com

doi:10.1016/j.cveq.2005.12.012
vetequine.theclinics.com

results. The colt's vaccination status was current for influenza, rhinopneumonitis, tetanus, eastern and western equine encephalitis, and Potomac horse fever.

Physical examination

At admission, the patient was depressed but responsive and occasionally
seemed anxious. The body condition score was 3/9 (Henneke scale [1]) with
a dull hair coat, and the body weight was 68 kg. The rectal temperature was
39.6°C (103.3°F), the pulse was 64 beats per minute, and the respiratory rate
was 48 breaths per minute. The oral membranes were pale pink and slightly
tacky, with a capillary refill time of 2 to 3 seconds. The remainder of the oral
examination was normal. Dehydration was estimated at 5%. A soft, decre-
scendo, grade II/VI systolic murmur was auscultated on the left side, with
a point of maximal intensity (PMI) over the mitral valve. A quiet, decre-
scendo, grade II/VI diastolic murmur was also heard on the left side, with
a PMI over the pulmonary valve. Neither jugular pulses nor peripheral
edema was detected, and the cardiac rhythm was normal on auscultation.
Thoracic auscultation of all fields was normal. Gastrointestinal (GI) sounds
were present in all quadrants. Because of the colt's small size, the rectal
examination was limited to a digital examination that revealed normal feces
in the rectum. Both testicles were descended and palpated within normal
limits. The packed cell volume (PCV) was 23%, and total solids (TS) were
10.1 g/dL.

Case assessment

The colt's primary problems included poor appetite, depression, fever,
weight loss, dull hair coat, tachycardia, tachypnea, mild dehydration, heart
murmurs, anemia, and elevated total solids. The differential diagnosis for
persistent fever, in conjunction with depression, poor appetite, and weight
loss as well as a dull hair coat, includes chronic infections of any body system (pulmonary, GI, hepatobiliary, renal, cardiovascular, and nervous systems) or neoplasia with secondary tumor necrosis and local infection. Based
on historical neutrophilia, hyperproteinemia, and the young age of the patient (although some neoplastic diseases may affect young horses), chronic
sepsis was considered more likely than neoplasia. The affected body system
could not yet be ascertained.

Weight loss with chronic infection is typically a consequence of a negative
energy balance. Other potential causes of severe weight loss include GI malabsorption and/or maldigestion, neoplasia, renal failure, endocrine disease,
and poor nutrition. Dentition problems must also be suspected as a contributing factor. Pneumonia was a possible cause, although normal lung sounds
were heard in all fields and nasal discharge and coughing were not historical
complaints. Thoracic or abdominal abscessation was also considered as
a cause. Other intestinal diseases, such as lymphosarcoma, parasitism (large

and small strongyles), granulomatous and/or eosinophilic enteritis, and pro-liferative enteropathy (*Lawsonia intracellularis* infection) were considered, although diarrhea or colic is often observed with these illnesses [2]. Potential renal diseases included renal neoplasia, congenital anomaly, and abscessa-tion and/or pyelonephritis [3,4]. Endocrine disease in 2-year-old previously healthy equids is rare [5]. In addition, the colt's diet provided adequate nutrition.

Anemia can result from blood loss, hemolysis, or inadequate red blood cell production. The patient did not have a history of any of these conditions and showed no evidence of blood loss. Additionally, there was no evidence to support hemolysis (ie, pigmenturia, icterus). Anemia with chronic illness can be attributed to bone marrow suppression (decreased erythropoiesis) as well as to a shortened erythrocyte life span because of premature clearance by the reticuloendothelial system (when red blood cells have been coated with antigen or antibody) [6].

Increased TS may result from dehydration or increased globulin produc-tion, such as occurs with chronic infection or neoplastic diseases. The colt's history suggested that infection and dehydration were likely causes. When the total protein concentration is estimated by determining plasma TS via refractometry, other particulates in plasma (eg, triglycerides, hemoglobin) can artifactually increase this estimate of protein concentration. The plasma was neither lipemic nor discolored pink in this patient, however.

In a resting horse, tachycardia and tachypnea can result from anxiety, pain, dehydration, or heart disease. Physical examination findings pointed toward dehydration and anxiety as likely causes; no signs of discomfort were observed. Although murmurs were present, evidence of myocardial failure, including weak peripheral pulses, jugular distention, and ventral edema, were not found. Both murmurs may have been caused by valvular regurgitation or physiologic turbulent flow. In a 2-year-old horse, congenital valvular anomalies and physiologic murmurs were possible causes. With concurrent evidence of infection, valvular endocarditis was another impor-tant differential.

Diagnostic procedures

The CBC on day 1 showed anemia, mature neutrophilia, and an elevated fibrinogen concentration (Table 1). A decrease in mean corpuscular volume (MCV) corresponded with a nonregenerative anemia and lack of immature larger red blood cells. The mild increase in mean corpuscular hemoglobin concentration (MCHC) could accompany hemolysis as a result of hemoglo-bin release into circulation. In the absence of other evidence of hemolysis, the elevated MCHC was considered clinically insignificant. Potential expla-nations for the neutrophilic response included chronic infection, a physio-logic response to stress, and, less likely, neoplasia. The concurrent elevation in fibrinogen strongly suggested that the primary disease process

Table 1
Complete blood cell count results on day 1 and day 53 at referral clinic recheck examination

Date/hospital day	Day 1	Day 53	Normal values
PCV(%)	22	24	30–45
RBC $\times$ 10^6/μL	6.15	7.13	6.91–10.36
MCV(fL)	33.1	33.0	38.1–52.7
MCH(pg)	12.8	12.4	12.7–18.8
MCHC(%)	38.6	37.0	32.6–37.2
RBC morphology	Normal	1 + echinocytes	
White blood cells/μL	38,150	14140	5100–13,120
Segmented neutrophils/μL	32,430	7370	1940–7400
Lymphocytes/μL	5340	5230	960–5740
Monocytes/μL	380	700	10–350
Eosinophils/μL	0	50	0–1070
Basophils/μL	0	50	30–260
Leukocyte morphology	Few Dohle bodies, few reactive lymphocytes	Normal	
Platelets/μL	308,000	304,000	97,000–309,000
Fibrinogen(g/dL)	1.1	0.1	0–0.4

Abbreviations: MCH, mean corpuscular hemoglobin; MCHC, mean corpuscular hemoglobin concentration; MCV, mean corpuscular volume; PCV, packed cell volume; RBC, red blood cell.

was an infection. Fibrinogen, an acute-phase protein, can remain elevated even in chronic infections because of persistent inflammation.

Chemistry profile results showed hyperglobulinemia, hypoalbuminemia, and hypoglycemia as well as marginally decreased calcium, phosphorus, and magnesium concentrations (Table 2). The iron concentration was extremely low. Elevated globulins may be attributable to dehydration, but one would expect a concurrent increase in the albumin concentration as well. Dehydration was present in this case; as such, the albumin level in the euhydrated state would have been expected to be even lower. Other causes for high globulins include chronic infection and neoplasia.

The low albumin concentration suggested hastened loss or poor production. Without concomitant signs of liver disease, such as icterus, decreased synthesis was considered a less likely primary cause but could have been a contributing factor because of the negative energy balance. Hypoalbuminemia can result from gastrointestinal or renal loss in addition to increased capillary permeability, secondary to inflammation, and loss into the interstitial space. Low blood glucose was most likely attributable to decreased feed intake coupled with increased use (sepsis). Other explanations include excess plasma insulin attributable to overdose or tumor. The calcium, phosphorous, and magnesium decreases were marginal and considered to be a consequence of inadequate intake with continued losses in sweat, urine, and feces. In addition, hypoalbuminemia decreases the available protein-binding sites for calcium, thus leading to a low total serum calcium concentration. Ionized calcium was normal, suggesting that the low total calcium was caused

Table 2
Chemistry profile and venous blood gas results on day 1 and day 53 at referral clinic recheck examination

Date/hospital day	Day 1	Day 53	Normal values
BUN mg/dL	10	20	11–31
Creatinine mg/dL	0.8	0.9	0.8–1.8
Alk Phos IU/L	222	177	90–295
AST IU/L	115	168	210–380
ID/SDH IU/L	9.8	9.9	4.1–20.4
CK IU/L	91	136	156–417
Total bilirubin mg/dL	1.1	0.7	0.1–2.1
Direct bilirubin mg/dL	Not available	Not available	No reference range
Glucose mg/dL	70	94	75–119
Na mEq/L	127	132	128–158
K mEq/L	3.3	3.8	2.6–4.9
Cl mEq/L	94	99	91–110
Ca mg/dL	10.0	10.4	10.1–13.7
P mg/dL	1.1	4.5	1.2–4.6
Mg mg/dL	1.1	1.8	1.3–2.1
Osmolarity (calculated) mOsm/L	261.5	276.4	No reference range
Total protein g/dl	9.6	9.1	6.1–8.9
Albumin g/dL	1.8	2.5	3.5–4.7
Globulin g/dL	7.8	6.6	2.4–4.2
Cholesterol mg/dL	90	89	51–117
Venous blood gas			
pH	7.482		7.345–7.433
Po$_2$ venous mm Hg[a]	34.3		37–56
Pco$_2$ venous mm Hg[a]	36.9		38–48
HCO$_3$ mmol/L	27.8		22–29
Base excess mmol/L	4.9		−3–4

Abbreviations: ALK phos, alkaline phosphatase; AST, aspartate aminotransferase; BUN, blood urea nitrogen; CK, creatine kinase; ID, inositol dehydrogenase; SDH, sorbitol dehydrogenase.

[a] Slightly out of reference range, but were considered clinically insignificant.

by inadequate albumin binding sites. The low iron level was consistent with the chronic anemia.

Thoracic and abdominal radiographs showed normal lung fields and coarse ingesta in the large colon; no other significant findings were described. Transabdominal ultrasonography was performed to assess intestinal motility and wall thickness, shape and size of the kidneys and liver, and the presence of effusion or masses. The examination revealed normal GI motility and no peritoneal effusion. The left kidney was subjectively enlarged (150% of the size of a normal left kidney), however, although normal size ranges are not published for Miniature Horses. It had a thin cortex and heterogeneous and echogenic areas throughout the medulla. Differentials include renal abscessation and/or pyelonephritis, neoplasia (including nephroblastoma, teratoma, and adenocarcinoma), a congenital anomaly, or parasitism (Dioctophyma renale). The size, shape, and echogenicity of the right kidney were considered to be within normal limits. Abdominocentesis was performed, and the fluid appeared grossly normal. The fluid had a mildly elevated white blood cell (WBC) count and total protein concentration and was defined as an exudate without evidence of sepsis. These findings were consistent with an active intra-abdominal inflammatory process.

Voided urine was collected and submitted for urinalysis and bacterial culture and sensitivity testing. Urinalysis results showed no evidence of proteinuria, indicating that hypoalbuminemia was not caused by protein-losing nephropathy (Table 3). Findings supported a diagnosis of a urinary tract infection, with an increased WBC count. Urine concentrating ability was still present. No bacterial growth was isolated from the sample. Based on the test results at this point, renal abscessation or neoplasia was considered the most likely diagnosis.

On day 2, a needle aspirate of the left kidney was performed. Sampling yielded a green-yellow mucoid material. A renal biopsy was also pursued, but only more mucoid material was recovered on several attempts. Thus, a tissue sample was not submitted for histologic examination. A gram-positive organism was cultured and eventually identified as an *Actinomyces* species. Final species identification was never made, although the isolate shared characteristics with a swine pathogen, *Actinomyces hyovaginalis*. On day 4, cystoscopy revealed normal bladder mucosa. Urine flow from the right ureteral opening had regular frequency, volume, and appearance, but left ureteral urine flow was decreased and the scant urine produced was turbid yellow. In addition, the left ureteral opening was hyperemic and swollen. Because of the small size of the patient, a small-diameter

Table 3
Urinalysis reports on day 1 and day 53 at referral clinic recheck examination

Date/hospital day	Day 1	Day 53	Normal values
Source	Voided	Voided	
Color	Yellow	Orange	
Appearance	Hazy	Cloudy	
Specific gravity	1.023	1.037	1.001–1.027
pH	7.4	8.5	5.5–8.0
Protein	Negative	Negative	Negative through +30
Glucose	Negative	Negative	Negative
Acetone	Negative	Negative	Negative
Bilirubin	Negative	Negative	Negative
Blood	Negative	negative	Negative
Casts	None	None	None
Leukocytes/HPF	3–5	15–20	0–2
Epithelial cells/HPF	Few transitional	Occasional squamous	Occasional
Erythrocytes/HPF	None	None	None
Crystals	Moderate amorphous	Many amorphous	Moderate to many
Bacteria	Moderate	None	None
Other	Mucous strands		

Abbreviation: HPF, high-power field.

endoscope was used, which precluded collection of urine from each ureteral opening. Cystoscopic examination findings suggested minimal function of the left kidney. A nuclear scintigraphic imaging study to evaluate split renal function further was declined by the owner because of the expense.

These findings supported a diagnosis of unilateral pyelonephritis or renal abscessation, although neoplasia with secondary infection had not been ruled out. Intra-abdominal neoplastic conditions reported in young equids include nephroblastoma, granular lymphocyte tumor, teratoma, fibroma, adenocarcinoma, and lymphangioma [3,7–12]. Although these differentials were considered, they were ruled out based on the colt's inflammatory and/or infectious leukogram, ultrasonographic findings, and histopathologic findings.

Possible causes for renal infection include bacterial endocarditis or periodontal disease, with subsequent bacteremia and renal seeding, and idiopathic ascending urinary tract disease [13,14]. In small animal species, actinomycosis is typically associated with oropharyngeal damage and entry of the organism or with bite wounds [13]. To rule out valvular disease, echocardiography was performed and revealed normal heart valve anatomy and function, although mild regurgitation of the pulmonic valve was found on color-flow Doppler examination. Contractility was excellent. By day 2, the systolic murmur heard at admission was no longer detectable, suggesting that the murmur was likely associated with dehydration. A thorough dental examination was also performed. No wounds or gingival lesions were observed. Mild hooks and points on the upper and lower second premolars and third molars were found and corrected with manual dental floats.

Treatment and clinical outcome

To correct dehydration on day 1, the patient received a 3-L crystalloid fluid bolus with 23% calcium borogluconate added (calcium, 250 mg/kg) at admission. Empirically, broad-spectrum antimicrobial treatment was started with ampicillin (20 mg/kg administered intravenously every 8 hours) and gentamicin (6.6 mg/kg administered intravenously every 24 hours). Anti-inflammatory and antipyretic medication consisted of flunixin meglumine (0.5 mg/kg administered intravenously every 12 hours). In addition, the colt was offered water and timothy-alfalfa hay ad libitum and 1 kg of a complete pelleted feed every 12 hours.

The patient showed steady clinical improvement during 5 days of hospitalization. Further treatment options discussed with the owner included a left nephrectomy or long-term antibiotic treatment. If true unilateral renal infection can be confirmed using scintigraphic imaging, a unilateral nephrectomy may be the most successful means of treatment [14,15]. Because of financial concerns on the part of the owner, surgery was not an option, and the colt was discharged on day 5. Based on the drug sensitivity profile of the isolated *Actinomyces* species, antimicrobial treatment was changed to enrofloxacin (5 mg/kg administered orally every 24 hours). The patient slowly improved at home, with a gradual return of appetite and regular weight gain.

At a follow-up examination 7 weeks after discharge, the colt was active and alert, had gained 9 kg, and had an improved CBC. Anemia, with a low MCV and mean corpuscular hemoglobin, persisted but was less severe. A mildly elevated WBC count and monocytosis were also present, all of which were indicative of chronic but resolving infection (see Table 1). The chemistry profile showed low aspartate aminotransferase (AST) and creatine kinase (CK) activity (likely insignificant), resolving hypoalbuminemia, and elevated but decreasing total protein and globulin concentrations (see Table 2). Renal ultrasonography showed that the left kidney had decreased in size but still contained multifocal, small, fluid-filled pockets in the medullary region. These images were interpreted as resolving abscessation. Urinalysis showed high WBC numbers but no bacteria (see Table 3). Urine culture was again negative for bacterial growth. The favorable response to antibiotic treatment further supported a diagnosis of renal abscessation and eliminated neoplasia as a differential diagnosis.

Again, because of financial concerns, enrofloxacin therapy could not be continued. Based on the antimicrobial susceptibility profile, ability to concentrate in urine, and affordability, trimethoprim-sulfamethoxazole (25 mg/kg administered orally every 12 hours) was prescribed for another 30 to 60 days, depending on clinical response and resolution of CBC and chemistry profile abnormalities. The colt was maintained on this drug for approximately 50 days until CBC results had normalized and the serum globulin concentration was only minimally outside the reference range. The referring veterinarian performed periodic evaluations, and more than 1 year later, the patient continued to thrive.

References

[1] Henneke DR, Potter GD, Kreider JL, et al. Relationship between condition score, physical measurements and body fat percentage in mares. Equine Vet J 1983;15(4):371–2.
[2] Jones SL, Blikslager AT. Disorders of the gastrointestinal system. In: Reed SM, Bayly WM, Sellon DC, editors. Equine internal medicine. 2nd edition. St. Louis (MO): WB Saunders; 2004. p. 769–801, 937–49.
[3] Schott HC, Van Metre DC, Divers TJ. Disease of the renal system. In: Smith BP, editor. Large animal internal medicine. 3rd edition. St. Louis (MO): Mosby; 2002. p. 825–51.
[4] Schott HC. Urinary tract infection and bladder displacement. In: Robinson NE, editor. Current therapy in equine medicine 5. St. Louis (MO): WB Saunders; 2003. p. 837–9.
[5] Toribio RE. Disorders of the endocrine system. In: Reed SM, Bayly WM, Sellon DC, editors. Equine internal medicine. 2nd edition. St. Louis (MO): WB Saunders; 2004. p. 1295–379.
[6] Sellon DC. Disorders of the hematopoietic system. In: Reed SM, Bayly WM, Sellon DC, editors. Equine internal medicine. 2nd edition. St. Louis (MO): WB Saunders; 2004. p. 721–68.
[7] Jardine JE, Nesbit JW. Triphasic nephroblastoma in a horse. J Comp Pathol 1996;114(2): 193–8.

[8] Grindem CB, Roberts MC, McEntee MF, et al. Large granular lymphocyte tumor in a horse. Vet Pathol 1989;26(1):86–8.

[9] Wilson TD, Sykes GP. Fibroma in the abdomen of a horse. Vet Rec 1981;108(15):334.

[10] Turk JR, Gallina AM, Liu IM, et al. Cystic lymphangioma in a colt. J Am Vet Med Assoc 1979;174(11):1228–30.

[11] Kirchhof N, Steinhauer D, Fey K. Equine adenocarcinomas of the large intestine with osseous metaplasia. J Comp Pathol 1996;114(4):451–6.

[12] Shaw DP, Roth JE. Testicular teratocarcinoma in a horse. Vet Pathol 1986;23(3):327–8.

[13] Edwards DF. Actinomycosis and nocardiosis. In: Greene CE, editor. Infectious diseases of the dog and cat. Philadelphia: Elsevier; 1998. p. 303–10.

[14] Schott HC. Urinary tract infections. In: Reed SM, Bayly WM, Sellon DC, editors. Equine internal medicine. 2nd edition. St. Louis (MO): WB Saunders; 2004. p. 1253–8.

[15] Irwin DH, Howell DW. Equine pyelonephritis and unilateral nephrectomy. J S Afr Vet Assoc 1980;51(4):235–6.

ELSEVIER
SAUNDERS

VETERINARY
CLINICS
Equine Practice

Vet Clin Equine 22 (2006) 219–227

Polydipsia and Polyuria in a Weanling Colt Caused by Nephrogenic Diabetes Insipidus

Michael Brashier, DVM, MS

College of Veterinary Medicine, PO Box 6100, Mississippi State University,
Starkville, MS 39762–6100, USA

History

This colt was obtained from a breeding operation by the current owner 2 weeks before presentation. Historically, the colt had been weaned at 3 months of age and dewormed at that time with fenbendazole. Neither a vaccination nor nutritional history was available. After acquisition, the new owner dewormed the colt with an ivermectin-based anthelmintic. During the past 2 weeks, the colt had been receiving one-half gallon of a corn, oats, and calf manna mixture and one flake of alfalfa hay twice daily, with free access to grass pasture during the day. A salt block was available. The colt's appetite was reported as being normal, because it would consume grain, but the colt had not seemed to gain weight. The colt was seen to drink large amounts of water, spending increased time at the water trough. The owner's impression was that the colt was not grazing or eating adequate amounts of hay because of the amount of water it was consuming. None of the new owner's other three horses were exhibiting any abnormal signs. According to the current owner, all other foals at the breeding farm had seemed normal.

Case assessment

Except for a thin body condition, small stature, and rough hair coat, the colt seemed to be normal. As part of the initial physical examination, the colt was observed over the weekend in a controlled environment to assess the volume of water ingested and urination. The colt drank an average of 58 L/d (568 mL/kg/d). Urination was frequent, but the colt exhibited

E-mail address: brashier@cvm.msstate.edu

doi:10.1016/j.cveq.2005.12.010   *vetequine.theclinics.com*

a normal micturition process with normal stance, stream, and volume per urination. The colt's appetite seemed to be normal.

The primary problems were polyuria and polydipsia as well as poor body condition. Primary rule-outs for polyuria and polydipsia include psychogenic water drinking, psychogenic salt consumption, pituitary dysfunction, diabetes mellitus, diabetes insipidus, and acute or chronic renal failure. Primary rule-outs for poor body condition are extensive but include many of the previously listed conditions, with the addition of an inadequate plane of nutrition and excessive parasitism.

An initial complete blood cell count, serum chemistry, urinalysis, and fecal flotation test were performed.

The white blood cell differential and fibrinogen were normal, making chronic infection unlikely. All red blood cell parameters were within normal limits, making chronic renal failure less likely. The blood glucose level was normal, eliminating diabetes mellitus as the cause of the polyuria and polydipsia. The serum creatinine and blood urea nitrogen levels were also within normal limits, indicating adequate glomerular function. Serum sodium (149 mEq/L), chloride (108 mEq/L), and osmolality (298 mOsm/kg) were slightly elevated and could be attributable to an inability to conserve water by urine concentration or perhaps to an adaptation by the body to maintain circulating volume.

Urinalysis and electrolyte fractional excretions showed no glucose or protein loss in the urine and normal electrolyte fractional excretions, indicating that most renal tubular function was intact. Normal fractional excretion of sodium (0.2%) and chloride (0.5%) also indicated that excessive salt consumption and subsequent excretion were not the cause of the polyuria and polydipsia. The only abnormality noted on the urinalysis was a specific gravity of 1.004 and an osmolality of 76 mOsm/kg. Urine osmolality is generally 900 to 1200 mOsm/kg or three to four times that of serum unless there is excessive fluid intake.

The results of fecal flotation were negative, as was expected, because of the recent treatment with ivermectin, but the test was run to ensure adequate dosage and administration and to rule out the possibility of acquisition of a resistant parasite burden. Even though a parasite burden was unable to be documented because of the recent anthelmintic therapy, parasites were still considered to be a likely contributor to the poor body condition because of a history of inadequate deworming.

The initial battery of diagnostic tests narrowed down the differential list for the polyuria and polydipsia to three primary rule-outs of primary polydipsia, central diabetes insipidus, and nephrogenic diabetes insipidus. To determine which of the three was the cause, water deprivation, exogenous vasopressin (also known as antidiuretic hormone) administration, and Hickey-Hare (hypertonic saline infusion) tests were performed.

The duration of the water deprivation test was based on assessment of hydration and weight loss. Baseline and end deprivation serum and urine samples were submitted for osmolality and electrolyte concentrations, but the results were not immediately available. Plasma collected at the beginning and end of the water deprivation test was submitted for arginine vasopressin radioimmunoassay. A body weight loss of 11.2% occurred in 12 hours. This was a greater weight loss than was intended, although, clinically, the colt did not seem to be dehydrated, nor did the packed cell volume (PCV) or total plasma protein (TPP) change significantly, increasing by 2% and 0.2 g/dL respectively. Had serum osmolality been more readily available, water deprivation could have been discontinued when an increase in osmolality of greater than 5% was attained. Serum sodium increased from 140 to 164 mEq/L, chloride increased from 101 to 119 mEq/L, and osmolality increased from 283 to 326 mOsm/kg during the water deprivation test. Urine specific gravity did not change significantly during the water deprivation test, beginning at 1.003 and ending at 1.004. The arginine vasopressin concentration increased from an already high 7.4 to 11.1 pg/mL in the face of dehydration, indicating appropriate hypothalamic response to dehydration [1].

The colt was allowed to rehydrate. Initially, water was provided at a rate of 3 L/h for the first 2 hours and then at 4 L/h until the colt was sated before being provided free-choice water. Although the development of cerebral edema on rehydration seemed unlikely because of the short duration of the dehydration and hypernatremia, it was deemed prudent to err on the side of caution. A period of normal hydration was allowed before further testing.

To rule out renal medullary washout as a complicating factor that could affect the colt's ability to respond appropriately to antidiuretic hormone, a Hickey-Hare test was performed [2]. A Hickey-Hare test involves infusion of a hypertonic saline solution with subsequent following of urine volume production and osmolality. An indwelling urinary catheter was placed the evening before the test to avoid the alterations in glomerular filtration rates induced by the use of acepromazine for penile relaxation. Hypertonic saline (2.5%) was administered at a dose of 0.25 mL/min/kg for 45 minutes. The bladder was emptied every 15 minutes, and the volume was measured. Serum and urine osmolality were assessed at the beginning and end of the period. One hour after the end of the administration of hypertonic saline, a dose of aqueous arginine vasopressin (0.20 U/kg) diluted in sodium chloride (NaCl) was administered over a period of 60 minutes. Urine collection continued as before until 1 hour after the end of the administration of vasopressin. Urine and serum electrolytes and osmolality were measured at the beginning, end, and 1 hour after the end of the vasopressin infusion. The dose of vasopressin is that which has been shown to cause urine concentration in ponies and horses with neurogenic diabetes insipidus [3,4].

Serum sodium increased from 134 to 143 mEq/L in response to the administration of hypertonic saline. Urine volume increased from 600 mL per 15 minutes to 900 mL per 15 minutes as the sodium load was excreted.

A positive test result, indicating renal medullary washout, would have been for the urine volume to decrease in response to the re-establishment of the renal medullary interstitial osmotic gradient. There was no response to exogenous vasopressin, indicating lack of an appropriate renal tubular response to antidiuretic hormone, which would have been compatible with nephrogenic diabetes insipidus. Urine osmolality increased to 156 mOsm but only by an amount that could be accounted for by excess sodium excretion and did not begin to approach serum osmolality.

Ultrasound examination of the kidneys was performed, which appeared normal. An ultrasound-guided biopsy of the left and right kidneys was performed. The histopathology report showed nephrotic changes consisting of severe vacuolization and intracytoplasmic eosinophilic granular changes in the epithelium of the distal collecting ducts. Glomeruli were relatively normal, with a possible slight increase in cellularity occasionally. No changes were noted in the proximal tubules.

Case management and follow-up

A vaccination protocol was initiated. The colt was maintained on 0.75 lb of sweet feed given twice daily for the first month, 1 lb given twice daily for the second month, and 1.5 lb given twice daily for the third month. Unlimited access to alfalfa hay was allowed. Access to salt was limited to that available in the sweet feed and hay. Water was provided at a rate of 30 L/d divided into five or six aliquots. Ivermectin-based anthelmintics were administered at a 4-week interval. The colt gained 0.76 kg/d (1.66 lb/d) and weighed 170 kg (375 lb) at the end of 3 months. Because nephrogenic diabetes insipidus is a sex-linked heritable trait based on the X chromosome in other species and is also thought to be so in horses, it was recommended that the colt be gelded [4]. Follow-up laboratory values remained within normal limits, except for a continued low urine concentration. Follow-up renal ultrasound and histopathologic examination of biopsies showed no evidence of the lesions noted on the previous submission.

Discussion

The primary problems associated with this case were polydipsia and polyuria as well as poor body condition with retarded growth and poor coat quality. Rule-outs for polyuria and polydipsia include renal insufficiency (acquired or congenital), primary polydipsia (psychogenic water drinking), psychogenic salt consumption, diabetes mellitus, and diabetes insipidus (central or nephrogenic). Many of the congenital renal defects, such as renal agenesis, renal dysplasia, or polycystic kidneys, were considered unlikely as the cause of the polyuria and polydipsia. These are severe enough to cause azotemia or uremia or oliguria, for example, or are detected as an incidental finding. Ultrasound examination further ruled them out. Acquired renal insufficiency (eg, from thromboembolic or bacteremic showering associated with neonatal sepsis), ingestion of a nephrotoxic substance (eg, oxalate), or iatrogenically induced toxicity (eg, aminoglycoside toxicity) was not considered likely for the same reasons and was ruled out in the face of normal glomerular function as demonstrated by a normal serum creatinine concentration and normal urinalysis, indicating normal tubular resorption of electrolytes, glucose, and albumin. Failure to concentrate urine during water deprivation and a Hickey-Hare test allowed the elimination of primary polydipsia and primary salt consumption and led to a diagnosis of diabetes insipidus.

Diabetes insipidus can be of neurogenic or nephrogenic origin. Neurogenic diabetes insipidus results from injury or dysfunction of the hypothalamus or pituitary gland. Possible causes include a pituitary abscess, a pituitary adenoma, neoplasia, encephalitis, aberrant parasite migration, traumatic injury, or a congenital defect [4,5]. Neurogenic diabetes insipidus was ruled out because of the patient's ability to produce an appropriate vasopressin response during water deprivation. Nephrogenic diabetes insipidus is a failure of the collecting ducts to respond to vasopressin and may be congenital or acquired. The congenital form is sex linked and is almost always seen in male members of all species investigated [6,7]. Acquired nephrogenic diabetes insipidus can be caused by anything that results in renal tubular damage. Although cases of acquired nephrogenic diabetes insipidus may exhibit histologic damage as a result of the inciting cause, cases of congenital nephrogenic diabetes insipidus generally do not have histologic changes [4,7,8]. Although the list of causes of renal tubular damage can be extensive, some of the more common causes include aminoglycoside toxicity, nonsteroidal anti-inflammatory drug toxicity, pyelonephritis ascending or caused by bacteremia as a neonate, oxalate toxicity, tetracycline toxicity, and blister beetle toxicity. Tetracycline has particularly been associated with the induction of nephrogenic diabetes insipidus [7], but no history of exposure to any of these substances could be elucidated in the case reported here. Because of the intimate association between tubular cells and the interstitium, damage to one usually means damage to the other; thus, the term *tubulointerstitial nephrosis* or *tubulointerstitial nephritis*. In this case, all changes seemed to be restricted to the tubular cells alone because of the lack of influx of any inflammatory cells or the development of fibrosis and seemed to be consistent with cellular necrosis. Renal tubular epithelial cells can regenerate themselves, and damage limited to the renal tubular epithelium is generally considered reversible [8]. In this case, however, restitution of a histologically normal renal tubular epithelium did not result in a return to normal function. Finally, no history of related animals developing polyuria and polydipsia could be obtained from the breeder. Because of the histologic anomaly on the first histopathologic sample, an absolute diagnosis of hereditary or congenital nephrogenic diabetes insipidus could not be made. Considering the animal's young age, lack of historical risk factors, and lack of resolution of signs accompanying restitution of the renal tubular epithelium, this still seems to be the most likely diagnosis, however.

It is believed that the elevation seen in the day 1 serum sodium level and osmolality may have been real and reflected an alternative attempt by the body to maintain normal circulating volume. This is supported by normal clinical hydration, a normal initial serum creatinine level, and the fact that psychogenic salt consumption was not the cause of the problem. Antidiuretic hormone (vasopressin), angiotensin, aldosterone, atrial natriuretic hormone, blood pressure, and other factors have complex interrelations in the maintenance of normal fluid and electrolyte balance. When the equilibrium is changed by the loss of one of these control mechanisms, the others adjust to compensate. If renal medullary osmotic pressure is normal, antidiuretic hormone–induced increased permeability to water in the collecting tubules and ducts results in the retention of water for the maintenance of arterial blood pressure. When fluid cannot be retained via normal antidiuretic hormone activity, it may be retained by increasing serum electrolyte concentrations, thereby, increasing osmotic pressure. The down side to this can be an increase in extracellular fluid volume, which may lead to an increase in the diuresis at the new point of equilibrium [9]. Partial control of nephrogenic diabetes insipidus has been reported by limiting salt and water intake and administering thiazide diuretics. This produces a mild negative salt balance contracting the extracellular fluid volume. The overall effect is to reduce the glomerular filtration rate (GFR), enhancing proximal renal tubular resorption of sodium, chloride, and water as well as reducing the volume of fluid delivered to the distal tubules. Reduced fluid flow may also decrease any effect of renal medullary washout. A reduction in urine output of 50% to 85% has been reported [7,10]. With access to salt limited to that in the diet, serum electrolytes and osmolality returned to within normal limits in this patient, and the volume of water consumption was able to be safely decreased by approximately half. Although this still resulted in a urine osmolality significantly less than that of the serum, it allowed the colt to maintain homeostasis and grow at a normal rate. It is possible that addition of a thiazide diuretic may have had additional benefits.

This colt only weighed 102 kg (224 lb) at 5 months of age. Assuming that the colt weighed somewhere in the neighborhood of 45 kg (100 lb) at birth, it had only gained 0.38 kg/d (0.83 lb/d). An average weight at weaning should have been approximately 175 to 200 kg (385–440 lb), with a moderate rate of gain from weaning to 6 months of 0.85 kg/d (1.87 lb/d) and 0.65 kg/d (1.43 lb/d) from 6 to 12 months of age, for an average 454- to 500-kg (1000–1100-lb) adult horse [11]. The differential diagnosis for poor body condition can be extensive but can be broken down to the basics of lack of intake, maldigestion, malassimilation, increased metabolic needs, or increased losses. Malnutrition (lack of adequate intake) and parasite problems (increased losses) are the most common causes and were highest on a differential list that also initially included chronic renal failure and diabetes mellitus because of the signs of polyuria and polydipsia. Although the colt's current nutritional plane was adequate, this had only been provided for the past 2 weeks. Before that, poor observation of the weanlings at the breeding farm made it impossible to determine the adequacy of the colt's nutritional level. Even if the nutritional level for the group of weanlings as a whole had been sufficient, early weaning and the small size of this colt may have prevented it from adequately competing for the provided feed. The colt's deworming had been markedly inadequate, especially for a breeding farm, where there is generally high traffic and mixing of horses with different and unknown parasite burdens. Fenbendazole given at the standard dose does not provide systemic larvicidal concentrations. *Parascaris equorum* and the large strongyle species would have been in the migratory phase at 3 months and would have been unaffected. Additionally, many small strongyles have become resistant to fenbendazole.

Other differentials that would encompass the clinical signs of polyuria and polydipsia as well as poor body condition could include acute or chronic renal failure, diabetes mellitus, and pituitary disease. Acute or chronic renal disease can result in a diminished ability to reabsorb filtered solutes, such as electrolytes, glucose, and protein, resulting in an osmotic diuresis. This can be an effect of greater flow rate per surviving nephron such that tubular resorptive capacity is exceeded and there is diminished resorptive capacity because of tubular damage, decreased renal medullary tonicity because of renal medullary washout, and diminished vasopressin responsiveness. Diminished numbers of nephrons also result in retention of normally filtered waste products, such as creatinine and urea. Examination of the serum chemistry revealed normal serum creatinine and blood urea nitrogen levels. The urinalysis was normal, except for a low specific gravity, showing no glucosuria or proteinuria. Fractional excretion of electrolytes was normal, indicating normal tubular function. Although chronic renal disease can result in vasopressin insensitivity, it is highly unlikely that chronic renal disease could result in that alone. Chronic renal disease also often presents with mild anemia because of the diminished renal production of erythropoietin, which was not present in this colt [6].

Type I diabetes mellitus or insulin-dependent diabetes is a rare condition in horses [12]. When glucose exceeds the renal threshold for resorption, it acts as an osmotic diuretic and has been reported to result in water consumption exceeding 80 L/d in horses [6]. Type II diabetes mellitus results from insulin resistance [13]. A similar syndrome in horses has recently been referred to as omental Cushing's disease or equine metabolic syndrome. To achieve polyuria and polydipsia with this syndrome, glucose again must exceed the renal threshold for reabsorption. Although a battery of confirmatory diagnostic tests for this syndrome remains to be defined, insulin levels generally greatly exceed normal.

The most common pituitary disorder in horses is equine Cushing's disease, pituitary adenoma, or pars intermedia hypertrophy. The underlying pathophysiology seems to be an age-related decrease in hypothalamic dopamine production. As the inhibitory effect of the dopamine wanes, the pars intermedia hypertrophies, ultimately resulting in increased cortisol production by the adrenal glands and increased responsiveness to the cortisol by peripheral tissues because of the release of other mediators from the pars intermedia. Polyuria and polydipsia may occur by one of several mechanisms with this disease. Hyperglycemia that can exceed the renal threshold is often a component of this disease. Nevertheless, some animals that are not excessively hyperglycemic still exhibit the sign of polyuria and polydipsia. Other contributing factors include compression of the pars nervosa, the site of release of vasopressin, by the expanding pars intermedia within the sella turcica. Glucocorticoids also induce an increase in the glomerular filtration rate that may contribute to diuresis [12]. One of the most common diagnostic tests used for determination of this disease is the low-dose dexamethasone suppression test [14]. Successful therapy has been achieved in some horses using the dopamine agonist pergolide [15].

Making an absolute diagnosis of congenital nephrogenic diabetes insipidus in this case was confounded by the initial finding of distal renal tubular epithelial histologic abnormalities. Lesions were strictly restricted to the distal tubular epithelium and restitution of a histologically normal renal tubular epithelium did not result in a return to normal function. Additionally, no history of related animals developing polyuria and polydipsia could be obtained from the breeder. Considering the animal's young age, lack of historical risk factors, and lack of resolution of signs accompanying restitution of the renal tubular epithelium, congenital nephrogenic diabetes insipidus still seems to be the most likely diagnosis, however.

References

[1] Houpt KA, Thornton SN, Allen WR. Vasopressin in dehydrated and rehydrated ponies. Physiol Behav 1989;(45):659–61.

[2] Chew DJ, Dibartola SP. Diagnosis and pathophysiology of renal disease. In: Ettinger SJ, editor. Textbook of veterinary internal medicine. Philadelphia: WB Saunders; 1989. p. 1893–961.

[3] Breukink HJ, Van Wegen P, Schotman AJ. Idiopathic diabetes insipidus in a Welsh pony. Equine Vet J 1983;15(3):284–7.

[4] Schott HC II, Bayly WM, Reed SM, et al. Nephrogenic diabetes insipidus in sibling colts. J Vet Intern Med 1993;7(2):68–72.

[5] Wallace CE, Kociba FJ. Diabetes insipidus in a cow. J Am Vet Med Assoc 1979;175(8): 809–11.

[6] Schott HC II, Bayly WM. Disorders of the urinary system. In: Reed SM, Bayly WM, Sellon DC, editors. Equine internal medicine. St. Louis (MO): WB Saunders; 2004. p. 1169–294.

[7] Robertson GL, Berl T. Pathophysiology of water metabolism in the kidney. In: Brenner BM, Rector FV, editors. The kidney. Philadelphia: WB Saunders; 1991. p. 677–736.

[8] Maxie MG, Prescott JF. The urinary system. In: Jubb KVF, Kennedy PC, Palmer N, editors. Pathology of domestic animals. San Diego (CA): Academic Press; 1993. p. 447–538.

[9] Guyton AC, Hall JE. The kidneys and body fluids. In: Textbook of medical physiology. Philadelphia: WB Saunders; 1996. p. 297–424.

[10] Polzin D, Osborne C, O'Brien T. Diseases of the kidneys and ureters. In: Ettinger SJ, editor. Textbook of veterinary internal medicine. Philadelphia: WB Saunders; 1989. p. 1962–2046.

[11] Ott EA, Baker JP, Hintz HF, et al. Nutrient requirement of horses. Fifth edition. Washington, DC: National Academy Press; 1989. p. 100.

[12] Toribio RE. Disorders of the endocrine system. In: Reed SM, Bayly WM, Sellon DC, editors. Equine internal medicine. St. Louis (MO): WB Saunders; 2004. p. 1295–379.

[13] Ruoff WW, Baker JP, Morgan SJ, et al. Type II diabetes mellitus in a horse. Equine Vet J 1986;18(2):143–4.

[14] Dybdal NO, Hargreaves KM, Madigan JE, et al. Diagnostic testing for pituitary pars intermedia dysfunction in horses. J Am Vet Med Assoc 1994;204(4):627–32.

[15] Donaldson MT, LaMonte BH, Morresey PM, et al. Treatment with pergolide or cyproheptadine of pituitary pars intermedia dysfunction (equine Cushing's disease). J Vet Intern Med 2002;16:742–6.

ELSEVIER
SAUNDERS

VETERINARY
CLINICS
Equine Practice

Vet Clin Equine 22 (2006) 229–237

Type 1 Renal Tubular Acidosis in a Broodmare

Tamara Gull, DVM

Department of Veterinary Pathobiology, Texas A&M University, TAMU 4467,
College Station, TX 77843–4467, USA

History

An 11-year-old, 455-kg, multiparous Quarter Horse broodmare with a 2-month-old foal was presented to the referral hospital for lethargy and inappetence of 5 days' duration. A veterinarian had examined the horse 4 days before presentation and had reported a normal physical and rectal examination and a 30-day pregnancy. No treatment had been administered. The mare's prior history included a bout of severe diarrhea 5 months before presentation. The diarrhea had resolved with symptomatic therapy and supportive care from the farm veterinarian, and no specific cause had been determined.

The mare and foal had been shipped from the breeding farm to the home farm 2 weeks previously. They were housed on coastal Bermuda and prairie grass pasture with one other mare and foal pair. These horses were reported to be normal. The mare's diet consisted of free-choice pasture supplemented with alfalfa hay and a 14% protein sweet feed. Current vaccinations included tetanus; Venezuelan, eastern, and western encephalitis; equine influenza; and rhinopneumonitis. The mare had been dewormed 6 weeks previously with ivermectin. A Coggins test drawn 6 weeks before presentation was negative.

Physical examination

On presentation to the hospital, the mare was quiet but alert and in good body condition. The mare's temperature was 37.8°C (100.0°F), the heart rate was 40 beats per minute with normal pulse quality, and the respiratory rate was 12 breaths per minute. The mucous membranes were slightly tacky,

E-mail address: tgull@cvm.tamu.edu

pink, and icteric, with a capillary refill time of 2 seconds. The skin over the neck remained tented when pinched. The horse was clinically assessed to be 5% to 6% dehydrated. The physical examination, including an oral examination and a rebreathing examination, was otherwise unremarkable. Nasogastric intubation yielded no reflux. Examination per rectum revealed normal feces and no palpable abnormalities. Ultrasound of the reproductive tract per rectum revealed a viable pregnancy of approximately 30 to 35 days' gestation.

Case assessment

Problems identified included lethargy, inappetence, icterus, and dehydration. There are many differential diagnoses for lethargy and inappetence because these are usually associated with systemic disease of many causes. Respiratory, cardiovascular, and reproductive diseases were considered unlikely based on the lack of corresponding clinical signs. Physical examination could not rule out gastrointestinal, hepatic, renal, endocrine, metabolic, or hemolymphatic disease. The differential diagnoses for dehydration include decreased consumption, third space sequestration, and increased losses to include renal failure, diarrhea, hemorrhage, excessive sweating, polyuria, and gastric reflux. Of these, only gastric reflux and diarrhea could be ruled out via physical examination. The differential diagnosis for icterus includes anorexia, hepatocellular disease, cholestasis, and hemolysis, none of which could be immediately ruled out.

Procedures

A complete blood cell count (CBC), plasma biochemical profile, abdominocentesis, and urinalysis were performed at presentation. The CBC revealed a mild neutrophilia. Serum chemistry analysis revealed a profound hyperchloremic metabolic acidosis with an increased anion gap, moderate azotemia, mild hyperbilirubinemia, mild hyperproteinemia, and hyperalbuminemia (Table 1). The bilirubin consisted entirely of unconjugated bilirubin. The urinalysis showed concentrated alkaline urine (pH 8.5, specific gravity of 1.035). Urine gamma-glutamyltransferase (GGT) and creatinine (Cr) concentrations were also determined. A bacteriologic culture of urine was negative. Abdominocentesis yielded normal fluid.

Causes of neutrophilia include physiologic, corticosteroid-induced, inflammation, hemorrhage, hemolysis, endotoxemia, and malignancy. Given the otherwise normal CBC, normal fibrinogen, and low normal lymphocyte count, a corticosteroid-induced (stress) response was considered most likely. The increased chloride (Cl^-) concentration probably reflected the severe acidosis (decreased HCO_3^-), because plasma chloride concentrations typically follow plasma sodium concentrations and vary inversely with the

Table 1
Serum chemistry values

	Normal	Day 1	Day 2	Day 3	Day 4	Day 6	Day 8	Day 9	Day 11	Day 14	Day 28
BUN	7–28 mg/dL	38		29	22	18			26	18	19
Creatinine	1.1–2.0 mg/dL	3.3	2.9	3.6	2.2	1.7			1.9	1.5	1.5
tBilirubin	0.1–4.1 mg/dL	4.5							1.9		
Na	132–141 mmol/L	134	139	140	135	133			133	134	135
K	3.0–4.2 mmol/L	3.8	3.2	2.3	2.1	3.5			4.2	4.2	4.0
Cl	98–105 mmol/L	116	121	111	99	98			98	104	101
Ca	11.0–13.0 mmol/L	11.4			11.7	13.0			13.0		
Anion gap	0–13	16	12	13	10	10			6	9	11
pH	7.38–7.42		7.086	7.259	7.408	7.396	7.425	7.422	7.427		
Po_2	37–56 (venous), 80–112 (arterial)		108.1 (arterial)	35.2 (venous)	37.7 (venous)	40.0 (venous)	42.8 (venous)	45.9 (venous)	40.6 (venous)		
Pco_2	38–48		26.2	39.7	43.2	44.8	45.2	45.6	43.7		
HCO_3	21–27		7.7	17.5	26.9	27.0	32.6	33.3	35.0		
Total CO_2	24–31 mmol/L	6.0	9.0	19	28	28	34	34.9	33	25	27
Base excess	−3 to 4		−19.8	−8.2	2.6	2.5					

Abbreviations: BUN, blood urea nitrogen; tBilirubin, total bilirubin.

bicarbonate concentration to preserve electroneutrality. Some causes of metabolic acidosis, such as diarrhea, strangulating bowel obstruction, and renal insufficiency, may result in loss or sequestration of Na^+ and Cl^-, which was not seen here. Other causes of metabolic acidosis include grain overload, exertional rhabdomyolysis, peritonitis, and hypovolemic shock. All these causes usually manifest with a high anion gap because of accumulation of unidentified anions (eg, lactic acid, salts of uremic acids). Although a mildly increased anion gap was present, this mare failed to show signs consistent with any of these etiologies. Hyperalbuminemia can contribute to an increased anion gap and is usually seen with dehydration. Mild renal insufficiency could not be ruled out because of the azotemia, but the urine was concentrated and the azotemia was attributed to prerenal causes (dehydration). This assessment was supported by a urine Cr/serum Cr ratio of greater than 50:1, which suggested prerenal azotemia. The urine GGT/Cr ratio was normal at 12.2 (reference value <25). Because this ratio is a sensitive indicator of proximal renal tubular damage, indications were that tubular damage was unlikely. The dehydration was attributed to decreased intake, because other causes seemed unlikely based on the history, examination, and laboratory values. Based on the severe hyperchloremic metabolic acidosis, alkaline urine, and lack of other localizing clinical signs, a presumptive diagnosis of type 1 (distal) renal tubular acidosis (DRTA) with concurrent dehydration was made. Because of a lack of laboratory evidence of hepatic disease or hemolysis, the icterus was attributed to fasting hyperbilirubinemia.

This mare's evaluation suggested type 1 DRTA based on the presence of alkaline urine as well as the profound acidosis. In DRTA, the distal tubules are unable to excrete hydrogen ions (H^+), which results in alkaline urine. This is contrasted with type 2, or proximal, rental tubular acidosis (RTA), in which bicarbonate cannot be reabsorbed and is lost in urine. In type 2 RTA, the tubules retain the ability to excrete H^+, so urine is acidified [1,2]. This distinction between types 1 and 2 RTA may be difficult to determine in herbivores because of the normally alkaline urine found in these species, but treatment is the same for either type. Horses with RTA are not usually azotemic, because urine concentrating ability is preserved. The azotemia in this mare was attributed to lack of water intake, with continued losses resulting in dehydration, a decreased glomerular filtration rate, and prerenal azotemia. Hyperalbuminemia is usually seen only with dehydration (relative increase), which would support this hypothesis. Causes of RTA in other species include primary (idiopathic) or secondary to other systemic disease, such as hypergammaglobulinemia, multiple myeloma, interstitial nephropathy, hepatitis, systemic lupus erythematosus, altered calcium metabolism, toxins, or drug reactions [1–4]. Clinical and laboratory evaluation made all these diagnoses unlikely, although toxins could not be entirely ruled out. This mare did not seem to have other concurrent systemic disease but did have a history of diarrhea several months previously. The mare had also been shipped recently and had a change in environment, which may have caused predisposing stress.

Treatment and outcome

The goals of therapy for this mare were rehydration, diuresis, and normalization of acid-base and electrolyte balance. Speed of correction of the acid-base imbalance in RTA seems to influence hospitalization time, and no problems have been reported with administration of the entire calculated base deficit over 24 hours [5]. Fluid deficit and maintenance requirements were calculated, and the mare was started on physiologic saline solution with potassium chloride (KCl), 20 mEq/L, and HCO_3^-, 60 mEq/L, at a fluid rate of 100 mL/kg/d (2 L/h). The total bicarbonate deficit was calculated at 2870 mEq (455 kg × base deficit [mEq/L] × 0.3 [extracellular fluid volume]). Because the mare had arrived in the evening, reassessment was planned for the morning. As a result, half of the calculated bicarbonate deficit (1435 mEq) was added to the fluids for overnight administration. In addition, the mare was given baking soda ($NaHCO_3$), 25 g, administered orally every 4 hours (at an HCO_3^- concentration of 12 mEq/g) for additional bicarbonate (1800 mEq). In the morning (day 2), the mare was brighter and less lethargic and ate a small amount of hay. The horse seemed to be well hydrated and was urinating and defecating normally. Laboratory results revealed continued hyperchloremia and acidosis. The anion gap was normal. Azotemia was still present. Serum bile acids were measured to assess liver function and were normal, making significant hepatic disease unlikely. Ultrasonographic evaluation of the kidneys and liver revealed no abnormalities. Urinalysis showed dilute alkaline urine. A blood gas analysis revealed metabolic acidosis with respiratory compensation. The calculated deficit of HCO_3^- (2460 mEq) was added to physiologic saline at an HCO_3^- concentration of 70 mEq/L. This was administered at a total fluid rate of 80 mL/kg/d (1.5 L/h). In addition, KCl, 40 mEq/L, was added to fluids because of the decreasing serum K^+ concentration. RTA frequently results in whole-body K^+ depletion, because intracellular K^+ is exchanged for extracellular H^+ in acidemic states and K^+ is wasted through kaliuresis. Potassium is shifted from the extracellular space back to the intracellular space during corrective alkalinization, resulting in serum hypokalemia. Although this mare was normokalemic at admission, normokalemia in the presence of severe acidosis is suggestive of whole-body K^+ depletion. Thus, the decreasing serum K^+ concentration was expected. Oral bicarbonate supplementation was increased to 35 g administered orally every 4 hours. The mare continued to improve clinically and ate hay with an increasing appetite. On day 3, laboratory results indicated improving acidosis and hyperchloremia, but hypokalemia was now present. Azotemia was improved from day 2. Hyperproteinemia was present. The calculated HCO_3^- deficit of 1092 mEq was added to physiologic saline at a concentration of 33 mEq/L, and fluids were administered at a rate of 80 mL/kg/d for continued diuresis. KCl, 60 mEq/L, was added to fluids, and oral KCl, 20 g, was given three times daily to address hypokalemia. Oral bicarbonate supplementation was continued. The mare began to show a good appetite. On day 4, the mare was bright, active, and hungry. Laboratory parameters indicated resolution of the hyperchloremia and acidosis. Hypokalemia was still present, as was mild azotemia. A blood gas analysis showed a positive base excess and normocapnia. The results of a CBC were normal. Fluid therapy was changed to lactated Ringer's solution supplemented with KCl, 60 mEq/L, administered at a rate of 50 mL/kg/d. Oral KCl was increased to 40 g administered orally every 8 hours. Oral bicarbonate was continued at a rate of 35 g administered orally every 4 hours.

Although hypokalemia can have severe consequences, including cardiac arrhythmias and muscular weakness, none were noted in this mare. An electrocardiogram was not done, so subtle electrocardiographic abnormalities may have been missed. By day 6, the mare seemed to be clinically normal and her appetite was excellent. The icterus had resolved. Laboratory parameters showed resolution of hypokalemia and azotemia with persistent mild hyperproteinemia. A serum protein electrophoresis was submitted to determine the source of the hyperproteinemia, and results indicated that all classes were within reference ranges. This ruled out hypergammaglobulinemia and polyclonal gammopathy as causes of the RTA. Urinalysis showed dilute alkaline urine. Fluid therapy and oral KCl were discontinued. Oral bicarbonate therapy was continued but changed to $NaHCO_3$, 70 g, administered orally every 8 hours for the same total daily dose (2520 mEq/d). Between days 8 and 11, the mare became mildly alkalotic; oral bicarbonate supplementation was decreased to 90 g administered orally every 12 hours (2160 mEq/d). By day 14, the mare's bicarbonate level was within normal limits. The mare and foal were discharged on day 15 with instructions to continue oral bicarbonate supplementation (90 g administered orally every 12 hours) indefinitely and to monitor for recurrent lethargy or inappetence, particularly during high-stress periods.

Two weeks after discharge, the mare was reported to be clinically normal by the owner and the referring veterinarian. Laboratory values submitted from the referring veterinarian, including serum chloride and total carbon dioxide, were within normal limits. Continued bicarbonate supplementation was recommended. A recheck examination was declined by the owner. Telephone follow-up 3 months after discharge indicated that the mare remained clinically normal and was still receiving bicarbonate. The foal had been weaned without difficulty 6 weeks after discharge. No further laboratory data were available.

Discussion

RTA is an uncommon syndrome that has been reported in many species. The syndrome is characterized by alterations in renal tubular ion handling that result in increased renal conservation of chloride ions and a subsequent hyperchloremic metabolic acidosis, which is the hallmark of this disease. Three types of RTA are described, including distal (type 1), proximal (type 2), and hyperkalemic distal (type 4) [1,2]. Only types 1 and 2 have been described in veterinary species to date, and both have been reported in horses [6–11]. Type 1 RTA results when the distal tubules are unable to excrete hydrogen ions and, subsequently, cannot produce acidic urine. Type 2 RTA occurs when proximal tubular reabsorption of bicarbonate is inadequate and the bicarbonate ions are lost in the urine. Because excretion of hydrogen ions occurs simultaneously with reabsorption of bicarbonate ions, both types of RTA result from decreased excretion of hydrogen ions. Hyperchloremia results from conservation of chloride in lieu of bicarbonate so that electroneutrality may be preserved.

There is no apparent breed or sex predilection for RTA in horses, and its pathogenesis is unknown [5]. Several different genetic mutations in ion transport genes have been implicated in heritable forms of RTA in human beings [2], but there is no evidence of an inherited form of the disease in veterinary species. Also in people, RTA has been linked to drug administration as well as to other systemic diseases, including autoimmune disease, calcium disorders, dysproteinemic disorders, and other types of renal disease. Diet has not been linked with development of RTA in equine species. In horses, one retrospective study reported the average age at onset of RTA to be 7 years [5], although several cases of horses affected at 2 years or younger are found in the literature [5,9]. Clinical signs exhibited by horses with RTA include lethargy, depression, inappetence, poor performance, weight loss, and mild colic. Dehydration is variable. Clinicopathologic abnormalities are generally restricted to electrolyte and acid-base status. Typical cases of RTA demonstrate a striking hyperchloremia (> 105 mEq/L) and a profound metabolic acidosis (plasma bicarbonate < 13 mEq/L and venous blood pH < 7.25). Respiratory compensation may be evident on blood gas analysis. Horses may be presented in a normokalemic or hypokalemic condition, but hypokalemia is common during bicarbonate replenishment. Potassium loss in urine (in lieu of hydrogen ion) and anorexia contribute to the hypokalemia.

More than half of the horses with RTA are reported to have some degree of renal disease or damage, and abnormal urinalysis results are common [5]. It is not known if renal damage predisposes horses to the development of RTA; however, a canine model has demonstrated that renal ischemia may impair distal tubular acidification [12]. The mare in this report was dehydrated and azotemic at presentation, and the azotemia persisted for several days despite diuresis. Additional renal tubular dysfunction may have been present in this case, but a renal biopsy was not pursued after the mare's acid-base status was normalized. A diagnosis of DRTA may be confirmed with an ammonium chloride tolerance test. In this test, oral ammonium chloride (0.1 g/kg) is converted to urea by the liver with formation of glutamine and hydrogen chloride (HCl). HCl is buffered by HCO_3^-, lowering the plasma HCO_3^- concentration [13]. Normal horses excrete the fixed acid and acidify urine to less than pH 7.0 within 2 to 3 hours after administration [8]. Horses with DRTA fail to acidify urine despite acidemia. Although the diagnosis of DRTA in this mare was not confirmed with challenge testing, the metabolic abnormalities were characteristic and the mare responded to therapy. Fractional excretions of electrolytes in horses with DRTA typically show increased clearance of Na^+ (normal value <1%) with normal Cl^- and K^+ clearances (normal values <1.6% and 15%–65%, respectively) [8]. In proximal RTA, fractional excretion of potassium is decreased, whereas sodium and chloride clearances are normal [11]. Urine net charge (UNC, also known as urine anion gap) is reported to be low or even negative in horses with RTA (normal value: 111–189) [5]. UNC is calculated as follows: Urine Na^+ + Urine K^+ − Urine Cl^-. Many of the other tests used for diagnosis of RTA in human beings are misleading in horses because of a lack of appropriate reference values and the alkaline urine of herbivorous species [5].

Treatment of RTA is centered around aggressive bicarbonate supplementation by intravenous and oral routes [2,4], and the entire deficit can be administered over each 24-hour period. Frequent reassessment (daily to every other day) is necessary to adjust the rate of administration while the patient is on intravenous bicarbonate. Isotonic (1.3%) bicarbonate solution and isotonic (0.9%) or half-strength (0.45%) sodium chloride with added 5% or 8.4% sodium bicarbonate are acceptable fluids for intravenous administration; additional KCl should be supplemented if the patient is normo- or hypokalemic at presentation (20–80 mEq/L, not to exceed 0.5 mEq/kg/h). The patient's serum chloride normalizes as acidosis is corrected, despite administration of chloride-containing fluids. Bicarbonate should not be added to calcium-containing fluids (eg, lactated Ringer's solution) because of the potential for calcium carbonate precipitation. Oral supplementation of bicarbonate may be started with $NaHCO_3$, 100 to 150 g, administered every 12 hours, and KCl may also be orally supplemented. Transient diarrhea may occur with large-volume oral bicarbonate supplementation in anorectic horses [5]. Clinical improvement is closely correlated with normalization of acid-base status. Relapses may occur when the patient is transitioned from intravenous to oral bicarbonate. Proximal (type 2) RTA is also treated with bicarbonate therapy, although some proximal RTA patients may attain a steady-state acidemia without treatment [2]. Treatment should be pursued in both types of RTA to minimize the risks of nephrocalcinosis, osteomalacia, renolithiasis, or muscle wasting as seen in human beings [2,14,15]. Spontaneous resolution of DRTA in horses has been reported 16 to 28 months after initial recognition, but more than half of the reported cases experience relapses when oral bicarbonate is refused or discontinued. Relapses occurred more frequently in horses with renal disease in addition to RTA [5]. Lifelong bicarbonate supplementation may be necessary in horses with RTA to control clinical signs.

No studies have been done on the effects of long-term oral sodium bicarbonate supplementation in horses. Human RTA patients are typically treated with oral potassium bicarbonate or potassium citrate, which is converted to bicarbonate once ingested [15]. Neither potassium bicarbonate nor potassium citrate treatment has been studied in horses.

In summary, RTA is an uncommon disease that can manifest with nebulous clinical signs, including lethargy, inappetence, poor performance, and weight loss. Its classic presentation is a hyperchloremic metabolic acidosis, and many affected horses have concurrent renal disease. RTA is treated with intravenous and oral bicarbonate supplementation, and cases usually respond quickly to therapy. Affected horses may require lifelong oral bicarbonate, but spontaneous resolution has been reported.

References

[1] Battle D. Renal tubular acidosis. Med Clin North Am 1983;67:859–78.
[2] Soriano JR. Renal tubular acidosis: the clinical entity. J Am Soc Nephrol 2002;13:2160–70.
[3] Hemstreet BA. Antimicrobial-associated renal tubular acidosis. Ann Pharmacother 2004; 38(6):1031–8.
[4] Nicoletta JA, Schwartz GJ. Distal renal tubular acidosis. Curr Opin Pediatr 2004;16(2): 194–8.
[5] Aleman MR, Kuesis B, Schott HC, et al. Renal tubular acidosis in horses (1980–1999). J Vet Intern Med 2001;15(2):136–43.
[6] Hansen TO. Renal tubular acidosis in a mare. Compend Contin Educ Pract Vet 1986;8: 864–6.
[7] Trotter GW, Miller D, Parks A, et al. Type II renal tubular acidosis in a mare. J Am Vet Med Assoc 1986;188(9):1050–1.
[8] Ziemer EL, Parker HR, Carlson GP, et al. Renal tubular acidosis in two horses: diagnostic studies. J Am Vet Med Assoc 1987;190(3):289–93.
[9] Ziemer EL, Parker HR, Carlson GP, et al. Clinical features and treatment of renal tubular acidosis in two horses. J Am Vet Med Assoc 1987;190(3):294–6.
[10] van der Kolk JH, Kalsbeek HC. Renal tubular acidosis in a mare. Vet Rec 1993;133(2):43–4.
[11] MacLeay JM, Wilson JH. Type-II renal tubular acidosis and ventricular tachycardia in a horse. J Am Vet Med Assoc 1998;212(10):1597–9.
[12] Winaver J, Agmon D, Harari R, et al. Impaired renal acidification following acute renal ischemia in the dog. Kidney Int 1986;30(6):906–13.
[13] Shaw DH. Acute response of urine pH following ammonium chloride administration to dogs. Am J Vet Res 1989;50(11):1829–30.
[14] Polzin DJ, Osborne CA, Bell FW. Canine distal renal tubular acidosis and urolithiasis. Vet Clin North Am Small Anim Pract 1986;16(2):241–50.
[15] Morris RC Jr, Sebastian A. Alkali therapy in renal tubular acidosis: who needs it? J Am Soc Nephrol 2002;13:2186–8.

VETERINARY
CLINICS
Equine Practice

ELSEVIER
SAUNDERS

Vet Clin Equine 22 (2006) 239–246

Rhodococcus equi Pneumonia in a Foal

Bonnie S. Barr, VMD

Rood and Riddle Equine Hospital, 2150 Georgetown Road, Lexington, KY 40580, USA

History

A 3-month-old Thoroughbred colt was presented with a history of fever and tachypnea of 1-day duration. The foal was housed with other mares and foals of similar age. Recently a foal of similar age had presented to the hospital in acute respiratory distress and died 12 hours later. The foal had been dewormed every 30 days, but had not received any vaccinations.

Physical examination

The foal's temperature was 40.3°C (104.5°F), heart rate was 72 beats/minute, and respiratory rate was 44 breaths/minute. Auscultation of the lung fields identified generalized crackles and wheezes bilaterally, with the cranioventral lung field seeming to be the most severely affected. There was a mild increase in respiratory effort with no evidence of nasal discharge. Auscultation of the heart and intestinal tract failed to detect any abnormalities. No lameness or joint effusion was detected.

Case assessment

The most common causes of fever and tachypnea in a foal include diseases of the upper respiratory tract, diseases of the lower respiratory tract, gastrointestinal disorders, and musculoskeletal disorders. Musculoskeletal disorders in a foal this age would include septic arthritis, osteomyelitis, and physitis. No evidence of musculoskeletal disorders was seen on the initial physical examination. The foal was not lame, nor did it have any joint distension. Common gastrointestinal diseases associated with fever and tachypnea in a foal include enteritis, enterocolitis, peritonitis, ruptured viscous, and strangulating lesions. In this case there was no history of any signs of colic. Physical examination did not identify any abdominal

E-mail address: bbarr@roodandriddle.com

distension; therefore a gastrointestinal disorder was ruled out. Common upper airway disorders that cause fever and tachypnea in a foal would include pharyngeal cysts, progressive ethmoidal hematomas, sinus cysts, retropharyngeal abscesses, and guttural pouch tympany/empyema. There was equal airflow through both nostrils, and no evidence of an inspiratory or expiratory stridor was noted. In addition, there was no submandibular lymphadenopathy; thus, upper airway disorders were ruled out. Diseases involving the lower respiratory tract that can cause fever and tachypnea in the foal include viral and bacterial pneumonia, pleuropneumonia, and acute respiratory distress syndrome. The most likely diagnosis at this time was disease of the lower respiratory tract. Diagnostics performed included complete blood cell count, serum chemistry profile, thoracic radiography and ultrasonography, and transtracheal aspiration.

Procedures

Laboratory abnormalities identified a leukocytosis and hyperfibrinogenemia. No abnormalities were noted on the clinical chemistry. Abnormalities in the white blood cell count and fibrinogen are indicative of an inflammatory process. Thoracic radiographs identified radiographic changes and patchy, dense alveolar opacities suggestive of lung abscesses (Fig. 1). Thoracic ultrasound was performed using a 6.0-MHz microconvex probe (a 5.0-MHz probe or a 3.0-MHz probe could also be used). The ultrasound identified consolidated lung in the mid-thorax (Fig. 2).

A percutaneous transtracheal aspirate was performed using the following procedure: the foal was sedated with xylazine (0.2 mg/kg intravenously) and butorphenol (0.02 mg/kg intravenously) to perform a percutaneous transtracheal aspirate safely. The author has found that BD Intracath made by

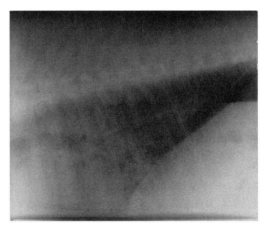

Fig. 1. Thoracic radiograph. Patchy focal opacities indicate multiple abscesses.

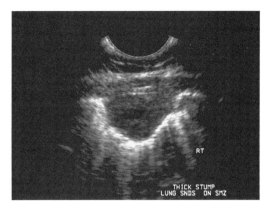

Fig. 2. Ultrasound image: peripheral region of consolidation with central hypoechoic fluid pocket in the lung.

Becton Dickinson is a convenient kit to use to perform this procedure. Briefly, the procedure is as follows. The ventral neck was divided into thirds, and a small area was clipped at the junction of the first and second third of the ventral neck. The area was blocked with lidocaine and aseptically prepared. A needle, or cannula, is passed through the skin, between tracheal rings, and into the tracheal lumen. A sterile polypropylene catheter is passed approximately to the area of tracheal bifurcation. Six mL of saline is infused into the catheter and then aspirated. If little fluid is obtained with the first aspirate, a second 6 mL can be infused. After the sample is obtained, the catheter is withdrawn. Possible complications include subcutaneous emphysema or subcutaneous infection from leakage of exudate while the catheter is removed. Another method for obtaining a sample is through the endoscope using a protected aspiration catheter. The biggest complication with this technique is the potential for contamination by the upper airway. The best way to prepare the slide is to centrifuge the sample and make the slide from the sediment pellet. Air-dried smears can be stained with Diff Quick (or Gram's stain), allowed to dry then examined under oil emersion. In this case, cytologic evaluation identified gram-positive coccobacilli that which were suggestive of *Rhodococcus equi*. The diagnosis was confirmed 48 hours later when culture results were available.

Discussion of differential diagnosis

Other causes of bacterial pneumonia in a foal that need to be considered include *Streptococcus equi ss zooepidemicus*, *S equi ss equi*, and other bacteria such as *Escherichia coli*, *Klebsiella spp*, or *Actinobacillus spp*. *S zooepidemicus* is a beta-hemolytic streptococcus species that is commonly found in the upper respiratory tract of healthy horses [1–3]. It can cause bronchopneumonia, pleuritis, or pleuropneumonia in sucklings and weanlings

[4,5]. Common clinical signs include depression, nasal discharge, cough, fever, and increased respiratory effort. Adventitial lung sounds vary, ranging from diffuse crackles and wheezes to decreased or absent lung sounds ventrally. The organism is a common inhabitant of the upper airway and is unable to invade intact mucous membranes; pre-existing damage is necessary for infection [1–3]. Viral respiratory infections or environmental stressors such as overcrowding, poor nutrition, or transportation can lead to impairment of the normal defense mechanism of the respiratory tract and allow the establishment of disease. Thoracic radiographs and ultrasound identify lung pathology, but culture and cytology of a transtracheal aspirate is necessary to make a definitive diagnosis.

S equi is a beta-hemolytic organism that is known to cause strangles. It is typically a disease of the upper respiratory tract and lymph nodes, although lower respiratory tract disease can occur. It is more commonly a disease of yearlings through 3-year-olds [6–10]. Clinical signs include depression, fever, purulent nasal discharge, cough, swelling, and tenderness of the intramandibular area where abscesses eventually form in the submandibular and submaxillary or retropharyngeal lymph nodes. Bronchopneumonia can result from aspiration of the purulent material or metastatic spread of the organism to the lungs [6–10]. Radiographs and ultrasound identify lung pathology. Diagnosis is based on clinical signs of upper respiratory involvement and results of a transtracheal aspirate culture and cytology.

Other bacteria that can cause pneumonia in a 3-month-old foal include E coli, Klebsiella species, and A equi, to name a few [4,5]. Physical examination findings include adventitial lung sounds and a cough. Thoracic radiographs and thoracic ultrasound indicate varying degrees of lung pathology. Once again, a definitive diagnosis is made only by transtracheal aspirate with cytologic analysis and culture of the fluid.

R equi can cause subacute to chronic bronchopneumonia in foals less than 6 months of age [11,12]. It is a pleomorphic gram-positive bacterium that has been frequently isolated from soil samples throughout the world, even in areas never inhabited by horses [13]. Despite this widespread environmental distribution, R equi infection is endemic to some farms, occurs occasionally on others, or may never by found on a farm. Several factors may influence the incidence of the disease, including the environment, management of the farm, and virulence of the organism [13–16]. Clinical signs can include fever, increased respiratory rate, lethargy, and tachypnea. Physical examination findings may include localized wheezes to diffuse crackles noted on auscultation of the thorax. Often, in addition to pulmonary involvement, lesions may be found in other organ systems including the gastrointestinal tract, musculoskeletal system, and neurologic system. Thoracic radiographic changes include a diffuse increase in interstitial pattern, to diffuse alveolar opacities. Ultrasound of the thorax is helpful if the lesions extend to the periphery, but generally radiographs are more useful. Definitive diagnosis is based on a transtracheal aspirate in which cytologic analysis identifies gram-positive, coccobacilli-shaped organisms, and culture confirms the diagnosis (Table 1).

Extrapulmonary lesions may be associated with pneumonia or independent of pneumonia [11]. Gastrointestinal involvement may consist of ulcerative colitis, abdominal lymphadenitis, typhlitis, or a single large abdominal abscess. Clinical signs of intestinal involvement include colic, diarrhea, weight loss, and poor growth. Diagnostic procedures include abdominal ultrasound and abdominocentesis. Polysynovitis has been reported in foals with R equi pneumonia and is caused by an immune complex deposition within the synovial structures [11]. Lameness is rarely apparent, and cytologic evaluation of the synovial fluid reveals a nonseptic, mononuclear pleocytosis. Bacteremia occasionally results in septic arthritis or osteomyelitis; these foals are lame, and analysis of synovial fluid reveals a septic process. Other manifestations, including uveitis, anemia, and thrombocytopenia, may arise from an immune-mediated response [11]. Neurologic signs may be associated with R equi vertebral body osteomyelitis.

Treatment and outcome

The most common antimicrobial combination used to treat R equi is erythromycin and rifampin. This combination is able to penetrate abscesses and cells because of its lipophilic nature [16]. Azithromycin and clarithromycin are two additional macrolides that are used to treat R equi pneumonia. Azithromycin is administered daily, often in conjunction with rifampin. Clarithromycin is most often used in cases not responding well to erythromycin or azithromycin but is expensive (Table 2). A recent report, however, has suggested that the combination of clarithromycin and rifampin is superior to the combinations of erythromycin and rifampin or azithromycin and rifampin [17].

The initial treatment for this foal included azithromycin and rifampin. The foal's vital signs were closely monitored, and an antipyretic (a nonsteroidal anti-inflammatory drug) was administered as needed for fevers.

Table 1
Microscopic features of common bacteria from foals with pneumonia

Bacteria	Morphology	Other Features	Gram reaction
Streptococcus zooepidemicus (and other *streptococcus* spp)	Cocci	Single pairs and short chains	Positive
Rhodococcus equi	Coccobacilli	Chinese figures or watermelon seed appearance	Positive
Escherichia coli	Rods		Negative
Klebsiella sp	Rods		Negative
Actinobacillus sp	Rods		Negative

Table 2
Common drug dosages for treatment of *Rhodococcus equi* pneumonia in foals

Drug	Dose	Route	Frequency
Erythromycin phosphate	37.5 mg/kg	po	Q 12 hours
Erythromycin ethylsuccinate	10–25 mg/kg	po	Q 8 hours
Erythromycin stearate	10–30 mg/kg	po	Q 6 hours
Erythromycin lactobionate	10 mg/kg	iv	Q 6 hours
Azithromycin	10 mg/kg	po	Q 24 hours for 5 days, then every other day
Clarithromycin	7.5 mg/kg	po	Q 12 hours
Rifampin	5 mg/kg	po	Q 12 hours

This author typically administers omeprazole to all sick foals, especially those receiving nonsteroidal anti-inflammatory drugs. Response to treatment is noted with resolution of clinical signs, normalization of blood work, and resolution of radiographic lesions. In this case, treatment extended over 4 weeks. In general, treatment usually ranges from 4 to 9 weeks. Treatment of extrapulmonary lesions includes the previously mentioned antimicrobial agents plus additional supportive measures such as fluids, blood transfusions, and nonsteroidal anti-inflammatory agents. Aggressive joint lavage and local therapy may be required if septic arthritis or osteomyelitis is diagnosed. Clinical signs that result from an immune-mediated response resolve once the systemic disease is under control. Occasionally, erythromycin can cause changes in the foal's fecal consistency or thermoregulation [18]. In addition *Clostridium difficile* enterocolitis has been reported in mares of foals being treated with erythromycin and is suspected to be caused by inadvertent ingestion of erythromycin from the foal's feces or material contaminated with feces, which disrupts the mare's intestinal flora [19]. In the author's experience, the thermoregulatory problem has not been observed in foals treated with azithromycin, but changes in fecal consistency have been observed. Prognosis for survival is reported to be around 70% to 80%, with death more likely in foals that have severe respiratory signs, severe thoracic radiographic changes, lameness, and joint effusion [20]. Appropriate therapy needs to be instituted; even more importantly, preventative and control measures must be taken to prevent the disease, especially on endemic farms. Appropriate management factors to decrease the size of infective challenges are important and include avoiding overcrowding, decreasing the amount of dirt or sandy areas, rotating pastures, housing in well-ventilated and dust-free areas, and grouping/isolating of foals with clinical signs together because they have the more virulent form in their feces [1,21,22]. Foals should be closely monitored for early recognition of disease. Monitoring should include daily rectal temperature, peripheral white blood cell and plasma fibrinogen levels weekly or every 2 weeks, and physical examination. Currently the mainstay of protection for endemically infected farms has been the administration of hyperimmunized plasma to provide passive immunization. The ideal amount and time for plasma administration are still not known, but current recommendations include 1 L within the first week of life and then another liter 25 to 30 days later [1,21]. A single administration at 10 to 21 days may be adequate for farms with lower morbidity [1,21]. The administration of hyperimmunized plasma should be combined with the appropriate management factors to provide the best protection in an endemic area.

Summary

This foal's therapy extended for a period of 4 weeks. Over this time the foal's clinical signs improved, and the abnormalities on the blood work resolved. Twelve months later this foal/yearling is doing well.

References

[1] Barr BS. Pneumonia in weanlings. Vet Clin North Am Equine Prac 2003;19:35–49.

[2] Beech J. Streptococcus equi spp zooepidemicus. In: Colahan PT, Mayhew IG, Merritt AM, et al, editors. Equine medicine and surgery. 5th edition. Philadelphia: Mosby; 1999. p. 530.

[3] Anzai T, Walker JA, Blair MB, et al. Comparison of the phenotypes of Streptococcus zooepidemicus isolated from tonsils of healthy horses and specimens obtained from foals and donkeys with pneumonia. Am J Vet Res 2000;61(2):162–6.

[4] Lavoie JP, Fiset L, Laverty S. Review of 40 cases of lung abscesses in foals and adult horses. Equine Vet J 1994;26(5):348–52.

[5] Paradis MR. Pneumonia in foals. In: Smith BP, editor. Large animal internal medicine. 3rd edition. Philadelphia: Mosby; 2002. p. 496–9.

[6] Sweeney C, Benson C, Whitlock R, et al. Streptococcus equi infections in horses—part 1. Compend Equine 1987;9(6):689–93.

[7] Sweeney C, Benson C, Whitlock R, et al. Streptococcus equi infections in horses—part 2. Compend Equine 1987;9(8):845–51.

[8] Timoney J. Strangles. Vet Clin North Am Equine Pract 9(2):365–73.

[9] Sweeney C. Strangles: Streptococcus equi infection in horses. Equine Vet Educ 1996;8(6): 317–22.

[10] Timoney JF. Equine strangles. In: Proceedings of the 45th annual convention of the American Association of Equine Practitioners. 1999. p. 31–7.

[11] Giguere S. Rhodococcus equi infections. In: Wilkins PA, Palmer JE, editors. Recent advances in equine neonatal care. Ithaca (NY): International Veterinary Information Services; 2001.

[12] Zink MC, Yager JA, Smart NL. Corynebacterium equi infections in horses, 1958–1984: a review of 131 cases. Can J Vet Res 1986;27:213–7.

[13] Hughes KL, Sulaiman I. The ecology of Rhodococcus equi and physicochemical influences on growth. Vet Microbiol 1987;14:241.

[14] Takai S, Fujimori T, Katsuzaki K, et al. Ecology of Rhodococcus equi in horses and their environment on horse-breeding farms. Vet Microbiol 1987;14:233.

[15] Takai S, Narita K, Ando K, et al. Ecology of Rhodococcus (Corynebacterium) equi in soil on a horse-breeding farm. Vet Microbiol 1986;12:169.

[16] Lakritz J, Wilso WD. Erythromycin and other macrolide antibiotics for treating Rhodococcus equi pneumonia in foals. Compend Cont Educ Prac Vet 2002;24:256–61.

[17] Giguere S, Jacks S, Roberts GD, et al. Retrospective comparison of azithromycin, clarithromycin, and erythromycin for the treatment of foals with Rhodococcus equi pneumonia. J Vet Intern Med 2004;18:568–73.

[18] Stratton-Phelps M, Wilson WD, Gardner IA. Risk of adverse effects in pneumonic foals treated with erythromycin versus other antibiotics: 143 cases (1986–1996). J Am Vet Med Assoc 2000;217(1):68–73.

[19] Baverud V, Franklin A, Gunnarsson A, et al. Clostridium difficile associated with acute colitis in mares when their foals are treated with erythromycin and rifampin for Rhodococcus equi pneumonia. Equine Vet J 1998;30(6):482–8.

[20] Ainsworth D, Eicker S, Yeagar A, et al. Associations between physical examination, laboratory, and radiographic findings and outcome and subsequent racing performance of foals with Rhodococcus equi infections: 115 cases (1984–1992). J Am Vet Med Assoc 1998; 213(4):510–5.

[21] Giguere S, Prescott JF. Strategies for the control of Rhodococcus equi infections on enzootic farms. In: Proceedings of the 43rd annual convention of the American Association of Equine Practitioners. 1997. p. 65–70.

[22] Prescott JF. Epidemiology of Rhodococcus equi infection in horses. Vet Microbiol 1987;14: 211–4.

ELSEVIER
SAUNDERS

VETERINARY
CLINICS
Equine Practice

Vet Clin Equine 22 (2006) 247–254

Pneumonia and Pleuritis in a Mare

Jonathan H. Magid, DVM, MS

Dr. T's Equine Clinic, 586 Lonesome Dove Lane, Salado, TX 76571, USA

History

A 3-year-old Appaloosa mare was presented for evaluation of respiratory disease. The mare, which had never been off the owner's farm, had been moved to a stable and started in training as a western pleasure horse 3 weeks before presentation. The horse began to cough 6 days before presentation. The trainer started treating the mare with trimethoprim-sulfa 5 days before presentation. This treatment continued for 2 days without improvement. Three days before presentation, the referring veterinarian examined the mare, which had a fever of 39.4°C (103°F) and was diagnosed with pneumonia. Previous treatment was stopped; flunixin meglumine, 10 mL, administered intramuscularly twice daily (every 12 hours); albuterol, 5 tablets, administered orally every 12 hours; and ceftiofur, 1 g, administered intramuscularly once daily were prescribed. This treatment continued until presentation. On the morning of presentation, the mare's temperature was 40.2°C (104.4°F) and it was anorectic and refused to drink. The mare had been vaccinated for eastern equine encephalomyelitis, western equine encephalomyelitis, tetanus, rhinopneumonitis, and influenza on arrival at the training stable. It had never been vaccinated for *Streptococcus equi*. It had been dewormed 8 weeks before presentation with ivermectin and was routinely dewormed with ivermectin at 8-week intervals. The mare had received a negative Coggin's test result for equine infectious anemia (EIA) 3 weeks before presentation. The horse was housed in an unheated stall and bedded on shavings. The diet was grass hay and one cup of sweet feed pellets twice daily. The mare had never been bred.

Physical examination

The rectal temperature was 38.6°C (101.5°F), the heart rate was 68 beats per minute with no pulse deficits, and the respiratory rate was 60 beats per minute. The body weight was 431 kg. The mare seemed to be depressed and

E-mail address: jmagid@twoalpha.net

stood with a lowered head. The body condition was good. The skin tent was prolonged. The gums were pink, hyperemic, and tacky. The eyes and conjunctiva were normal. The limbs were cool without swelling. The digital pulses were within normal limits. The peripheral lymph nodes were normal. The nostrils were flared, and respiratory effort was increased. Serous nasal discharge was present. There was no abnormal odor to the mare's breath. The horse seemed to resent pressure applied to the thorax. Crackles and wheezes were ausculted in both lungs. No pleural friction rubs were ausculted. There was an area of diminished lung and heart sounds on the right side of the thorax below the level of the elbow. Percussion of the thorax (using a rubber examination hammer and an inexpensive spoon) revealed an area of dullness at the level of the elbow on the right hemithorax but not on the left side. No coughing was observed. Heart sounds and rhythms were normal. Gut sounds were diminished and heard only on the lower left quadrant. Feces were dry. No signs of colic were present, and rectal palpation was not performed. Dehydration was estimated at 3% to 5%.

Case assessment and management

The primary problems identified were respiratory disease, hyperemic mucous membranes, fever, historical anorexia, and dehydration. The respiratory disease was most likely pneumonia or pleuropneumonia of bacterial, fungal, mycoplasmal, or viral origin, although thoracic neoplasia [1] and abscessation were also differentials. The history and physical examination did not support heart disease, trauma, aspiration pneumonia, ruptured esophagus, or allergic lung disease as differentials. The fact that the horse was no longer coughing is consistent with pleuritis; some pleuritis patients attempt to avoid coughing because they seem to find it painful. Hyperemic mucous membranes suggested septicemia or endotoxemia. Hyperemic mucous membrane* and fever were assumed to be secondary to the respiratory disease. Anorexia and dehydration often occur in animals with pulmonary disease and may be secondary to dyspnea or fever.

The initial workup included a complete blood cell count, fibrinogen assessment, serum chemistry, arterial and venous blood gases, and transtracheal wash. Transtracheal wash samples were submitted for cytology and aerobic and anaerobic culture testing. Chest radiographs were not taken, because no radiologist was available until the next day. While awaiting results of the blood tests, thoracic ultrasonography was performed using a portable ultrasound machine with a 5-mHz linear reproductive probe. This showed a hypoechoic area within the chest consistent with a fluid line just below the elbow in the right hemithorax. No abnormalities were seen in the left hemithorax. This was consistent with the percussion findings. The total white blood cell count (WBC) and neutrophil count were normal, but immature and toxic neutrophils were present (Table 1). There was mild lymphopenia. Serum chemistry (Table 2) showed mild hypoproteinemia, mild

Table 1
Complete blood cell count values

Date/hospital day	Normal values	3/22/98 Day 1	3/27/98 Day 5	4/13/98 Day 50
PCV (%)	32–53	43.5	26.6	30.4
RBC $\times 10^6/\mu L$	7–13	10.4	6.26	7.16
MCV (fL)	37–59	41.9	42.4	42.4
MCH (pg)	12–20	15.7	15.9	15.3
MCHC (%)	31–38	37.5	37.5	36.2
Hemoglobin (g/dL)	11–19	16.3	9.96	11.0
White blood cells/μL	5.5–12 k	7090	9320	3950
Band neutrophils/μL	0–100	141.8	0	0
Segmented neutrophils/μL	3–7 k	5601	6990	2488.5
Lymphocytes/μL	1.5–5 k	921	2050	1343
Monocytes/μL	0–1 k	425	0	79
Eosinophils/μL	0–1 k		280	40
Leukocyte morphology		2 + toxic granulocyte		
Platelets/μL	1–6 (100k)	325,000		
Fibrinogen (mg/dL)	100–400	700	900	200
OSPT (seconds)	10–20			
APTT (seconds)	<60			

Abbreviations: APTT, activated partial thromboplastin time; k, 1,000; MCH, mean corpuscular hemoglobin; MCHC, mean corpuscular hemoglobin concentration; PCV, packed cell volume; RBC, red blood cells.

hyponatremia, hyperglycemia, and hyperbilirubinemia. Serum bicarbonate concentration, a measure of total carbon dioxide, was normal. Arterial and venous blood gases were normal (Tables 3 and 4). Fibrinogen was elevated at 700 mg/dL. The transtracheal wash sample had abundant gray mucus; because it was submitted on a Sunday, results of the cytologic examination were not available until the following day. The left shift and toxic changes in the leukon suggested bacterial infection. Lymphopenia was consistent with bacterial infection, septicemia, endotoxemia, or acute viral disease. Because liver enzymes and albumin were normal and fibrinogen was elevated, normal liver function could be assumed. Protein loss into urine and feces was unlikely based on the physical findings and history. Hypoproteinemia was thus probably attributable to loss of protein into a body cavity or to consumption of immunoglobulins used in combating infection. Hyponatremia was unremarkable. Hyperglycemia was probably attributable to a stress response from transport and illness, mediated by endogenous glucocorticoids and catecholamines. Other causes of hyperglycemia, such as severe colic [2], Cushing's syndrome [3], exogenous glucocorticoids [4], and xylazine administration [5,6], could be ruled out by the physical examination and history. Normal serum bicarbonate and blood gas values suggested that respiratory compromise was not severe, was adequately compensated, or both.

A working diagnosis of bacterial pneumonia and mild pleuritis was made. Bacterial pneumonia is often a sequela of viral infection of the lungs. The

Table 2
Chemistry profile values

Date/hospital day	Normal values	3/22/98 Day 1
BUN mg/dL	14–26	14.3
Creatinine mg/dL	0.9–1.7	1.2
Alk phos IU/L	0–239	116
SGOT (AST) IU/L	160–300	199
SDH IU/L	0–9	5.4
CPK IU/L	120–350	271
GGT IU/L	4–20	11
Total bilirubin mg/dL	0.6–2.6	4.7
Glucose mg/dL	65–129	193
Na mEq/L	137–148	134
K mEq/L	2.9–5.3	3.3
Cl mEq/L	98–110	99
Ca mg/dL	9–13	10.2
P mg/dL	1.9–4.5	3.9
Total protein gm/dL	5.5–7.5	5.3
Albumin gm/dL	2.5–3.5	2.6
Globulin gm/dL	2.0–5.0	2.7
Cholesterol mg/dL	52–104	92
HCO_3 mEq/L	24–34	26.7

Abbreviations: Alk phos, alkaline phosphatese; AST, aspartate aminotransferase; BUN, blood urea nitrogen; CPK, creatine kinase; GGT, γ-glutamyltransferase; SDH, sorbitol dehydrogenase; SGOT, serum glutamin-oxaloacetic transaminase.

most common viral agents in respiratory disease are influenza and equine herpesvirus type 1. Infection with these viruses is common in young horses, and there is controversy about the protection afforded by vaccination [7,8]. These pathogens damage the lung tissue and defenses, paving the way for bacterial invasion. Inflammation and infection spread from the parenchyma to the pleura, and effusion occurs. The effusion can be septic or nonseptic. A foul odor to the breath or an effusion is associated with anaerobic infection and is a bad prognostic sign [9]. The most common aerobic bacterial isolates from adult equine pneumonia and pleuropneumonia are β-hemolytic *Streptococcus*, *Actinobacillus*, *Pasteurella*, *Escherichia coli*, *Klebsiella*, and

Table 3
Arterial blood gas values

Date/hospital day	Normal values	3/22/98 Day 1
pH	7.347–7.475	7.44
$Paco_2$ (mm Hg)	36–46	32
Pao_2 (mm Hg)	80–112	83
HCO_3 (mEq/L)	22–29	23.8
Total CO_2 (mEq/L)		21.9
Base excess (mEq/L)	−2 to 4	−2.2
O_2 saturation (%)	90–100	96.8

Table 4
Venous blood gas values

Date/hospital day	Normal values	3/22/98
pH	7.345–7.433	7.4
P$\bar{v}$co$_2$ (mm Hg)	38–48	41
P$\bar{v}$o$_2$ (mm Hg)	37–56	39
HCO$_3$ (mEq/L)	22–29	24.8
Total CO$_2$ (mEq/L)		26.0
Base excess (mEq/L)	−3–4	−0.3
O$_2$ saturation (%)		68

Abbreviations: P$\bar{v}$co$_2$, partial pressure of carbon dioxide; P$\bar{v}$o$_2$, partial pressure of oxygen.

Enterobacter. Anaerobic bacteria isolated from pleuropneumonia cases include *Bacteroides*, *Fusobacterium*, and *Clostridium*. Multibacterial infections are common [10]. Because of the variety of bacteria potentially involved in this disease, broad-spectrum antimicrobials were indicated pending transtracheal wash culture results. Nonsteroidal anti-inflammatory drugs (NSAIDS) were indicated to treat pain, prevent and treat endotoxemia, and reduce fever and pleural inflammation. Intravenous fluid therapy was initiated, with lactated Ringer's solution (10 L) given over 2 hours to replace the estimated 7- to 12-L deficit. The horse was treated with ceftiofur, 2 mg/kg, administered intramuscularly once daily; gentamicin, 6.6 mg/kg, administered intramuscularly once daily; and metronidazole, 15 mg/kg, administered orally four times daily. Flunixin meglumine was given intravenously at an antiendotoxic [11] dose of 0.5 mg/kg twice daily, and phenylbutazone, 1 g, was given orally twice daily 6 hours after flunixin meglumine to control musculoskeletal pain [12,13]. Flunixin meglumine is thought to be better than phenylbutazone at preventing endotoxemia and treating visceral pain, but phenylbutazone is thought to be more effective at treating musculoskeletal pain, pleurodynia in this case. Lactated Ringer's solution was continued at a maintenance rate of 1.5 L/h (80 mL/kg/d) as supportive care to maintain hydration and minimize nephrotoxicity from NSAIDS and aminoglycosides. Pleural drainage was not done because of the small amount of fluid present. Mineral oil was given by nasogastric tube to prevent fecal impaction secondary to dehydration.

The mare was intermittently tachypneic, tachycardic, and febrile throughout day 1; however, the horse's attitude improved and it ate a small amount of grass hay. On day 2, the temperature was 37°C (99.8°F), the heart rate was 60 beats per minute, and the respiratory rate was 40 beats per minute. The mare's attitude improved and the respiratory effort lessened. Transtracheal wash cytology showed large amounts of mucus, moderate numbers of neutrophils, and some bacteria. The area of dullness on the right lung field extended higher up the chest than on the previous day. Chest radiographs showed increased parenchymal density and a soft tissue density ventral to the vena cava, consistent with consolidation of the ventral lung or pleural effusion. An ultrasound scan to differentiate these findings could not be repeated until the next day. Antimicrobial treatment was unchanged, but flunixin meglumine was discontinued. On day 3, the mare's temperature was 38.2°C (100.8°F), the heart rate was 56 beats per minute, the respiratory rate was 52 beats per minute, and the respiratory effort was increased. The right lung field had an area of dullness identified by auscultation and percussion from the level of the shoulder ventrally. Increased adventitial lung sounds were noted bilaterally. A transtracheal wash culture showed growth of *Streptococcus zooepidemicus zooepidemicus*, which is sensitive to ceftiofur and gentamycin. Gentamycin was discontinued. A thoracic ultrasound examination demonstrated moderate to severe bilateral pleural effusion. More fluid was noted on the right side. Pleural drainage was indicated because of respiratory compromise. After aseptic preparation and local anesthesia, bilateral skin incisions were made in the seventh intercostal space at the level of costochondral junction, and a 28-French chest tube was introduced into each hemithorax. First, the right side was drained of 8 L of inoffensive smelling fluid, and less than 1 L of fluid was then drained off the left side. Both chest tubes were fitted with Heimlich valves and left indwelling under sterile bandages. Pleural fluid was submitted for cytology and aerobic and anaerobic culture and sensitivity testing. The pleural fluid had a total protein level of 3.3 g/dL, specific gravity of 1.023, 7000 white cells/μL (60% of which were macrophages and 40% neutrophils), and did not appear septic. No cytologic evidence of neoplasia was observed [14]. Pleural fluid could have been collected anaerobically and tested for pH, P_{CO_2}, bicarbonate, lactate, and glucose. If the pleural effusion had been septic, these values would have been lower than the same values in a simultaneously drawn venous blood sample [15]. This would not, however, have changed treatment; thus, it was not performed. After drainage, the mare's breathing was less labored. On day 4, the temperature was 38.2°C (100.8°F), the heart rate was 44 beats per minute, and the respiratory rate was 32 beats per minute. During the day, the horse developed a plaque of ventral edema, which resolved gradually. On day 5, the temperature was 37.8°C (100.1°F), the heart rate was 48 beats per minute, and the respiratory rate was 52 beats per minute. The mare was lying down in the stall but easily rose to its feet. Pleural friction rubs, increased large airway sounds, and crackles and wheezes were ausculted above a line of dullness 2 cm above the elbow bilaterally. The ultrasound examination was repeated, showing nearly complete resolution of pleural fluid. The drains were removed. Phenylbutazone was increased to 2 g administered orally every 12 hours to relieve respiratory discomfort. A complete blood cell count (see Table 1) showed a normal WBC count with mild neutrophilia, no toxic changes, and mild anemia. No bacteria were isolated from the pleural fluid. Fluids were discontinued, and the catheter was removed. Phenylbutazone was reduced to 1 g administered orally every 12 hours on day 7. On day 9, radiographs of the lungs showed lessening of the ventral lung field opacity and an area at the cranial aspect of the heart that seemed to be fluid or consolidated lung. The mare was discharged on day 12. The horse was to be stall rested with daily hand walking; given metronidazole, 15 mg/kg, orally three times daily; ceftiofur, 1 g, intramuscularly daily; and phenylbutazone, 0.5 g, orally twice daily. At a recheck on day 23, the temperature was 37.8°C (100.2°F), the heart rate was 44 beats per minute, and the respiratory rate was 40 beats per minute. Mildly increased lung sounds were noted on physical examination. Pleurodynia was absent. Radiographs showed less ventral opacity in the lung field, but air bronchograms were noted, indicating unresolved parenchymal disease. Phenylbutazone and metronidazole were discontinued. On day 50, the body weight was 415 kg and the physical examination was unremarkable. Leukopenia, neutropenia, lymphopenia, and mild anemia were present. These were attributed to chronic inflammation and may reflect an underlying etiology of infection viral or immune deficiency. Radiographs showed improvement in the generalized lung pattern, but there were two soft tissue density opacities dorsal to the heart. The owner was informed that these might be lung abscesses, scar tissue, or bronchial mucus plugs. Tumors were considered to be a remote possibility. Ceftiofur and stall rest were continued until the mare was rechecked. On day 80, radiographs showed no changes from day 50. Scarring of the lung seemed to be the most probable source of the opacities, because 30 days of treatment did not affect them. Ceftiofur was discontinued. The owner was advised to return the horse to work gradually. The horse was reported to be in training without further problems on day 125.

References

[1] Mair TS, Brown PJ. Clinical and pathological features of thoracic neoplasia in the horse. Equine Vet J 1993;(3):220–3.
[2] Parry BW, Gay CC, Anderson GA. Assessment of the necessity for surgical intervention in cases of equine colic: a retrospective study. Equine Vet J 1983;15(3):216–21.
[3] Schott HC II. Pituitary pars intermedia dysfunction: equine Cushing's disease. Vet Clin North Am Equine Pract 2002;18(2):237–70.
[4] French K, Pollitt CC, Pass MA. Pharmacokinetics and metabolic effects of triamcinolone acetonide and their possible relationships to glucocorticoid-induced laminitis in horses. J Vet Pharmacol Ther 2000;23(5):287–92.
[5] Thurmon JC, Steffey EP, Zinkl JG, et al. Xylazine causes transient dose-related hyperglycemia and increased urine volumes in mares. Am J Vet Res 1984;45(2):224–7.
[6] Greene SA, Thurmon JC, Tranquilli WJ, et al. Effect of yohimbine on xylazine-induced hypoinsulinemia and hyperglycemia in mares. Am J Vet Res 1987;48(4):676–8.
[7] Mumford EL, Traub-Dargatz JL, Carman J, et al. Occurrence of infectious upper respiratory tract disease and response to vaccination in horses on six sentinel premises in northern Colorado. Equine Vet J 2003;35(1):72–7.
[8] Townsend HGG. Strategic use of equine vaccines. In: Proceedings of the 22nd Annual American College of Veterinary Internal Medicine Forum. Minneapolis, MN, 2004. p. 207–9.
[9] Reimer JM, Spencer PA. Ultrasonography as a diagnostic aid in horses with anaerobic bacterial pleuropneumonia and of pulmonary abscessation: 27 cases (1984–1986). J Am Vet Med Assoc 1989;94(2):278–82.

[10] Sweeney CR, Holcolmbe SJ, Beech J. Aerobic and anaerobic isolates from horses with pneumonia or pleuropneumonia and antimicrobial sensitivity of the aerobes. J Am Vet Med Assoc 1991;198(5):839–42.

[11] Semrad SD, Hardee GE, Hardee MM, et al. Low dose flunixin meglumine: effects on eicosanoid production and clinical signs induced by experimental endotoxaemia in horses. Equine Vet J 1987;19(3):201–6.

[12] Foreman J.H. Does stacking of non-steroidal anti-inflammatories work? In: Proceedings of the 22nd Annual American College of Veterinary Internal Medicine Forum. Minneapolis; 2004. p. 146–7.

[13] Semrad SD, Sams RA, Harris ON, et al. Effects of concurrent administration of phenylbutazone and flunixin meglumine on pharmacokinetic variables and in vitro generation of thromboxane B2 in mares. Am J Vet Res 1993;54(11):1901–5.

[14] Garber JL, Reef VB, Reimer JM. Sonographic findings in horses with mediastinal lymphosarcoma: 13 cases (1985–1992). J Am Vet Med Assoc 1994;205(10):1432–6.

[15] Brumbaugh GW, Benson PA. Partial pressures of oxygen and carbon dioxide, pH, and concentrations of bicarbonate, lactate, and glucose in pleural fluid from horses. Am J Vet Res 1990;51(7):1032–7.

ELSEVIER
SAUNDERS

VETERINARY
CLINICS
Equine Practice

Vet Clin Equine 22 (2006) 255–266

Diaphragmatic Hernia in a 19-year-old Thoroughbred Broodmare

Pamela A. Wilkins, DVM, MS, PhD

University of Pennsylvania School of Veterinary Medicine, New Bolton Center,
382 West Street, Kennett Square, PA 19348, USA

History

A previously normal, multiparous pregnant broodmare experienced an episode of apparent shock approximately 3 weeks before presentation. She had been kept in a large field with several other horses and was found shaking, hypothermic, and weak in the field following a storm. She was brought in the barn, placed in a stall, and covered with blankets and coolers. Medical treatment at that time included intravenous administration of large volumes of warmed isotonic crystalloid fluids. The mare remained tachycardic and depressed for 3 days following the episode, after which she displayed increasing respiratory rate and effort. At the time of referral, at 322 days' gestation, the mare was exhibiting persistent tachypnea and dyspnea and was approximately 3 weeks from her estimated parturition date at approximately 348 days of gestation based on previous pregnancies.

Physical examination

At presentation the mare was quiet, alert, and responsive. Her body condition was judged to be 4.5/9. She was afebrile (37.8°C; 100.0°F) with a normal heart rate (30 beats/minute) and was tachypneic (30 breaths/minute). Her mucous membranes were pink and moist with a capillary refill time of less than 1 second. Examination of the cardiovascular system revealed normal sinus rhythm, strong synchronous pulses peripherally, and good vascular tone. No murmurs were appreciated. Auscultation of the thorax revealed increased harshness bilaterally without wheezes or crackles. Rebreathing examination was similar. The lung fields appeared to be

---

E-mail address: pwilkins@vet.upenn.edu

doi:10.1016/j.cveq.2005.12.018   *vetequine.theclinics.com*

compressed craniodorsally, more so on the right, but percussion of the thorax was unremarkable, and the basic shape of the lung fields had been preserved. No heave line was noted, and more effort was present for inspiration than for expiration. No abnormal upper airway sounds were present. Borborygmi were consistently heard during thoracic auscultation in the ventral thorax bilaterally. Examination of her urogenital tract revealed an intact episioplasty. Palpation of her uterus per rectum revealed that she was indeed pregnant. The fetus was very active. Uterine tone was normal for this stage of gestation, but the cervix was relaxed. The remainder of her physical examination was unremarkable except for minor dermatitis and scarring of her limbs.

Case assessment

Initial clinical chemistry, hematology, and arterial blood gas results were unremarkable except for a mild-to-moderate decrease in Pao_2 at 72 mm Hg (temperature corrected) and a mild increase in $Paco_2$ of 48 mm Hg. In older horses, the more common causes of respiratory distress accompanied by abnormalities in arterial blood gas samples such as seen here include problems such as heaves (recurrent airway obstruction), interstitial pneumonia (idiopathic, granulomatous, viral, or other causes), and bacterial pneumonia with and without pleural fluid accumulation. These diseases were considered less likely given her normal hematology and fairly unremarkable thoracic auscultation. Less common causes of respiratory problems include pneumothorax and diaphragmatic hernia, but these diagnoses were placed high on the differential list because of her history of acute-onset shock and respiratory difficulties after a storm, making trauma to the contents of thorax more plausible. Hemothorax was also considered but was considered less likely because of her normal packed cell volume.

In the late-term pregnant mare, important physiologic changes primarily associated with the cardiovascular and respiratory systems may make interpretation of some routine testing more difficult. Late-term pregnant mares have a reduced functional residual capacity in their lungs accompanied by an increase in minute volume, resulting in increased respiratory rates at rest that, when combined with increased alveolar ventilation, produces chronic respiratory alkalosis [1]. Cardiac output is also increased, associated with higher resting heart rates and stroke volumes. These changes make pregnant mares more susceptible to problems associated with blood loss or hypovolemia. Late-term pregnant mares have an increased plasma volume and a relative (physiologic) anemia. The enlarged uterus limits lung expansion, contributing to the reduction in functional residual capacity and ventilation–perfusion mismatching. The reduction in oxygen reserve and higher rate of oxygen consumption (20%–25% increase compared with nonpregnant mares) results in an intolerance of apnea and a propensity for hypoxemia [2]. It was determined that additional testing was necessary, and thoracic ultrasonography and radiography were chosen as imaging modalities.

Procedures

A sonogram of the right hemithorax revealed the large colon to be visible in the thorax, ventral to the ventral tip of the lung and dorsal to the diaphragm throughout the entire hemithorax at the level of the point of the shoulder. The diaphragm was incomplete and could be visualized only ventrally, where the colon was visible both dorsal and ventral to the collapsed diaphragm (Fig. 1). The ventral tip of the lung was displaced dorsally, and the range of respiratory motion was decreased. The findings were similar in

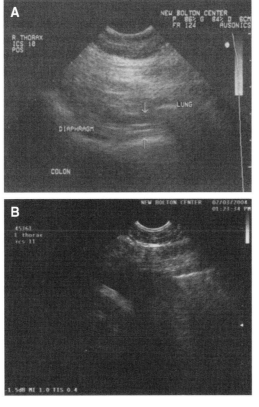

Fig. 1. (*A*) Ultrasonographic appearance of the right lung, diaphragm, and colon within thorax at time of admission at the tenth intercostal space just dorsal to the level of the point of the shoulder. (*B*) Ultrasonographic appearance of the left lung, diaphragm, and colon within thorax at the eleventh intercostal space just dorsal to the level of the point of the shoulder, 7 years after diagnosis.

the left hemithorax, except that the diaphragm was intact on the left. Normally aerated pulmonary parenchyma was seen gliding smoothly in both hemithoraces. The sonogram was consistent with a large diaphragmatic hernia associated with a large tear in the right crus of the diaphragm and entrapment of the large colon within the thorax. Radiographs of the thorax revealed increased radiodensity throughout the ventral thorax and a gas-filled structure extending from the diaphragm through the visible portions of the dorsal thorax, consistent with a diagnosis of diaphragmatic hernia (Fig. 2).

Transabdominal ultrasonographic evaluation of the fetus and uterine environments revealed a single live fetus in anterior presentation in the right uterine horn. The fetal heart rate (FHR) ranged from 83 to 86 beats/minute in normal sinus rhythm. Regular breathing motions were observed throughout the examination, as was good fetal tone, although the fetus was minimally active. An area of placental folding and cystic structures was seen at the base of the nonpregnant horn.

Discussion of differential diagnoses

There are relatively few common causes of respiratory distress accompanied by abnormalities in arterial blood gas samples as seen in this mare [3]. Clinical signs representative of heaves or recurrent airway obstruction range from mild exercise intolerance to crisis respiratory distress. The clinical signs are associated with increased resistance to flow in the airways caused by diffuse bronchoconstriction affecting the entire pulmonary parenchyma. This increased resistance affects both the inspiratory and expiratory phases of the respiratory cycle. Observation of a horse with recurrent airway obstruction gives the clinical picture of cough, serous to mucoid nasal discharge, and increased respiratory rate and effort with weight loss apparent in severe cases, along with a heave line. Severely affected horses in crisis manifest respiratory distress with nostril flaring and with greatly increased rate and abdominal effort associated with breathing. In this case, the classic abnormal auscultation finding in heaves (wheezes and crackles throughout the lung) was not present, nor was there a history of previous respiratory difficulties.

Interstitial pneumonia (idiopathic, granulomatous, viral, or other causes) is an uncommon problem of the horse. Horses affected with interstitial pneumonia frequently present with fever, cough, weight loss, nasal discharge, exercise intolerance, severe dyspnea, cyanosis, and a restrictive breathing pattern. A heave line is frequently present; nostril flare and an anxious expression are usual. The history can be acute or chronic; horses may be bright and alert with a variable appetite. The disease proceeds with progressive respiratory compromise toward death in many cases, although some may slowly improve with time.

The primary differential diagnosis of heaves may be excluded by the leukocytosis and hyperfibrinogenemia that commonly occur in horses with

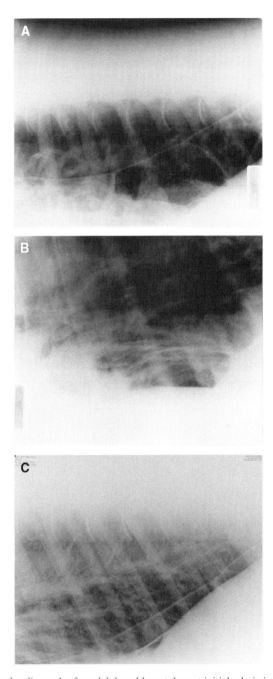

Fig. 2. (*A*) Lateral radiograph of caudal dorsal lung taken at initial admission. There is an increased bronchointerstitial pattern, and the outline of the gas-filled colon can be seen traversing the diaphragm. (*B*, *C*) Lateral radiograph of caudal dorsal lung taken at last admission, 7 years after initial evaluation. There is an increased bronchointerstitial pattern, and the outline of the gas-filled colon can be seen traversing the diaphragm, essentially unchanged from the radiograph in 2A.

interstitial pneumonia and fibrosis but are unusual in horses with heaves. These abnormal features are common in horses with infectious broncho-pneumonia, however, and thoracic radiography is of paramount importance in establishing a definitive diagnosis. Typically, thoracic radiographs reveal extensive interstitial and bronchointerstitial pulmonary patterns in interstitial pneumonia. Nodular infiltrates may be present and may be either large or miliary but are always diffusely distributed. Thoracic radiographs obtained in this mare effectively ruled out this problem.

Typically, the horse with bacterial pneumonia, with or without pleural fluid accumulation pleuropneumonia, has fever, lethargy, and exercise intolerance. Pleuropneumonia should be suspected in any horse that has been transported any significant distance and shows these clinical signs. Nasal discharge is a variable finding, as is cough. Thoracic auscultation may initially be unremarkable, but as the disease progresses abnormal lung sounds become apparent, particularly during an examination performed using a rebreathing bag. Horses with pleuropneumonia of any duration invariably have hyperfibrinogenemia. Leukocytosis is variable, as is neutrophilia. Some horses with severe infection may have leukopenia and neutropenia. In this case, the history, clinical signs, and laboratory findings were not consistent with a diagnosis of bacterial pleuropneumonia.

Pulmonary neoplasia is uncommonly reported in horses. Reports exist of both primary lung tumors and metastatic tumors in the lungs of horses, however, and neoplasia should be on the differential diagnosis list for any horse presenting with clinical signs referable to the lower respiratory tract. Pulmonary granular cell tumors are the most commonly discussed primary tumors of the lung of horses. These tumors commonly surround bronchi and bronchioles and can invade the airways, resulting in airway occlusion and the clinical signs of cough and exercise intolerance. Fungal pneumonia is an uncommon primary complaint in the geographic region where this mare presented (the northeastern United States). This differential would be more common in other geographic regions.

Pneumothorax/hemothorax has been reported secondary to trauma, suspected to have occurred in this mare during the storm. Pneumothorax can be closed, with air trapped in the pleural space, or open, with free communication between the pleural space and external environment. Tension pneumothorax occurs when air accumulates in the thorax until intrapleural pressure exceeds atmospheric pressure. This type of pneumothorax may lead to cardiovascular compromise (thoracic tamponade) because compression of the vena cava decreases venous return to the heart and, subsequently, cardiac output. Pneumothorax is frequently bilateral because of an incomplete mediastinum in horses. Clinical signs include dyspnea, tachypnea, and cyanosis. In cases secondary to trauma, wounds may be present, or a history of trauma may be elicited. Auscultation reveals absence of normal breath sounds in the dorsal thorax. If there is a concurrent hemothorax, normal lung sounds are absent ventrally also. Percussion reveals hyperresonance over the area of pneumothorax and hyporesonance ven-trally over the area of hemothorax. In this mare, hemothorax was consid-ered less likely because of her normal packed cell volume and lack of fluid seen on ultrasound examination.

Treatment and outcome

Perhaps the most important aspect of managing this case was frequent observation and development of a plan. A significant question posed to the owner at the outset was which was most important to the owner, the mare or the foal, because the answer would dictate the direction of the de-cision tree once labor began [4–7]. The owner stated that preservation of the life of the foal was paramount, but if the life of the dam could also be saved, the owner would retire her as a broodmare and let her live out her life at pasture.

Management of this case required a team approach and cooperation be-tween the intensivist, perinatologist, theriogenologist, surgeon, and anesthe-siologist. A conservative, nonsurgical approach was taken, and it was decided that elective induction of parturition would not be pursued because of potential complication for the foal. There were no reports in the literature describing management of a late-term pregnant mare with a large diaphrag-matic hernia, but reports of horses with respiratory distress and diaphrag-matic hernia and descriptions of their surgical management were available and were discussed [8–11]. The team managing the mare developed a plan for handling parturition once labor began and for fetal resuscitation follow-ing delivery. The mare would be allowed to deliver normally, and if the foal was not rapidly delivered vaginally, or if the mare developed worsening re-spiratory distress/failure, the team would pursue more aggressive means of delivery. All equipment that might be needed was readily available stall side, and a call sheet listing contact numbers for all involved was posted on the stall. The plan included a decision as to how to handle a complicated dys-tocia, should it occur, with permission for general anesthesia and cesarean section obtained before the event so that time would not be wasted. Permis-sion was also obtained for terminal cesarean section should it be deemed necessary.

The mare was observed at least hourly for evidence of early-stage labor and was constantly under video surveillance. To the equine neonatologist, opportunities for intervention may seem limited, and for many causes of fe-tal loss, this is true. Much, however, can be done to attempt to preserve the pregnancy and, in effect, treat the fetus. In a threatened pregnancy there are various ways of evaluating the fetus and its environment, and many poten-tial therapies can be used. Uterine blood flow is not autoregulated; it is di-rectly proportional to the mean perfusion pressure and is inversely proportional to uterine vascular resistance. Blood gas transport is largely independent of diffusion distance in the equine placenta, particularly in late gestation, and is more dependent on blood flow. Maternal hypoxemia can be quite threatening to the horse fetus. Information from other species cannot be extrapolated to the equine placenta because of its diffuse epitheliochorial nature and the arrangement of the maternal and fetal blood vessels within the microcotyledons [12,13]. Umbilical venous Po_2 is 50 to 54 mm Hg in the horse fetus, compared with 30 to 34 mm Hg in the sheep, whereas the difference in Po_2 in the maternal uterine vein and the umbilical vein is almost 0. Also unlike the sheep, the umbilical venous Po_2 values decrease by 5 to 10 mm Hg in response to maternal hypoxemia and increase in response to maternal hyperoxia [14,15]. Therefore the author and colleagues recommend that critically ill pregnant mares have arterial and venous blood gas evaluations performed early in their clinical course, with repeat measurements taken as indicated by their clinical course or following significant changes in management or condition. In this case, arterial blood gas analysis at admission revealed mild hypoxemia and hypercapnia associated with the additional respiratory compromise resulting from the diaphragmatic hernia. Intranasal oxygen insufflation of 10 to 15 L/minute to mares has been shown to increase significantly both Pao_2 and percent oxygen saturation of hemoglobin [16]. Combined with the finding of decreased fetal activity, it was decided to place the mare on intranasal oxygen insufflation at 15 L/minute, which increased her Pao_2 by 25 mm Hg (Fig. 3).

Fetal heart rate monitoring was also instituted. A companion to transabdominal ultrasonography, fetal ECGs can be measured continuously using telemetry or can be obtained using more conventional techniques several times throughout the day [17–19]. Electrodes are placed on the skin of the mare in locations aimed at maximizing the magnitude of the fetal ECG,

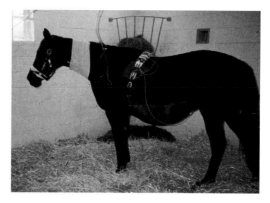

Fig. 3. Image of the mare with a large diaphragmatic hernia in the ICU. She is receiving intranasal oxygen insufflation (humidified oxygen) and having the fetal ECG monitored by telemetry. The telemetry unit is attached to the surcingle around her girth region. She also has an intravenous catheter in place. Her abdomen has been clipped for transabdominal evaluation of the fetus and uteroplacental unit.

but, because the fetus frequently changes position, multiple sites may be needed in any 24-hour period. The author and colleagues begin with an electrode placed dorsally in the area of the sacral prominence with two electrodes placed bilaterally in a transverse plane in the region of the flank. The maximal amplitude of the fetal ECG is low, usually 0.05 to 0.1 mV, and can be lost in artifact or background noise, so it is common to move electrodes to new positions to maximize the appearance of the fetal ECG (Fig. 4). The normal FHR during the last months of gestation ranges from 65 to 115 beats/minute, a fairly wide distribution. The range of heart rate of an individual fetus can be quite narrow, however. Recordings should be made over a 10- to 20-minute period of time and repeated several times daily if conventional techniques are used. If telemetry is used, paper recordings should be obtained at approximately 2-hour intervals to allow calculation of FHR and observation of rhythm. Bradycardia in the fetus is an adaptation to in utero stress, most usually thought to be hypoxia. By slowing the heart rate, the fetus prolongs exposure of fetal blood to maternal blood, increasing the time for equilibration of dissolved gas across the placenta and improving the oxygen content of the fetal blood. The distribution of fetal cardiac output is also altered in response to hypoxia, centralizing blood distribution [20,21]. Tachycardia in the fetus can be associated with fetal movement, and brief periods of tachycardia should occur in the fetus during any 24-hour period. Persistent tachycardia is a sign of fetal distress and represents more severe fetal compromise than bradycardia. Tachycardia

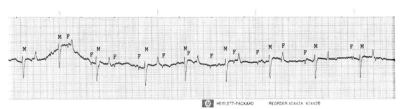

Maternal HR: 48 bpm; fetal HR 83 bpm

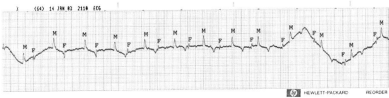

Maternal HR: 88-75 bpm; fetal HR 75 bpm

Fig. 4. Two fetal ECG tracings. It is easiest to find the maternal QRS complex and then locate the smaller-amplitude fetal complex. The fetal complex can occur during the maternal complex and alter its shape. The fetal rate is generally higher than the maternal rate but can be lower, depending on the health of the dam and the fetus. F, fetal QRS complexes; M, maternal QRS complexes.

followed by severe bradycardia can be observed terminally in some fetuses. During the last weeks of pregnancy, fetal foals usually have a baseline heart rate between 60 and 75 beats/minute. Of fetal foals that have a low FHR (40–75 beats/minute), 80% have a heart rate below 70 beats/minute, 55% have a heart rate below 60 beats/minute, and 14% have a heart rate below 50 beats/minute). Of fetal foals that have a high FHR (83–250 beats/minute), 86% have a heart rate higher than 100 beats/minute, 50% have a heart rate higher than 120 beats/minute, and 20% have a heart rate higher than 200 beats/minute) [22]. As indicated, transient low heart rates below 60 beats/minute are common and should not be considered ominous unless they are also recognized with no accelerations. Also, FHR transiently may be higher than 200 beats/minute. Transient FHR higher than 120 beats/minute are not threatening unless they are persistent and do not return to baseline levels. When FHR are below 60 or above 120 beats/minute throughout an observation period, repeat assessment within 24 hours or less is indicated. Beat-to-beat variability generally ranges from 0.5 to 4 mm, with most occurring in the range of 1 mm. This beat-to-beat variability requires an intact central nervous system and functioning sympathetic and parasympathetic systems. To measure the variation, periods when the heart rate is not accelerating or decelerating should be used for an accurate observation. The finding of no beat-to-beat variation in the absence of maternal drugs that may sedate the fetus is an indication of loss of fetal central nervous system input into cardiac function, and repeat observations are indicated [22].

The mare entered stage I labor in the evening of gestation day 350 when it was noted that she was restless and getting up and down frequently, dripping milk, and sweating. Stage II labor began shortly thereafter. Intranasal oxygen therapy was maintained. A vaginal examination performed with the mare standing revealed a normally positioned foal; however, the foal could not be extricated with the mare standing, and she was encouraged to lie down. The filly foal was delivered with assistance 11 minutes after the onset of stage II labor.

The foal demonstrated mild-to-moderate bradycardia and was briefly removed from the stall for administration of intranasal oxygen. The bradycardia resolved, and the foal was returned to the stall. Initial clinical chemistry, hematology, and arterial blood gas analyses were within normal limits for a newborn foal. The mare remained in lateral recumbency for 30 minutes following delivery. Her respiratory pattern was rapid and deep; because of concerns regarding hypovolemic shock secondary to the large intra-abdominal and intrathoracic volume changes associated with delivery, she received a 20-L bolus of isotonic crystalloid fluids intravenously. Flunixin meglumine was administered for pain. The mare passed her fetal membranes within 2 hours of delivery, and the foal stood unassisted and sucked from the dam, also within 2 hours of delivery. The mare's respiratory rate and effort gradually returned to normal, and an arterial blood gas obtained without oxygen supplementation was significantly improved over all previous measurements.

Radiographic and ultrasonographic evaluation of the mare's thorax post-foaling demonstrated significant improvement in the respiratory volume of her thorax, although the colon remained entrapped within her right hemi-thorax. The mare and foal were discharged 4 days following parturition. The foal became a successful racehorse. The mare was followed for 7 years after discharge, during which time she remained at pasture and comfortable, experiencing no episodes of respiratory distress or colic. She returned to the hospital to be euthanized following deterioration of a chronic musculoskel-etal condition. At necropsy, both her large colon and portions of her liver were entrapped within her thorax and adherent to the ventral aspect of the very large defect in the right crus of the diaphragm (Fig. 5).

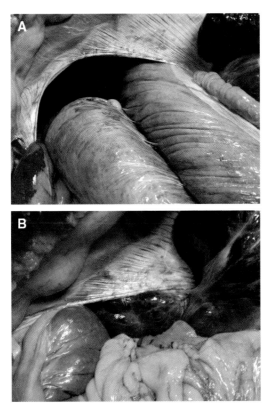

Fig. 5. (*A*) Postmortem image of large colon passing through large defect in right diaphrag-matic crus. (*B*) Postmortem image of liver lobe entrapped in thorax through a large defect in right diaphragmatic crus. (*Courtesy of* Dr. Fabio Del Piero, New Bolton Center, Kennett Square, PA)

References

[1] Hidebrand SV, Hill T, Vivrette S. Anesthesia in the late-term gravid mare. In: Proceedings of the 16th annual meeting of the American College of Veterinary Anesthesiologists. San Francisco (CA): College of Veterinary Anesthesiologists; 1991. p. 35.

[2] Wilson DV. Anesthesia and sedation for late-term mares. Vet Clin North Am Equine Pract 1994;10:219-36.

[3] Wilkins PA. Lower airway disease of adult horses. Vet Clin North Am 2003;19:101-22 [Equine Prac].

[4] Freeman DE, Hungerford LL, Schaeffer D, et al. Caesarean section and other methods for assisted delivery: comparison of effects on mare mortality and complications. Equine Vet J 1999;31:203-7.

[5] Embertson RM. Dystocia and caesarean sections: the importance of duration and good judgement. Equine Vet J 1999;31:179-80.

[6] Norton JL, Johnston JK, Palmer JE, et al. Retrospective study of dystocia in horses at a referral hospital. J Vet Intern Med 2005;19:428.

[7] Wilkins PA. Monitoring the pregnant mare in the ICU. Clinical Techniques in Equine Practice 2003;2:212-9.

[8] Everett KA, Chaffin MK, Brinsko SP. Diaphragmatic herniation as a cause of lethargy and exercise intolerance in a mare. Cornell Vet 1992;82:217-23.

[9] Perdrizet JA, Dill SG, Hackett RP. Diaphragmatic hernia as a cause of dyspnoea in a draft horse. Equine Vet J 1989;21:302-4.

[10] Goehring LS, Goodrich LR, Murray MJ. Tachypnoea associated with a diaphragmatic tear in a horse. Equine Vet J 1999;31:443-5.

[11] Santschi EM, Juzwiak JS, Moll HD, et al. Diaphragmatic hernia repair in three young horses. Vet Surg 1997;26:242-5.

[12] Samuel CA, Allen WR, Steven DH. Studies on the equine placenta. I. Development of the microcotyledons. J Reprod Fertil 1974;41:441-5.

[13] Bjorkman N. Fine structure of the fetal-maternal area of exchange in the epitheliochorial and endotheliochorial types of placentation. Acta Anat Suppl (Basel) 1973;61:1-22.

[14] Comline RS, Silver M. pO2 levels in the placental circulation of the mare and ewe. Nature 1968;217:76-7.

[15] Fowden AL, Forhead AJ, White KL, et al. Equine uteroplacental metabolism at mid- and late gestation. Exp Physiol 2000;85:539-45.

[16] Wilkins PA, Seahorn TL. Intranasal oxygen therapy in adult horses. Journal of Veterinary Emergency and Critical Care 2000;10:221.

[17] Vaala WE, Sertich PL. Management strategies for mares at risk for periparturient complications. Vet Clin North Am Equine Pract 1994;10:237-65.

[18] LeBlanc MM. Identification and treatment of the compromised equine fetus: a clinical perspective. Equine Vet J Suppl 1997;29:100-3.

[19] Buss DD, Asbury AC, Chevalier L. Limitations in equine fetal electrocardiography. J Am Vet Med Assoc 1980;177:174-6.

[20] Jensen A, Garnier Y, Berger R. Dynamics of fetal circulatory responses to hypoxia and asphyxia. Eur J Obstet Gynecol Reprod Biol 1999;84:155-72.

[21] Cohn HE, Piasecki GJ, Jackson BT. The effect of fetal heart rate on cardiovascular function during hypoxemia. Am J Obstet Gynecol 1980;138:1190-9.

[22] Palmer JE. Fetal monitoring. In: Proceedings of the Equine Symposium and Annual Conference. San Antonio (TX): International Veterinary Emergency and Critical Care; 2000.

**ELSEVIER
SAUNDERS**

Vet Clin Equine 22 (2006) 267–277

VETERINARY
CLINICS
Equine Practice

Index

Note: Page numbers of article titles are in **boldface** type.

0749-0739/06/$ - see front matter © 2006 Elsevier Inc. All rights reserved.
doi:10.1016/S0749-0739(06)00023-X   *vetequine.theclinics.com*